New Trends
in the Diagnosis and Therapy of
Non-Alzheimer's Dementia

Edited by
K. A. Jellinger and M. Windisch

Journal of Neural Transmission
Supplement 47

SpringerWienNewYork

Prof. Dr. Kurt A. Jellinger
L. Boltzmann Institute of Clinical Neurobiology, Lainz-Hospital,
Vienna, Austria

Dr. Manfred Windisch
EBEWE-Research Initiative, Graz, Austria

Product Liability: The publisher can give no guarantee for information about drug dosage and application thereof contained in this book. In every individual case the respective user must check its accuracy by consulting other pharmaceutical literature. The use of registered names, trademarks, etc. in this publication does not imply, even in the absence of a specific statement, that such names are exempt from the relevant protective laws and regulations and therefore free for general use.

Typesetting: Best-set Typesetter Ltd, Hong Kong
Printing: A. Holzhausens Nfg., A-1070 Wien
Printed on acid-free and chlorine-free bleached paper

With 61 partly coloured Figures

ISSN 0303-6995
ISBN-13:978-3-211-82823-6   e-ISBN-13:978-3-7091-6892-9
DOI: 10.1007/978-3-7091-6892-9

Foreword

Dementia is an acquired disorder of higher cerebral functions and cognition. Because of increasing life expectancy dementia poses a major health and socio-economic problem. Alzheimer's disease accounts for 70–90% of mental decline in the elderly. Degenerative non-Alzheimer's dementias are responsible for 7–30%. These include a variety of disorders clinically characterised by progressive cognitive dysfunction often combined with focal neurological deficits, e.g. Parkinson-plus syndromes, Lewy body dementia, lobar and multisystem atrophies, other neurodegenerative disorders, and prion diseases. Often it is difficult to distinguish these illnesses from Alzheimer's disease and vascular dementia.

In spite of considerable progress in molecular genetics, biochemistry, and neuropathology, the classification and pathogenesis of non-Alzheimer's dementias are still debatable. Diagnosis is frequently made only at postmortem. Because disease markers are not available for the majority of non-Alzheimer's dementias, consensus criteria for the identification of such diseases are warranted. These criteria could serve at a basis for early diagnosis and distinction from other dementing disorders.

The present volume includes the papers and posters presented at the 4th International Symposium of the Research Initiative EBEWE, held in October 13 to 15, 1995 in Vienna. This first international workshop on non-Alzheimer dementias was intended to provide an overview of the current classification, clinical features, pathomorphology, neuroimaging, and molecular biology of this important group of central nervous system disorders. The conference's aims were to ensure correct diagnosis and to give insight into the pathogenesis of these neurodegenerative diseases becoming increasingly important in neurobiology, clinical neuropsychiatry and neuropsychology, and, thus, to provide a basis for future treatment strategies. It is hoped that the data presented will promote research in the diagnosis, understanding, and treatment of dementing disorders.

Our thanks are due to Springer-Verlag Wien New York for excellent co-operation and technical performance that enabled a rapid publication of this volume.

Vienna, April 1996

K. A. Jellinger
M. Windisch

Contents

Jellinger, K. A.: Structural basis of dementia in neurodegenerative disorders 1

Dickson, D. W., Feany, M. B., Yen, S.-H., Mattiace, L. A., Davies, P.: Cytoskeletal pathology in non-Alzheimer degenerative dementia: new lesions in Diffuse Lewy body disease, Pick's disease, and Corticobasal Degeneration 31

Hauw, J. J., Duyckaerts, C., Seilhean, D., Camilleri, S., Sazdovitch, V., Rancurel, G.: The neuropathologic diagnostic criteria of frontal lobe dementia revisited. A study of ten consecutive cases 47

Pillon, B., Dubois, B., Agid, Y.: Cognitive deficits in non-Alzheimer's degenerative diseases 61

Gsell, W., Strein, I., Riederer, P.: The neurochemistry of Alzheimer type, vascular type and mixed type dementias compared 73

Gregory, C. A., Hodges, J. R.: Clinical features of frontal lobe dementia in comparison to Alzheimer's disease 103

Talbot, P. R.: Frontal lobe dementia and motor neuron disease 125

Kertesz, A., Munoz, D.: Clinical and pathological characteristics of primary progressive aphasia and frontal dementia 133

Aichner, F., Wagner, M., Kremser, Ch., Felber, S.: MR-imaging of non-Alzheimer's dementia 143

Brooks, D. J.: Functional imaging techniques in the diagnosis of non-Alzheimer dementias 155

Besthorn, C., Sattel, H., Hentschel, F., Daniel, S., Zerfaß, R., Förstl, H.: Quantitative EEG in frontal lobe dementia 169

Mielke, R., Kessler, J., Szelies, B., Herholz, K., Wienhard, K., Heiss, W.-D.: Vascular dementia: perfusional and metabolic disturbances and effects of therapy .. 183

Fischer, P.: The spectrum of depressive pseudo-dementia 193

Morris, C. M., Massey, H. M., Benjamin, R., Leake, A., Broadbent, C., Griffiths, M., Lamb, H., Brown, A., Ince, P. G., Tyrer, S., Thompson, P., McKeith, I. G., Edwardson, J. A., Perry, R. H., Perry, E. K.: Molecular biology of APO E alleles in Alzheimer's and non-Alzheimer's dementias 205

Brown, P.: Transmissible cerebral amyloidosis 219

Ironside, J. W.: Human prion diseases 231

Krieglstein, K., Maysinger, D., Unsicker, K.: The survival response of mesencephalic dopaminergic neurons to the neurotrophins BDNF and NT-4 requires priming with serum: comparison with members of the TGF-β superfamily and characterization of the serum-free culture system 247

Rösler, N., Wichart, I., Bancher, C., Jellinger, K. A.: Tau protein and apolipoprotein E in CSF diagnostics of Alzheimer's disease: impact on non-Alzheimer's dementia? 259

Hutter-Paier, B., Grygar, E., Windisch, M.: Death of cultured telencephalon neurons induced by glutamate is reduced by the peptide derivative Cerebrolysin® ... 267

Boado, R. J.: Molecular regulation of the blood-brain barrier GLUT1 glucose transporter by brain-derived peptides 275

VIII   Contents

Hutter-Paier, B., Frühwirth, M., Grygar, E., Windisch, M.: Cerebrolysin® protects
    neurons from ischemia-induced loss of microtubule – associated protein 2   276
Francis-Turner, L., Valouskova, V., Mokry, J.: The long-term effect of NGF, b-
    FGF and Cerebrolysin® on the spatial memory after fimbria-fornix lesion in rats   277
Gschanes, A., Windisch, M.: The influence of Cerebrolysin® and E021 on spatial
    navigation of young rats   278
Schwab, M., Antonow-Schlorke, I., Dürer, U., Bauer, R.: Effects of Cerebrolysin®
    on cytoskeletal proteins after focal ischemia in rats   279
Valouškova, V., Francis-Turmer, L.: The short-term influence of b-FGF, NGF and
    Cerebrolysin® on the memory impaired after fimbria-fornix lesion   280
Wojtowicz, J. M., Xiong, H., Baskys, A.: Brain tissue hydrolysate, Cerebrolysin®,
    acts on presynaptic adenosine receptors in the rat hippocampus   281
Subject Index   283

Listed in Current Contents/Life Sciences

J Neural Transm (1996) [Suppl] 47: 1–29

Structural basis of dementia in neurodegenerative disorders

K. A. Jellinger

L. Boltzmann Institute of Clinical Neurobiology, Lainz-Hospital, Vienna, Austria

Summary. Progressive dementia syndromes in adults are caused by a number of conditions associated with different structural lesions of the brain. In most clinical and autopsy series, senile dementia of the Alzheimer type is the most common cause of mental decline in the elderly accounting for up to 90%, whereas degenerative non-Alzheimer dementias range from 7 to 30% (mean 8–10%). They include a variety of disorders featured morphologically by neuron and synapse loss and gliosis, often associated with cytopathological changes involving specific cortical and subcortical circuits. These neuronal/glial inclusions and neuritic alterations show characteristic immunoreactions and ultrastructure indicating cytoskeletal mismetabolism. They are important diagnostic sign posts that, in addition to the distribution pattern of degenerative changes, indicate specific vulnerability of neuronal populations, but their pathogenic role and contribution to mental decline are still poorly understood. In some degenerative disorders no such cytopathological hallmarks have been observed; a small number is genetically determined. While in Alzheimer's disease (AD) mental decline is mainly related to synaptic and neuritic pathologies, other degenerative disorders show variable substrates of dementia involving different cortical and/or subcortical circuits which may or may not be superimposed by cortical Alzheimer lesions. In most demented patients with Lewy body disorders (Parkinson's disease, Lewy body dementia), they show similar distribution as in AD, while in Progressive Supranuclear Palsy (PSP), mainly prefrontal areas are involved. Lobar atrophies, increasingly apparent as causes of dementia, show fronto-temporal cortical neuron loss, spongiosis and gliosis with or without neuronal inclusions (Pick bodies) and ballooned cells, while dementing motor neuron disease and multisystem atrophies reveal ubiquitinated neuronal and oligodendroglial inclusions. There are overlaps or suggested relationships between some neurodegenerative disorders, e.g. between corticobasal degeneration, PSP and Pick's atrophy. In many of these disorders with involvement of the basal ganglia, degeneration of striatofrontal and hippocampo-cortical loops are important factors of mental decline which may be associated with isocortical neuronal degeneration and synapse loss or are superimposed by cortical AD pathology.

Introduction

Dementia, a syndrome of acquired global disturbances of higher cerebral functions and cognition sufficient to interfere with social and occupational performance without change of alertness, has become a major health problem because of worldwide increase in elder population. With the increase of life expectancy, the prevalence of dementia has risen exponentially from 1% in subjects aged 60 to 65 years to 20% up to over 40% of people over 85 years (Skoog et al., 1993; Katzman and Kawan, 1994). Dementia can be caused by many different conditions, particularly by chronic progressive and irreversible diseases, while the estimated incidence of reversible dementia varies from less than 1% to over 10% (Arnold and Kumar, 1993; Weytingh et al., 1995). The most widely used clinical classifications, the DSM-III-R and DSM-IV, and WHO ICD.10, distinguish several groups of progressive dementia disorders in adults, i.e. dementia in Alzheimer's disease (AD) (F00), vascular dementia (F01), dementia in otherwise classified disorders (F02), and unclassified forms (F04), that correlate with several groups of neuropathologically determined disorders. In most clinical and autopsy series, degenerative dementia of the Alzheimer type is the most common cause of mental decline in the elderly; it accounts for 65 to over 90% (Terry et al., 1994; Galasko et al., 1994), whereas degenerative non-Alzheimer's dementias range from 7 to 30% and, thus, represent the second most frequent form, exceeding vascular dementia that has been suggested to be next to AD (Roman et al., 1993; Jellinger and Bancher, 1994; Tatemichi et al., 1994; Kosunen et al., 1996); in less than 1% of elderly demented subjects no pathological CNS lesions are detected. The post mortem diagnoses in a personal consecutive 7-year autopsy series of aged individuals and of those with a clinical diagnosis of probable or possible AD (using the NINCDS-ADRDA criteria [McKhann et al., 1984]) are given in Tables 1 and 2. These data indicate that AD pathology with or without additional lesions was present in over 80 and 90% of all demented or clinical AD patients, while vascular dementia accounted for 8.5% of all dementias, but only for 0.9% of suggested AD cases. Other neurodegenerative disorders representing 8.2 and 10% of all demented and AD cases, respectively, are listed in Tables 3 and 4. No abnormal brain lesions beyond age were seen in 0.3 and 0.6% of demented patients, respectively.

Degenerative dementias of non-Alzheimer type are morphologically featured by neuronal degeneration and loss with accompanying astrocytosis involving specific, often disparate, cortical and subcortical populations or multiple circuits. They may or may not be associated with intracellular neuronal and/or glial inclusions/deposits, neuritic alterations or other cytopathological abnormalities that show characteristic immunoreactions and ultrastructure indicating cytoskeletal dysmetabolism (Table 5). Although the molecular basis and pathogenic relevance of these cytoskeletal abnormalities for most neurodegenerative disorders remain to be elucidated, they are important histological sign posts that are often pointing to the diagnosis (Fig. 1). Morphological and immunohistochemical overlaps between various types of

Table 1. Morphological diagnosis in consecutive autopsy series of demented aged individuals (1989–1995)

182 males/358 females (age 54–103 years)	n	percent
"Pure" AD (CERAD pos.; Braak V–VI)	194	35.9
AD "pure plaque type" (CERAD pos.)	10	1.9
"Limbic"/"neurofibrillary type" AD (CERAD neg.)	26	4.8
AD + CVD (lacunar state, infarcts)	80	14.8
AD + cerebral hemorrhage	16	3.0
Lewy body variant of AD	33	6.1
AD/DAT + Parkinson pathology	23	4.3
AD + nigral lesions/incidental Lewy bodies	25	4.6
MIX type dementia (AD + MIE/VaD)	22	4.0
AD + other pathology (tumors)	7	1.3
Alzheimer disease — total	**436**	**80.7**
Vascular dementia (VaD/MIE, SAE)	46	8.5
Other disorders	55	10.2
Nothing abnormal beyond age	3	0.6
Other pathologies	104	19.3
Total	**540**	**100.0**

Table 2. Consecutive autopsy series of patients with clinical diagnosis of probable or possible Alzheimer's disease (1989–1995) (108 males, 232 females; age 57–103 yrs)

Neuropathological diagnosis	n	percent	mean age
"Pure" AD (CERAD+; Braak V–VI)	155	45.6	82.1 ± 4.6
"Pure" probable AD (CERAD pos., Braak IV–V)	11	3.2	87.4 ± 2.3
AD "pure plaque type" (CERAD pos.)	8	2.4	78.0 ± 8.3
"Limbic" AD (CERAD neg.; Braak IV)	10	2.9	84.0 ± 2.0
"Neurofibrillary type" AD (CERAD neg.)	4	1.2	84.0 ± 4.0
AD + CVD (lacunar state, infarcts)	52	15.3	82.6 ± 5.5
AD + cerebral hemorrhage	10	2.9	83.4 ± 4.3
Lewy body variant of AD	22	6.5	81.4 ± 7.5
DAT + Parkinson pathology	8	2.4	75.4 ± 9.3
AD + nigral lesions (no Lewy bodies)	12	3.6	82.5 ± 6.3
AD + incidental subcort. Lewy bodies	7	2.0	79.4 ± 8.3
MIX dementia (AD + MIE/VaD)	7	2.0	83.6 ± 5.0
AD + other pathology (tumor)	2	0.6	78.5 ± 4.0
Alzheimer disease — total	**308**	**90.6**	81.3 ± 5.8
Vascular dementia (MIE, SAE)	3	0.9	84.0 ± 1.2
Other disorders	28	8.2	73.7 ± 8.3
Nothing abnormal	1	0.3	86.0
Other pathologies	32	9.4	81.2 ± 4.7
Total	**340**	**100.0**	81.3 ± 5.0

Table 3. Non-Alzheimer pathology in aged subjects with dementia

Vascular dementia (MIE, SAE)	46
Creutzfeldt-Jakob disease	12
Fronto-temporal degeneration	7
Huntington's disease	7
Parkinson's disease + other pathologies	5
Brain tumors (lymphomas)	3
Symmetric Ammons horn sclerosis	3
Corticobasal degeneration	3
Pick's disease	3
Multisystem atrophy	3
Wernicke's encephalopathy	3
Progressive Supranuclear Palsy	2
Symmetric thalamic sclerosis	1
Symm. Ammons horn + thalam. sclerosis	1
Chronic multiple sclerosis	1
Chronic HSV encephalitis	1
Nothing abnormal beyond age	3
Total	104

Table 4. Non-Alzheimer pathology in clinical cases probable or possible Alzheimer disease

Vascular dementia (MIE, SAE)	3
Fronto-temporal degeneration	7
Brain tumors (lymphomas)	3
Symmetric Ammons horn sclerosis	3
Corticobasal degeneration	2
Parkinson's disease (no AD lesions)	2
Pick's disease	2
Progressive Supranuclear Palsy	1
Creutzfeldt-Jakob disease	2
Multisystem atrophy	1
Huntington's disease	1
Symmetric thalamic sclerosis	1
Symm. Ammons horn + thalam. sclerosis	1
Chronic multiple sclerosis	1
Chronic HSV encephalitis	1
Nothing abnormal beyond age	1
Total	32

cytopathological hallmarks and the distribution pattern of neurodegeneration may result in difficulties in the differential diagnosis of some disorders, e.g. corticobasal degeneration (CBD), progressive supranuclear palsy (PSP), AD and Pick's disease, or suggest relationships between these entities (Feany et al., 1996). However, increasing use of modern molecular biological techniques has enabled a clear distinction between various dementing disorders that were previously unknown (Jellinger, 1995a; Feany et al., 1995; Buée-Scherrer et al.,1996; Dickson et al., 1996).

Table 5. Ultrastructural and immunohistochemical features of neuronal inclusions [modified after Jellinger (1995a)]

Type of inclusion	Ultrastructures	Immunohistochemistry								
		PHF	pNF	pTau	Ubi	ChrA	αBCrys	APP	αβTub	Trop
Pick bodies	15–18 nm SF + 24 nm LPCT	++	+++	++	++	++	+	+	–	+
Pick ballooned cells	same	+	+++°	++	++	+	+	?	–	+
AD-NFT	2 × 10 nm PHF + 18 nm SF	+++	+++	+/+++	++	–	–	+	–	+
PSP-NFT	12–15 nm SF + 10 nm PHF	±	+/+++	+++	++	–	–	+	–	+
PSP, ballooned cells	?	–	++	?	+	–	+	–	+	?
Lewy bodies (Parkinson dis.)	7–20 nm (mean 10 nm) SF	±	+++°°	±°°°	+++	+	+	–	+	?
"Pale" (Pre-Lewy) bodies	10 nm SF	?	+	–	++	?	?	?	?	?
LBD, cortical Lewy bodies[1]	~15 nm SF	+	+°	+	++	?	?	+	?	+
CBD inclusions (NFT-like)[2-4]	26–28 nm LPCT + 15 nm SF	+	+/++	++[+]	±/–	–	–	?	?	?
CBD, ballooned cells[5]	NF (10 nm SF) + 26 nm twisted tubules	–	++	±/+	–/++[8]	–	++	–	?	?
MND; FTD + MND	13–25 nm SF	–	+	–	+++	?	–	–	–	–
MSA, neuronal inclusions[6]	18–28 nm fibrils + 10 nm filaments	–	±	–	+++	–	?	?	–	?
MSA, oligodendroglial inclusions[7]	21–30 nm tubules	+	–	++	++	–	–	?	++	?
FTD, ballooned cells[9]		–	–	–	++	–	++	?	?	?

° persistent after phosphatase treatment, °° non persistent after phosphatase treatment, °°° but contain microtubule-associated protein 5 (MAP 5) (Gai et al., 1996), [+] different from AD and PSP. [1] Smith and Perry (1994), [2] Wakabayashi et al. (1994), [3] Ksiezak-Reding et al. (1994), [4] Feany et al. (1995), [5] Arima et al. (1994), [6] Arima et al. (1994), [7] Lantos and Papp (1994), [8] Halliday et al. (1995), [9] Cooper et al. (1995). PHF paired helical filaments, pNF phosphorylated neurofilament epitopes, pTau phosphorylated tau protein, Ubi ubiquitin, ChrA chromogranin A, αBCrys α-B crystallin, APP amyloid precursor protein, αβTub tubuline, Trop tropomyosin, SF straight filaments, LPCT long-period constricted tubules, LBD Lewy body dementia, CBD corticobasal degeneration, NF neurofilaments, MND Motor neuron disease, FTD Frontotemporal dementia

K. A. Jellinger

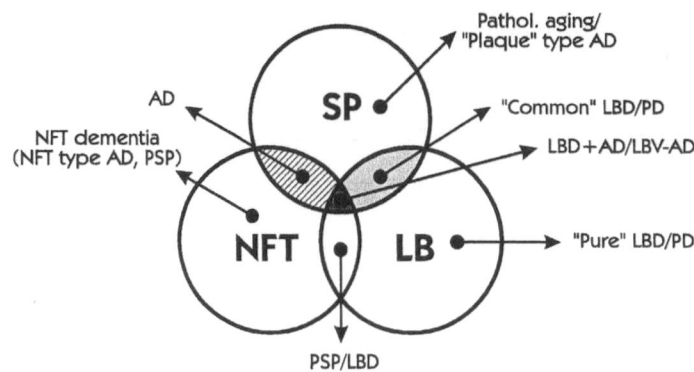

Fig. 1. Relationship between plaques, tangles, and Lewy bodies and classification of neurodegenerative disorders

Table 6. Non-Alzheimer degenerative dementias

1. Primary Lewy body disorders
   a) Parkinson's disease
   b) Diffuse Lewy body disease; Lewy body dementia

2. Neurofibrillary tangle/tau associated disorders
   a) Progressive supranuclear palsy — typical, atypical
   b) Corticobasal degeneration
   c) Dementia with argyrophilic grains
   d) Parkinson-dementia/ALS complex of Guam
   e) Postencephalitic parkinsonism

3. Other neuron inclusion disorders/lobar atrophies
   a) Pick's disease
   b) Frontal/Frontotemporal lobe atrophy/dementia (FLD)
   c) Motor neuron disease with dementia/FLD and motor neuron disease
   d) Primary progressive aphasia

4. Oligodendral inclusion diseases (Multisystem degeneration/MSA)
   a) Striatonigral degeneration
   b) Olivopontocerebellar atrophy
   c) Shy-Drager syndrome

5. Hereditary neurodegenerative diseases
   a) Huntington's disease
   b) Choreoacanthocytosis
   c) Pallidal degeneration and related variants
   d) Dentatorubropallidoluysian degeneration
   e) Machado-Joseph disease

6. Spongiform encephalopathies (Prion diseases)
   a) Creutzfeldt-Jakob disease
   b) Gerstmann-Sträussler-Scheinker disease
   c) Familial fatal insomnia/Thalamic dementia
   d) Famial progressive subcortical gliosis

Non-Alzheimer degenerative dementias can be classified according to established disease entities, e.g. Parkinson's, Pick's, Huntington's disease, multisystem atrophies (MSA), etc., or can be grouped according to cytoskeletal hallmarks and other criteria (Table 6). In addition to Lewy body-associated disorders related to neurofilament pathology, they include disorders related to microtubule associated tau protein pathologies with neuro-, and gliofibrillary tangles, neuropil threads, and argyrophilic grains, e.g. AD, PSP and CBD, and disorders associated with ubiquitinated inclusions, such as MSA and motor neuron disease. A number of dementing neurodegenerative disorders lack such pathognomonic cytopathological hallmarks or show only nonspecific neuritic pathology (Jackson et al., 1995) and, therefore, are currently classified according to the anatomical lesion patterns (Lantos, 1992; Hauw et al., 1994; Jellinger, 1995a). Recent studies on the reliability and validity of neuropathological diagnostic criteria for degenerative disorders of the extrapyramidal system revealed that histopathological examination alone was not fully adequate for the differentiation of some of these disorders, but the addition of clinical information improved the reliability of diagnosis (Litvan et al., 1996b). In a small number of degenerative dementia, e.g. Huntington's disease, a genetic defect or particular gene locus have been identified (Andrew and Hayden, 1995). Another group are infectious cerebral amyloidoses or prion diseases (see Budka et al., 1995; Brown, 1996; Ironside, 1996), while for the majority of neurodegenerative disorders the etiology and pathogenesis await further elucidation.

This paper gives a brief overview of the structural basis of mental decline in the degenerative non-Alzheimer dementias summarized in Table 6 in comparison to AD.

Alzheimer's disease

This neurodegenerative disorder representing the most common form of adult onset dementia is clinically characterized by progressive cognitive decline in which memory, initiation, learning and conceptualization are severely affected (Terry et al., 1994; Jellinger et al., 1994). Even though the accuracy of clinical diagnosis of AD using established criteria (McKhann et al., 1984; Corey-Bloom et al., 1995), is up to 90–96% in recent series (Tierney et al., 1988; Morris et al., 1988; Jellinger et al., 1990; Galasko et al., 1994; Gearing et al., 1995; Kosunen et al., 1996), the definite diagnosis of AD can only be established by histopathological examination of the brain (Mirra et al., 1993). The morphology of AD includes amyloid deposits (plaques), neuritic changes — neurofibrillary tangles (NFT), neuritic plaques, and neuropil threads — with deposition of paired helical filaments (PHF) containing phosphorylated tau proteins, extensive neuron and synapse loss, and disruption of the neuronal cytoskeleton with altered cortico-cortical connectivity (Terry et al., 1994; Braak and Braak, 1994; Larner, 1995; Trojanowski et al., 1995). However, its current morphological diagnosis is based on age-graded (semi)quantitative assessment of the classical AD markers — plaques and NFT — (Khachaturian,1985; Tierney et al., 1988; Mirra et al., 1991). It has been hypothesized that dementia in AD could be caused either by the presence of AD specific changes alone or by the synergistic effect of some or all of these lesions (Terry et al., 1991, 1994; Samuel et al., 1994; Masliah, 1995). While earlier studies have shown positive correlations between the degree of dementia as measured by psychological tests with neocortical plaques (Blessed et al., 1968; Wilcock and Esiri, 1982), recent reports have found more reliable relations between dementia scores and neuritic AD changes, in particular neocortical NFT (McKee et al., 1991; Jellinger et al., 1992; Arriagada et al., 1992; Samuel et al., 1994; Bierer et al., 1995b; Kosunen et al., 1996), and with cortical synapse density, as seen by electron microscopy (DeKosky et al., 1990; Scheff and Price, 1993) or by immunochemical quantification of synaptic proteins (Terry et al., 1991; Lassmann et al., 1992; Masliah, 1995; Dickson et al., 1995; Blennow et al., 1996). In contrast, large amounts of amyloid plaques are present in non-demented aged subjects (Crystal et al., 1988; Morris et al., 1991), and as "pathologic aging" have been distinguished from AD (Dickson et al., 1991). Both neuritic AD lesions and synapse loss appear earliest in the superficial parts of the entorhinal region of the hippocampal formation that is thought to be essential for memory and cognition (Hyman et al., 1986; Braak and Braak, 1991; Honer et al., 1992; Braak et al., 1994; Samuel et al., 1994a; Heinonen et al., 1995). It is correlated with abnormal expression of amyloid precursor protein (APP) (Masliah et al., 1994). The hierarchical spreading of neuritic AD pathology from the inferotemporal allocortex via hippocampus over areas of the association isocortex is independent of the pattern and quantity of β-A4 amyloid deposits (Braak and Braak, 1991, 1994). In human brain, the entorhinal region is the main gateway to the hippocampus from isocortical association areas and limbic circuits via the glutamatergic perforant pathway terminating in the hippocampal dentate gyrus, with output modules from interconnected CA1 and subiculum projecting to deep layers of the entorhinal region and multiple cortical and subcortical areas (Braak and Braak, 1991; Samuel et al., 1994a; Insausti et al., 1995). Damage to this circuit by early neuritic AD lesions in the entorhinal region correlates with early memory deficits in aging, AD and other disorders (Markowitsch, 1994). Later progression of neuritic AD pathology causing a bidirectional disconnection of the hippocampus from other target areas appears of relevance for the deterioration of mental functions (Samuel et al., 1994a), while a destructive process related to isocortical AD pathology and synapse loss causing deafferentation of cortico-cortical or intracortical connections is a major correlate of dementia in AD (Terry et al., 1991, 1994; Lassmann et al., 1993). Clinico-pathologic correlation studies of the staging of neuritic AD pathology (Braak and Braak, 1991) with mental status using Blessed test scores (Braak et al., 1993) and Mini-Mental state (MMS) (Folstein et al., 1975) in prospective cohorts of aged individuals showed a highly significant negative correlation between both parameters (Fig. 2a). It appears remarkable that the isocortical stages V and VI, featured by abundant neuritic involvement of cortical association areas, are almost exclusively seen in a cluster of severely demented patients (MMS 0–2), while the "limbic" stages III and IV are associated with a wide range of cognitive performance between intellectually almost normal to dementia (MMS 24–5). Although statistical evaluation of the relationship between psychostatus (MMS) and the current morphological criteria for the diagnosis of AD revealed a highly significant correlation for both Braak staging and CERAD criteria (Jellinger et al., 1995), these data confirm recent data showing that the Braak staging scheme does not reliably identify all cases clinically diagnosed as dementia (Xuereb et al., 1995). While a subgroup of AD cases with very little or no neuritic pathology referred to as "plaque-only" AD (Hansen et al., 1993) or "pathological aging" (Dickson et al., 1991) may display either dementia or only minimal cognitive changes, large numbers of isocortical neuritic AD lesions, particularly NFT, are only seen in severely demented subjects and are considered end stage markers of the AD degenerative process (Bancher et al., 1993, 1996). Although the majority of AD cases show "plaque and tangle" type pathology, another rare subtype occurring in very old subjects with moderate to severe dementia reveals abundant NFT mainly in the allocortex with no or only very few amyloid deposits in the absence of neuritic plaques ("neurofibrillary predominant" type) (Bancher and Jellinger, 1994).

Another marker of AD severity that parallels well with mental dysfunction is cortical synapse density in both midfrontal and temporal cortex that also significally correlates with neuritic AD pathology (Terry et al., 1991;

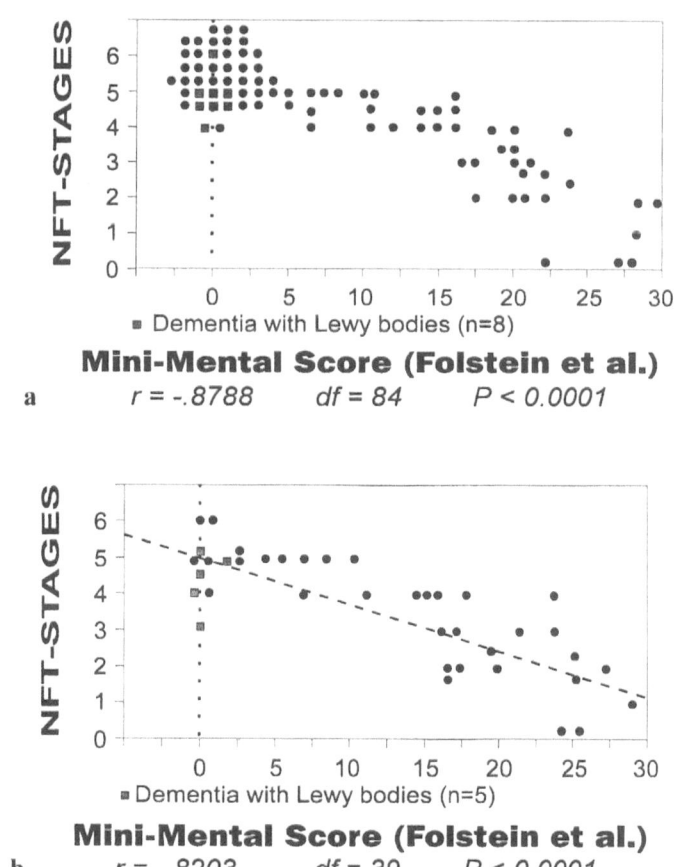

Fig. 2. a Correlation between neuropsychologically assessed psychostatus (Mini Mental-state) and neuritic Alzheimer stages in 84 consecutive autopsy cases of elderly subjects without parkinsonian symptoms (mean age 79.1 years) **b** Correlation between mental status and neuritic Alzheimer stages in 39 consecutive autopsy cases of Parkinson's disease (mean age 79.0 years)

Lassmann et al., 1992). However, all significances disappear after the exclusion of non-demented subjects with few or no pathology that could have been driving the strong correlations with pathologic markers (Lassmann et al., 1992; Dickson et al., 1995) while Blennow et al. (1996) found no correlation between synaptic pathology, SP, NFT, and the ApoE4 allele. Synapse loss in AD is accompanied by neuronal loss and aberrant sprouting, and studies in incipient AD cases have shown that this alteration occurs very early in the entorhinal region preceding tangle formation and causing early synapse loss in the hippocampal dentate gyrus that does not correlate with local amyloid accumulation (Masliah et al., 1994; Heinonen et al., 1995). The mechanism of synaptic pathology and neuronal degeneration that appear to play a central role in the multi-step pathogenesis of AD are not yet clear, but recent studies suggest that markers indicating cytoskeletal changes, e.g. NFT, neuritic plaques and PHF protein, may be better correlates of dementia than synapse markers (Dickson et al., 1995; Trojanowski et al., 1995). Other correlative studies indicate that neuritic pathology of the cholinergic nucleus basalis Meynert is a strong predictor of memory deficit in AD (Samuel et al., 1994b) reflecting disruption of the basal forebrain cholinergic system confirmed by many morphological and neurochemical studies (see Bierer et al., 1995a; Arendt et al., 1995).

Dementia with Lewy bodies (neurofilament associated disorders)

The most prominent cytoskeletal lesions associated with pathologically phosphorylated neurofilaments are Lewy bodies (LB), cytoplasmic inclusions occurring in many regions of the nervous system including brainstem and cortical areas. They are a morphological hallmark of Parkinson's disease (PD), and Lewy body disease (LBD) but are also found in a variety of neurodegenerative disorders either as an essential or coincidental feature (Pollanen et al., 1993; Dickson et al., 1996). Dementing disorders morphologically characterized by the presence of LB have been previously classified as PD + AD, Diffuse Lewy body disease (DLBD) (Kosaka et al., 1984; Burkhardt et al., 1988; Lippa et al., 1994), senile dementia of LB type (SLDT) (Perry et al., 1990) or LB variant of AD (LBV-AD) (Hansen et al., 1990). Since cortical LB are seen in almost all cases of PD (Hughes et al., 1992) and in many cases of AD (Kazee and Han, 1995), and nigral damage is frequently present in AD (Jellinger, 1987, 1995a; Kazee et al., 1995), the diagnostic criteria of Lewy body disease (LBD) and the question whether PD with concurrent AD, LBD with and without neuritic AD pathology, combined LBD and AD or LBV-AD, and AD with nigral lesions and occasional cortical LB represent separate disorders that can sometimes coexist, or whether they provide a spectrum of diseases with pure AD, LBD and PD with or without AD as poles and cases of "mixed pathology" (Table 7), are still under discussion (Lippa et al., 1994; Dababo et al., 1995). While Kosaka (1995) distinguishes 4 types of LBD — brain stem type or PD, transitional type, diffuse type or DLBD with a common and a pure form, and cortical type or DLBD/

Table 7. Morphological classification of Lewy Body Disorders (LBD) (Consortium of Dementia with Lewy bodies, Oct. 6, 1995)*

1. LBD, brainstem predominant, without diffuse plaques

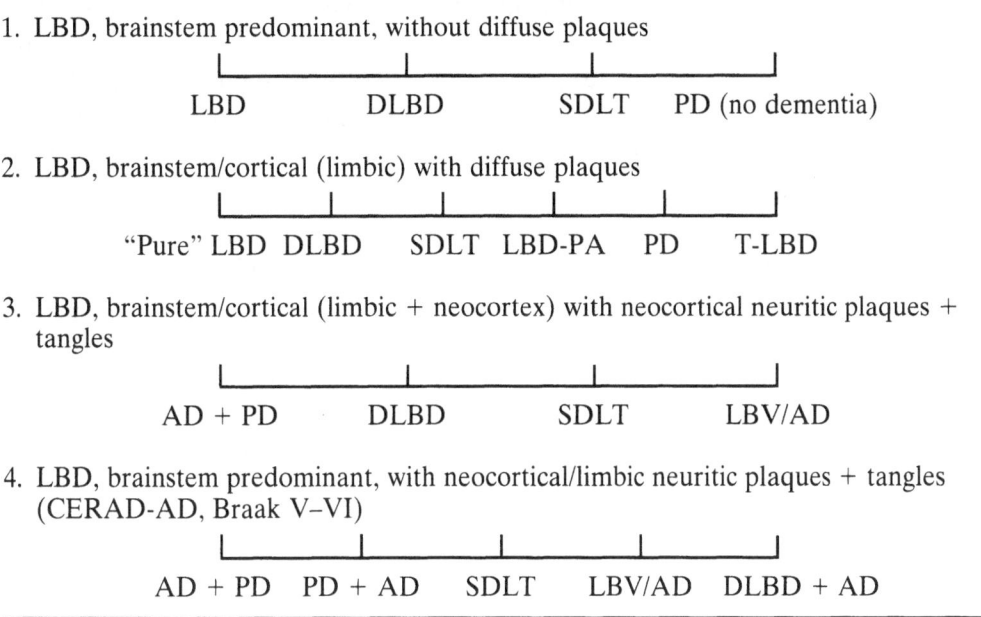

|LBD|DLBD|SDLT|PD (no dementia)|

2. LBD, brainstem/cortical (limbic) with diffuse plaques

"Pure" LBD   DLBD   SDLT   LBD-PA   PD   T-LBD

3. LBD, brainstem/cortical (limbic + neocortex) with neocortical neuritic plaques + tangles

AD + PD   DLBD   SDLT   LBV/AD

4. LBD, brainstem predominant, with neocortical/limbic neuritic plaques + tangles (CERAD-AD, Braak V–VI)

AD + PD   PD + AD   SDLT   LBV/AD   DLBD + AD

*Nigral cell loss rated according to CERAD criteria. *PA* pathological aging; *T* transitional; — previous terms

no PD — the recent suggestions of the Consortium of Dementia with Lewy bodies based on a semiquantitative assessment of LB in different brain regions and the CERAD morphological AD criteria are given in Table 8. While the recent demonstration of biochemical differences between cortical Lewy bodies in PD and LBD (Smith and Perry, 1995), the different distribution of neuritic AD pathology (Lippa et al., 1994; Jellinger and Bancher, 1995), of PHF and pathological tau proteins (Harrington et al., 1994), differences in cholinergic biochemistry (Perry et al., 1993), and in Apo E4 allele frequencies (Lippa et al., 1995; Martinoli et al., 1995; Morris et al., 1996) argue for a separation of LBD, PD, and AD, concurrence of these disorders with motor neuron disease (Hedera et al., 1995; Williams et al., 1995) and similar neurodegenerative "overlap" syndromes have been reported (Uitti et al., 1995). Although neither the frequency of cortical LB nor the intensity of cortical AD pathology have been shown to relate directly to the severity of dementia in many LBD patients (Jansen et al., 1995), the contribution of both types of lesions to cognitive impairment are under discussion.

In *Parkinson's disease* (PD), mental impairment is caused by dysfunction of neuronal networks in subcortical and cortical areas related to different CNS lesions (Jellinger et al., 1993; Jellinger and Bancher, 1995): 1. Degeneration of subcortico-cortical neuronal systems: a) striatonigral dopaminergic pathway due to neuronal loss in substantia nigra zona compacta causing deafferentiation of the striato-(pre)frontal loops and of the mesocorticolimbic dopamine system (Pillon et al., 1994a); b) degeneration of noradrenergic systems due to neuronal loss in locus coeruleus (Hoogendijk et al., 1995); c) degeneration of serotonergic systems resulting from damage to the dorsal raphe nuclei (Gai et al., 1995); d) degeneration of the ascending cholinergic system caused by cell loss and shrinkage in the substantia innominata and dorsolateral tegmental nuclei of the brainstem (Jellinger, 1987; Jellinger and Bancher, 1995; Perry et al., 1993); e) damage to the amygdala with a lesion pattern different from that in AD (Braak et al., 1994); f) combined degeneration of subcortical ascending systems that, however, is usually not sufficient by itself to produce overt dementia. In a chronic, slowly progressing model of PD in the monkey, however, specific cognitive deficits precede motor deficits, probably due to initially more extensive dopamine loss in the caudate inducing striato-frontal dysfunction, while the motor deficits result from later severe dopaminergic denervation of the putamen (Schneider and Pope-Coleman, 1995). 2. Cortical pathologies: a) limbic and/or neocortical AD lesions, b) cortical LB pathology and c) combined cortical lesions; 3. combination with other pathologies. In a consecutive autopsy series of 120 cases of clinically diagnosed parkinsonism, dementia seen in 38% of the total and in 30.8% of the cases with LBD of brainstem type (PD), was usually associated with AD or other pathologies, while only 1.8% of "pure" PD without additional brain pathologies had been demented (Table 9).

Dementia with Lewy bodies (LBD or SDLT) is distinguished from LBD of pure brainstem type (PD) by both clinical (Table 10) and morphological features (Table 8). In some recent autopsy series, it represents the second most frequent cause of dementia in the elderly, accounting from 7 to 30% (Harrington et al., 1994), and accounted for 11.7% in a personal consecutive autopsy series of 280 demented subjects or 28.3% of those with PD symptoms (Jellinger and Bancher, 1996). Correlative studies of Braak neuritic AD staging with psychostatus in 39 PD patients (mean age 79.0 years), displayed highly significant linear correlations (Fig. 2b). The results were similar to those in a cohort of age-matched non-PD subjects (Fig. 2a), although demented PD patients showed less frequently severe isocortical AD stages.

Table 8. Pathological classification of Lewy Body Disorders (LBD) [Consortium of Dementia with Lewy bodies, see McKeith et al., 1996]

Type of LBD	Cortical Lewy bodies					
	entorhinal	cingulate g.	temporal	frontal	parietal	total
Brainstem predominant	1	1	0	0	0	0–2
Transitional (limbic)	1–2	1–2	1	0	0	3–5
Cortical	2	2	1–2	1–2	1–2	6–10
CERAD-AD	−SP −NFT	+SP −NFT		+NP +NFT		
Combination neocortex	LBD + AD	LBD − AD ⟨ +SP (non-neuritic) / −SP				

0 = none   1+ = 1–5/region   2+ = >5/region

Table 9. Pathology of 120 consecutive autopsy cases of parkinsonism (1989–1994)

Neuropathology	total	with dementia n	dementia %
Park. disease LBtype (IPD)	54	1	1.8
IPD + lacunar state	10	0	0
IPD + cerebrovasc. lesions	7	0	0
IPD + AD/DAT	15	15	100.0
LB varient of AD	13	13	100.0
IPD + MIX (AD/MIE)	1	1	100.0
IPD + other pathology	4	2	50.0
Primary IPD	**104**	**32**	**30.8**
AD/DAT°	8	8	100.0
Prog. supranuclear palsy	3	2*	66.7
Multisystem atrophy	3	2*	66.7
Corticobasal degeneration	1	1	100.0
SAE Binswanger	1	1	100.0
Second. Park. Syndromes	**16**	**14**	**87.5**
Total	120	46	38.3

°with nigral lesion 4; *with AD

Table 10. Criteria for clinical diagnosis of dementia with Lewy bodies [LBD-Consortium, see McKeith et al., 1996]

1. Central feature: *progressive cognitive decline* of sufficient magnitude to interfere with social or occupational function (dementia — DSM-III-R, DSM-IV)

2. *Two* of the following features:
   a) Fluctuating cognition, with pronounced variations in attention and arousal
   b) Recurrent hallucinations which are typically visual, well formed and detailed
   c) Spontaneous extrapyramidal (parkinsonian) features

3. Features supportive of the diagnosis
   a) Repeated falls/syncope/orthostasis
   b) Transient losses of consciousness
   c) Systematised delusions

4. *Exclusion* by appropriate examination and investigation of any physical illness, or other brain disorder, sufficient to account for the clinical picture

Some severely demented cases with or without many cortical LB, however, were free of isocortical neuritic changes (Braak stage IV). These data suggest that although cortical AD pathology that may be superimposed on damage to other subcortico-cortical systems, is a major factor of overt dementia in a considerable proportion of LBD cases, it may not be the essential structural basis for mental decline in all instances of LBD. This is also illustrated by comparison of Braak neuritic AD staging in 100 consecutive autopsy cases of PD with or without dementia, 31 cases of LBD, 225 cases of AD and 50 age-matched controls showing considerable overlap between non-demented aged controls and PD patients on one hand, and between demented PD, LBD and AD cases on the other (Fig. 3). While almost 60% of the demented PD and about half of the LBD brains were "limbic" AD stages, corresponding to "plaque-predominant" or CERAD probable AD, about 40% of the demented PD and LBD brains as well as the majority of typical AD cases were isocortical stages meeting CERAD criteria of definite AD. About 70% of the LBD brains show subcortical lesions including severe nigral damage indistinguishable from PD, and the presence of ubiquitin-positive neurites in the CA2/3 region of hippocampus (Dickson et al., 1994) does not distinguish LBD from PD (Braak et al., 1994) but frequently coexists with cortical LB (Kim et al., 1995). In other cases of LBD mild diffuse nigral damage without LB resembles that seen in AD (Jellinger, 1987; Kazee et al., 1995). In addition to cortical AD and LB pathology, LBD, like AD and PD with dementia, reveals severe neuronal loss in the cholinergic nucleus basalis — 50 to 75% of controls — (Jellinger and Bancher, 1996). The accompanying decrease in cortical cholinergic markers is highly correlated with the severity of dementia in both LBD and AD with or without cortical LB (Perry et al., 1993, 1995; Bierer et al., 1995a). Decrease of synapse proteins in the hippocampal-entorhinal region in LBD and LBV is less severe than in AD (Wakabayashi et al., 1994), while its decrease in the isocortex is associated with neuritic AD pathology (Hansen, pers. comm.). These data suggest the importance of both cortical AD pathology and dysfuncion of the ascending cholinergic system for mental decline in LB dementia. Although synapse proteins appear to be involved in the formation of cortical LB, their significance for mental decline in LB

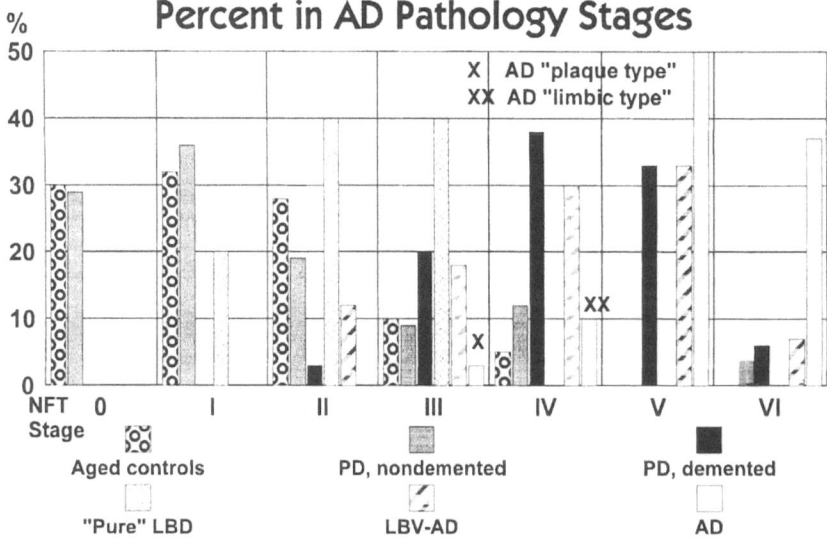

Fig. 3. Extent of neuritic Alzheimer changes using Braak stages in six diagnostic groups of the autopsy series given in Table 1: aged controls (n = 50), Parkinson's disease without/ with dementia (n = 66/34), "pure" Lewy body disease (LBD) (n = 5), Lewy body variant of Alzheimer's disease (LBV/AD) (n = 26), and Alzheimer's disease (AD) (n = 225). Incidence of neuritic AD pathology stages is expressed as percentage of cases in each diagnostic category

disorders and the pathogenic relationship between brainstem and diffuse LBD, and LBD + AD await further elucidation.

Pathological tau protein associated dementing disorders

A group of neurodegenerative disorders pathologically featured by widespread neuronal, glial and neuritic accumulation of abnormally phosphorylated tau proteins includes AD, PSP, CBD, and others (Table 6). Tau protein, occurring in NFT, neuropil threads or gliofibrillary tangles, may show different phosphorylation sites and involves different cell and axon populations (Ksiezak-Reding et al., 1994; Feany et al., 1995; Feany and Dickson, 1995).

Progressive supranuclear palsy (PSP), a sporadic parkinson-like dementing disorder with onset over 30 years of age, axial rigidity, akinesia, postural instability, vertical eye movement impairment, and frontal lobe symptoms (Tolosa et al., 1994; Collins et al., 1995; Daniel et al., 1995; Litvan et al., 1996a), is associated with variable neuronal loss and gliosis with widespread NFT and threads in basal ganglia, and brainstem including oculomotor complex, pontine basis, inferior olives, and dentate nucleus (Hauw et al., 1994). Involvement of the cerebral cortex mainly concerns (pre)frontal regions with sparing of the association areas predominantly involved in AD (Gearing et al., 1994), and there are both biochemical differences in tau protein isoforms and the distribution of cortical and subcortical lesions between PSP, AD, postencephalitic parkinsonism and Guam-PD dementia complex on Guam (Hauw et al., 1994; Vermersch et al., 1994; Hof et al., 1994; Buée-Scherrer et al., 1995). Mental decline in PSP suggested to be of subcortical type has been related to damage to striatofrontal circuits due to degeneration of the basal ganglia and prefrontal cortex (Pillon et al., 1994b, 1995) and/or to AD pathology in the allocortico-limbic system (Higuchi et al., 1994) and in some neocortical, mainly prefrontal, areas (Vermersch et al., 1994; Hanihara et al., 1995). However, neocortical AD changes in some PSP patients bear no clear relationship to the degree of cognitive impairment (DeBruin and Lees, 1994; Daniel et al., 1995). Since no histological distinction can be made between PSP with typical and atypical presentation, improved clinical and pathological criteria for "atypical" PSP and its distinction from other PD syndromes with NFT and "tufted glia" (Geddes et al., 1993; Handler et al., 1995; Feany et al., 1996) are needed.

Corticobasal degeneration, a rare sporadic late-onset dementing disorder with rigid-akinetic syndrome, asymmetric limb apraxia, dystonia, action tremor and myoclonus, clinically resembling PD or PSP (Lang et al., 1994a; Thompson et al., 1995), is associated with lobar frontal or parietal atrophy, swollen achromatic tau- and ubiquitin-positive cortical neurons, NFT-like neuronal inclusions, widespread neuropil threads and astrocytic plaques in the white matter (Horoupian and Chuy, 1994; Feany and Dickson, 1995). Although CBD may be difficult to be distinguished from PSP and Pick's disease with rare overlaps between these disorders (Feany et al., 1996) and coexistent cortical AD pathology (Schneider et al., 1995), biochemical tau profiles differ from those in AD, PSP, and Pick's disease (Feany et al., 1995; Buée-Scherrer et al., 1995). Mental decline associated with a dysexecutive syndrome probably due to degeneration of the basal ganglia and frontal cortex, and asymmetric praxis disorders, related to premotor and parietal lobe lesions (Pillon et al., 1995) are due to widespread tau-protein cytopathology related degeneration of cortical and subcortical gray and white matter (Feany and Dickson, 1995; Pollanen et al., 1995; Feany et al., 1996).

   Dementia with argyrophilic grains, a tau-related cytoskeletal abnormality mainly involving dendrospinal portions of neurons and oligodendroglia, may show morphological similarities with granular structures seen in CBD, PSP, and Pick's disease (Ikeda et al., 1995).

Fronto-temporal lobar atrophies (dementia)

The syndrome of fronto-temporal dementia (FTD) is clinically featured by progressive decline in personality, behavior, speech or other frontal lobe dysfunctions in the absence of severe amnesia, apraxia or perceptual spatial disorder (Brun et al., 1994) and may be preceded or followed by motor neuron disease (Talbot, 1996). This group of disorders accounting for 1 to 10% of dementias, also referred to as dementia lacking distinctive histopathology (Giannokopoulos et al., 1995), includes several morphological syndromes, the nosological position of which is under discussion (Jellinger, 1995b; Schmitt et al., 1995; Jackson and Lowe, 1996; Table II):

1. *Pick's disease*, a rare disorder, is featured by severe atrophy of the frontal and anterior temporal lobes, laminar cortical neuronal loss and gliosis, cortical neuronal inclusions (Pick bodies) and ballooned cells, both composed of tau, chromogranin A, ubiquitin and alpha B crystallin immunoreactive material, that are to be distinguished from LB and ballooned cells in PSP and CBD (see Table 5). Pick bodies are prominent in the prefrontal and temporal isocortex (layers II, III), in allocortex (granule cell layer of

Table 11. Differential diagnosis of frontotemporal lobar atrophies

Type of lesions	severity		
Fronto-temporal lobar atrophy	severe	mild	mild
Neuron loss	severe	mild	mild
Spongiosis cortical laminae I–III	absent/mild	present	present
Astrogliosis	severe	mild	mild
Subcortical involvement	often	occasional	severe
Neuronal inclusions	Pick bodies	absent	Ubi+/Tau neg.
	ballooned	ballooned	inclusions
	neurons	neurons	
	(Pick cells)	(αB cryst. pos.)	
	↓	↓	↓
	Pick's	Frontal Lobe	FLD +
	disease	Dementia (FLD)	MND

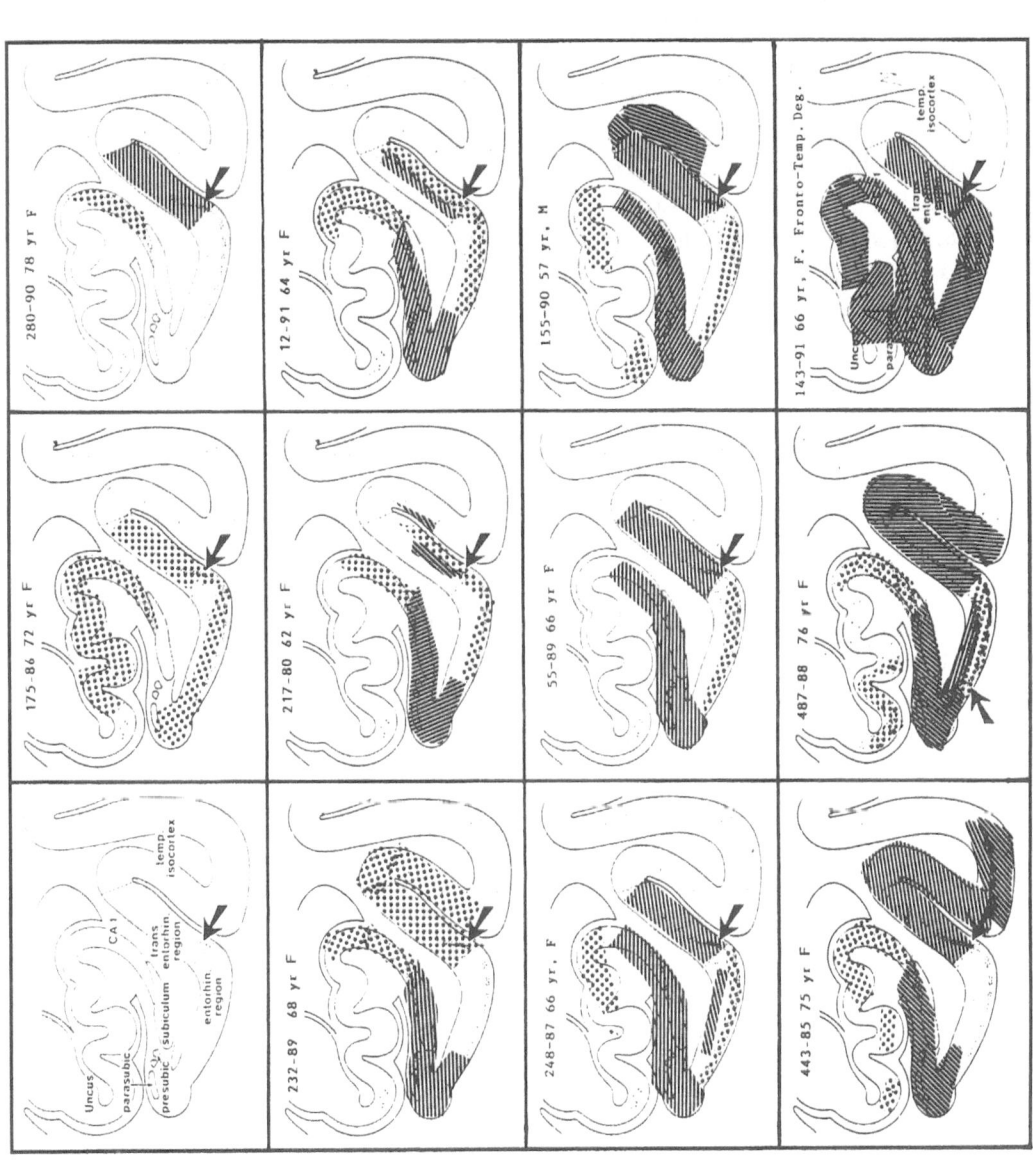

Fig. 4. Distribution of lesions in the hippocampal and parahippocampal formation in Pick's disease and one case of fronto-temporal degeneration. ▨ Spongy tissue destruction ▨ many Pick bodies/cells, — neurofibrillary tangles

dentate gyrus, CA 1 sector and entorhinal region), followed by neuron depletion and spongy changes in subiculum, transentorhinal region and temporal isocortex with relative sparing of entorhinal region and hippocampus. This pattern differs from both AD and non-Pick FLD (Fig. 3). While NFT are frequently present in Pick brain, pathologic tau proteins (55 and 64 kDa doublet) correlated with the presence of Pick bodies, differ from those in AD (55, 64, and 69 kDa) and in PSP (64 and 69 kDa doublet) (Delacourte et al., 1996; Tolnay et al., 1995; Buée-Scherrer et al., 1996); coexistence with AD and PSP is rare (Hof et al., 1994).

2. *Frontotemporal degeneration* (FTD) includes cases with frontotemporal atrophy, cortical spongiosis and neuron loss in the absence of neuronal inclusions but with swollen αB crystallin-reactive cortical neurons (Cooper et al., 1995; Jackson and Lowe, 1996) and variable subcortical lesions.

3. *Motor neuron disease type of FLD* (FLD + MND): reveals same lesions as FTD with spinal motor neuron degeneration and ubiquitin-positive, tau and αB crystallin negative inclusions in motor neurons, frontotemporal cortex and hippocampal dentate cells, and nigral lesion.

4. *Primary progressive aphasia* (PPA) may present lesion similar to FTD with or without Pick bodies, AD pathology or other non-specific changes with or without CBD-like bodies (Kertesz et al., 1994; Turner et al., 1996).

Whether Pick's disease and other lobar atrophies without neuronal inclusions, referred to as "atypical Pick's" (Hamada et al., 1995), represent distinct entities remains unclear; distinction is made from clinically similar syndromes in AD, PSP, and CBD by the lack of tau immunoreactivity, although pathological tau proteins have been detected in FTD and Pick's disease (Delacourte et al., 1996; Tolnay et al., 1995; Pollanen et al., 1995). The clinical symptoms of frontal dementia can be related to severe neuron and synapse loss in frontal cortex with no changes in parietal association areas severely affected in AD (Brun et al., 1995), while MND without dementia is not associated with significant loss of cortical synapse proteins (Ince et al., 1995).

Whereas in FTD and Pick's disease no prion protein (PrP) is observed (Owen et al., 1993), *familial progressive subcortical gliosis* (Neumann's disease), a rare disorder resembling Pick's (Lanska et al., 1994; Table 12), shows

Table 12. Familial progressive subcortical gliosis

Rare sporadic or familial (autosomal dominant) disorder	
Age at onset: 32–58 yrs; duration 3 months–37 years	
Clin. signs:	behavioral changes; memory decline; confusion; depression — severe dementia, decreased speech, extrapyramidal signs, mutism
Morphology:	cerebral atrophy (frontal, temporal lobes); marked astrogliosis in neocortex, subcortical white matter; less in basal ganglia, thalamus; spongy changes in superior cerebral cortex; neuronal loss in basal ganglia, thalamus, nigra, olivary nuclei; Pick and Lewy bodies absent
Protease resistant PRP plaques in cerebral cortex Linkage to chromosome 17 (Peterson et al., 1995)	

protease-resistant PrP in diffuse plaques (Petersen et al., 1995). Linkage to chromosome 17 differs from coding regions of PrP on chromosome 20.

Other inclusion diseases (Multisystem atrophies)

This group of sporadic or rarely autosomal dominant progressive disorders of middle-age onset presents with extrapyramidal-striatonigral degeneration (SND), cerebellar- olivopontocerebellar atrophy (OPCA), or autonomic symptoms, Shy-Drager syndrome (SDS), with rare dementia. The brain shows atrophy of discolorated striatum with neuron loss and deposition of lipofuscin-iron pigment, and secondary damage to lateral substantia nigra without and, rarely, with Lewy bodies, differing from the pattern in PD. SND may be associated with OPCA, while SDS shows neuronal loss in striatum, nigra, cerebellar cortex, olives, Westphal-Edinger nucleus, and intermediolateral columns of spinal cord. Specific histological hallmarks are cytoplasmic tau, ubiquitin, αB crystallin-positive inclusions in oligodendroglia and ubiquitinated neuronal nuclear or cytoplasmic inclusions (Table 5) partly related to neuronl loss (Papp and Lantos, 1994). Although the significance of these inclusions is unclear, they are diagnostic markers even in atypical cases (Wenning et al., 1995). Mental changes mainly include a dysexecutive syndrome, more severe for MSA than PD, although less severe than in PSP due to striato-frontal dysfunction (Gouider-Khounja et al., 1995).

Hereditary non-Alzheimer dementias

They include a group of autosomal dominant neurodegenerative disorders associated with expanding trinucleotide repeats located in coding regions of different genes: Huntington's disease, dentatorubropallidoluysian atrophy, and Machado-Joseph disease.

Huntington's disease, an autosomal dominant, fully penetrant progressive disorder, results from a genetic defect of an unstable polymorphic trinucleotide expanded repeat (CAG) in the coding region of the IT 15 gene on chromosome 4p (see Andreew and Hayden, 1995). Symptoms include personal change, chorea and dementia appearing at an average age of 45 years, with more severe progression in juvenile forms. The brain shows atrophy of the caudate nucleus with enlarged ventricles due to loss of GABAergic type II neurons with gliosis classified into 5 grades (Vonsattel, 1992). Neostriatal pathology starts with loss of GABA-ergic striosome neurons and gliosis producing hyperactivity of the nigrostriatal pathway and of thalamocortical feedback producing chorea, later involving both striosomes and matrix in a dorsoventral progression (Hedreen and Folstein, 1995). Damage to nucleus accumbens, pallidum, ventrolateral thalamus, subthalamus, and nigra lead to decreased motor activity and rigidity in later stages. Cognitive change is similar PD or PSP due to disorders of striatofrontal loops (Pillon et al., 1994); dementia results from severe cortical cell loss in primary sensory and association areas (layers III and V) (Heinsen et al., 1994) and in deep entorhinal cortex (Braak and Braak, 1992). Dystrophic ubiquinited neurites resembling CA 2/3 and brainstem Lewy neurites in LBD are seen in cerebral cortex and substantia nigra (Jackson et al., 1995; Soones et al., 1995). Their extent and the severity of morphological changes may be related to the severity of the genetic defect, the age of onset and the rate of progression of illness that correlate with CAG repeat length (Brandt et al., 1996), but appear independent of the CAG repeat length and the levels of IT15 in mRNA expression in neuronal systems (Claes et al., 1995; Landwehrmeyer et al., 1995). Widespread CNS expression of the HD gene product suggests that it may be involved in common cellular and, possibly, nerve terminal functions. The product of the expanded allel is expressed, consistent with a gain of functional mechanisms for HD at the protein level (Sharp et al., 1995). The mechanism of gene action causing a distinctive pattern of HD degeneration remains to be elucidated (Brandt et al., 1996).

Dentatopallidoluysian/nigral atrophy (DRPLA), a rare autosomal dominant disorder in Japan and Europe, is clinically presenting with choreoathetosis, ataxia, myoclonus, epilepsy, and dementia at various ages of onset and considerable intrafamilial variations (Uyama et al., 1995; Ikeuchi et al., 1995). Neuropathology shows multiple system atrophy involving dentatorubral, pallidofugal systems, subthalamus, (spino)cerebellar, and motor systems. Distinction from HD, OPCA and other multisystem degenerations is difficult (Warner et al., 1995). DRPLA shows clinical and genetic similarities with HD or spinocerebellar SCA1 disorders with apolymeric CAG trinucleotid repeat in a gene on the short arm of chromosome 12 (Komure et al., 1995; Ikeuchi et al., 1995).

Machado-Joseph disease (MJD), an autosomal dominant progressive ataxic disorder with external ophthalmoplegia and polyneuropathy, has several clinical subtypes with pyramidal, cerebellar, extrapyramlidal or distal amyotrophies and occasional dementia (Uitti, 1994). Pathology shows dentatonigrospinal degeneration with cell loss in dentate, subthalamic and brainstem nuclei, nigra, and spinal anterior horns. The disorder is linked to an unstable CAG repeat in a gene at chromosome 14q 32.1 which differs from the spinocerebellar locus SCA1 (Lang et al., 1994b; Kawaguchi et al., 1994; Watanabe et al., 1996) but shows linkage to spinocerebellar ataxia type 3 (SCA 3) (Haberhausen et al., 1995; Higgins et al., 1996).

In conclusion, most types of dementing neurodegenerative disorders, despite clinical and pathological overlaps, show characteristic pathologies with or without typical cytoskeletal sign posts or patterns of CNS lesions pointing to the correct diagnosis. Since in vivo markers for these disorders except for those with known genetic background are lacking, diagnosis, in general, depends on clinico-morphological features. Since some of these disorders share clinical and morphological features with other neurodegenerative disorders, comprehensive studies using modern molecular biological methods are needed to distinguish between the different disease entities. Dementia in the majority of these disorders is related to dysfunction of multiple cortico-subcortical neuronal populations and circults. In addition to disorders of striato-(sub)frontal and hippocampo-cortical loops, degeneration of cortico-cortical and intracortical loops due to nonspecific neuronal and synapse loss or superimposed AD pathologies are to be considered as major factors of mental decline, the latter lesions often differ in intensity and distribution pattern from those in AD. Further studies are warranted for the elucidation of the structural basis of dementia in these disorders in order to provide better insight into their pathogenesis and pathophysiology as a basis for future therapeutic strategies.

References

Andrew SE, Hayden MR (1995) Origins and evolution of Huntington's disease chromosomes. Neurodegeneration 4: 239–244

Arima K, Muramaya S, Oyanagi S, Akashi S, Inose T (1992) Presenile dementia with progressive supranuclear palsy tangles and Pick bodies. An unusual degenerative disorder involving the cerebral cortex, cerebral nuclei, and brain stem nuclei. Acta Neuropathol 84: 128–134

Arima K, Uesugi H, Fujita I, Oyanagi S, Andoh S, Izumiyama Y, Inose T (1994) Corticonigral degeneration with neuronal achromasia presenting with primary progressive aphasia: ultrastructural and immunocytochemical studies. J Neurol Sci 127: 186–192

Arnold SE, Kumar A (1993) Reversible dementias. Med Clin North Am 77: 215–230

Arriagada PV, Growdon JH, Hedley-Whyte T, Hyman BT (1992) Neurofibrillary tangles but not senile plaques parallel duration and severity of Alzheimer's disease. Neurology 42: 631–639

Bancher C, Braak H, Fischer P, Jellinger K (1993) Neuropathological staging of Alzheimer lesions and intellectual status in Alzheimer's and Parkinson's disease. Neurosci Lett 162: 179–182

Bancher C, Jellinger KA (1994) Neurofibrillary tangle predominant form of senile dementia of Alzheimer type: a rare subtype in very old subjects. Acta Neuropathol 88: 565–570

Bancher C, Jellinger K, Lassmann H, Fischer P, Leblhuber F (1996) Correlations between mental state and quantitative neuropathology in the Vienna longitudinal study on dementia. Eur Arch Psychiat Clin Neurosci 246: 137–146

Bierer LM, Haroutunian V, Gabriel S, Knott PJ, Carlin LS, Purohit DP, Perl DP, Schmeidler J, Kanof P, Davis KL (1995a) Neurochemical correlates of dementia severity in Alzheimer's disease: relative importance of the cholinergic deficits. J Neurochem 64: 749–760

Bierer LM, Hof PR, Purohit DP, Carlin L, Schneidler J, Davis KL, Perl DP (1995b) Neocortical neurofibrillary tangles correlate with dementia severity in Alzheimer's disease. Arch Neurol 52: 81–88

Blennow K, Bogdanovic N, Alafuzoff I, Ekman R, Davidsson P (1996) Synaptic pathology in Alzheimer's disease: relation to severity of dementia, but not to senile plaques, neurofibrillary tangles, or the ApoE4 allel. J Neural Transm 103: 603–618

Blessed G, Tomlinson BE, Roth M (1968) The association between quantitative measures of dementia and of senile change in the cerebral gray matter of elderly subjects. Br J Psychiatry 114: 797–811

Braak H, Braak E (1991) Neuropathological staging of Alzheimer-related changes. Acta Neuropathol 82: 239–259

Braak H, Braak E (1992) The human entorhinal cortex: normal morphology and lamina-specific pathology in various diseases. Neurosci Res 15: 6–31

Braak H, Braak E (1994) Pathology of Alzheimer's disease. In: Calne DB (ed) Neurodegenerative disease. Saunders, Philadelphia, pp 585–613

Braak H, Braak E, Mandelkow EM (1994) A sequence of cytoskeleton changes related to the formation of neurofibrillary tangles and neuropil threads. Acta Neuropathol 87: 554–567

Braak H, Braak E, Yilmazer D, De Ros RAI, Jansen ENH, Bohl J, Jellinger K (1994) Amygdala pathology in Parkinson's disesase. Acta Neuropathol 88: 493–500

Braak H, Duyckaerts C, Braak E, Piette F (1993) Neuropathological staging of Alzheimer-related changes correlates with psychometrically assessed intellectual status. In: Corain B, et al (eds) Alzheimer's disease. Advances in clinical and basic research. Wiley, Chichester, pp 131–137

Brandt J, Bylsma FW, Gross R, Stine OC, Ranen N, Ross CA (1996) Trinucleotide repeat length and clincial progression of Huntington's disease. Neurology 46: 527–531

Brown P (1996) Transmissible human amyloidosis. J Neural Transm [Suppl] 47: 219–229

Brun A, Englund B, Gustavson L, Passant U, Mann DMA, Neary D, Snowdon JS (1994) Clinical and neuropathological criteria for frontotemporal dementia. J Neurol Neurosurg Psychiatry 57: 416–418

Brun A, Liu X, Erikson C (1995) Synapse loss and gliosis in the molecular layer of the cerebral cortex in Alzheimer's disease and frontal lobe degeneration. Neurodegeneration 4: 171–177

Budka H, Aguzzi A, Brown P, Brucher J-M, Bugiani O, Gullotta F, Haltia M, Hauw J-J, Ironside JW, Jellinger K, Kretzschmar HA, Lantos PL, Masullo C, Scholte W, Tateishi J, Weller RO (1995) Neuropathological diagnostic criteria for Creutzfeldt-Jakob disease (CJD) and other human spongiform encephalopathies (prion diseases). Brain Pathol 5: 459–465

Buée-Scherrer V, Buée L, Hof PR, Leveugle-Giolles C, Loerzel AJ, Perl DP, Delacourte A (1995) Neurofibrillary degeneration in amyotrophic lateral sclerosis/parkinsonism dementia complex of Guam: immunochemical characterization of tau proteins. Am J Pathol 68: 924–932

Buée-Scherrer V, Hof PR, Buée L, Leveugle B, et al (1996) Hyperphosphorylated tau proteins differentiate corticobasal degeneration and Pick's disease. Acta Neuropathol 91: 351–359

Burkhardt CR, Filley CM, Kleinschmidt-DeMasters BK, de la Monte S, Norenberg MD, Schneck SA (1988) Diffuse Lewy body disease and progressive dementia. Neurology 38: 1520–1528

Collins SJ, Ahlskog JE, Parisi JE, Maraganore DM (1995) Progressive supranuclear palsy: neuropathologically based diagnostic clinical criteria. J Neurol Neurosurg Psychiatry 58: 167–173

Cooper PN, Jackson M, Lennox G, Lowe J, Mann DMA (1995) Tau, ubiquitin and alpha B crystallin immunohistochemistry define the principal causes of degenerative frontotemporal dementia. Arch Neurol 52: 1011–1016

Corey-Bloom J, Thal LJ, Galasko D, Folstein M, et al (1995) Diagnosis and evaluation of dementia. Neurology 45: 211–218

Crystal H, Dickson D, Fuld P, Masur D, Scott R, Mehler M, Masdeu J, Kawas C, Aronson M, Wolfson L (1988) Clinico-pathological studies in dementia: nondemented subjects with pathologically confirmed Alzheimer's disease. Neurology 38: 1682–1687

Dababo MA, Bigio EH, Hladik CL, White CL III (1995) Neuropathological evidence that the Lewy body variant of Alzheimer disease represents coexistence of Alzheimer disease and idiopathic Parkinson disease. J Neuropathol Exp Neurol 54: 429

Daniel SE, De Bruin VMS, Lees AJ (1995) The clinical and pathological spectrum of Steele-Richardson-Olszewski syndrome (progressive supranuclear palsy). Brain 118: 759–770

De Bruin VMS, Lees AJ (1994) Subcortical neurofibrillary degeneration presenting as Steele-Richardson-Olszewski and other related syndromes. A review of 90 pathologically verified cases. Mov Disord 9: 381–389

De Kosky ST, Harbaugh RE, Schmitt FA, et al (1992) Cortical biopsy in Alzheimer's disease: diagnostic occuracy and neurochemical. neuropathological and cognitive correlations. Ann Neurol 32: 625–632

Delacourte A, Robitaille Y, Sergeant N, Buée L, Hof PR, Wattez A, Laroche-Cholette A, Mathieu J, Chagnon P, Gavreau D (1996) Specific pathological tau protein variants characterizing Pick's disease. J Neuropathol Exp Neurol 55: 159–168

Dickson DW, Crystal HA, Bevona C, Honer W, Vincent I, Davies P (1995) Correlations of synaptic and pathological markers with cognition of the elderly. Neurobiol Aging 16: 285–304

Dickson DW, Feany MB, Yen SH, Matthiace LA, Davies P (1996) Cytoskeletal pathology in non-Alzheimer degenerative dementia. New lesions in Diffuse Lewy body disease, Pick's disease and Corticobasal Degeneration. J Neural Transm [Suppl] 47: 31–46

Dickson DW, Schmidt ML, Lee VMY, Zhao ML, Yen SH, Trojanowski JQ (1994) Immunoreactivity profile of hippocampal CA2/3 neurites in Diffuse Lewy body disease. Acta Neuropathol 87: 269–276

DSM-III-R (1987) Diagnostic and statistical manual of mental disorders, 3rd edn, revised. American Psychiatric Association, Washington

Feany MB, Dickson DW (1995) Widespread cytoskeletal pathology characterizes corticobasal degeneration. Am J Pathol 146: 1388–1396

Feany MB, Ksiezak-Reding H, Liu W-K, et al (1995) Epitope expression and hyperphosphorylation of tau protein in corticobasal degeneration; differentiation from progressive supranuclear palsy. Acta Neuropathol 90: 37–43

Feany MB, Mattiace LA, Dickson DW (1996) Neuropathologic overlap of progressive supranuclear palsy, Pick's disease, and corticobasal degeneration. J Neuropathol Exp Neurol 55: 53–67

Folstein MF, Folstein SE, McHugh PR (1975) "Mini-Mental State": a practical method grading the cognitive state of patients for the clinician. J Psychiatry Res 12: 189–198

Gai WP, Blessing WW, Blumbergs PC (1995) Ubiquitin-positive degenerating neurites in the brainstem in Parkinson's disesse. Brain 118: 1447–1459

Gai WP, Blumberg PC, Blessing WW (1996) Microtubule-associated protein 5 is a component of Lewy bodies and Lewy neurites in the brainstem and forebrain regions affected in Parkinson's disease. Acta Neuropathol 91: 78–81

Galasko D, Hansen LA, Katzman R, Widerholt W, Masliah E, Terry RD, Hill LR, Lessin P, Thal LJ (1994) Clinical-neuropathological correlations in Alzheimer's disease and related dementias. Arch Neurol 51: 888–895

Gearing M, Mirra SS, Hedreen JC, Sumi SM, Hansen LA, Heyman A (1995) The Consortium to Establish a Registry for Alzheimer's Disease (CERAD), part X. Neuropathology confirmation of the clinical diagnosis of Alzheimer's disease. Neurology 45: 461–466

Gearing M, Olson DA, Watts RL, Mirra SS (1994) Progressive supranuclear palsy: neuropathologic and clinical heterogeneity. Neurology 44: 1015–1024

Giannokopoulos P, Hof PR, Bours C (1995) Dementia lacking distinctive histopathology. Evaluation of 32 cases. Acta Neuropathol 88: 440–447

Gouider-Khouja N, Vidailhet M, Bonnet AM, Pichon J, Agid Y (1995) "Pure" striatonigral degeneration and Parkinson's disease: a comparative clinical study. Mov Disord 10: 288–294

Haberhausen G, Damian MS, Leweke F, Müller U (1995) Spinocerebellar ataxia type 3 (SCA 3) is genetically identical to Machado-Joseph disease. J Neurol Sci 132: 71–75

Halliday GM, Davies L, McRitchie DA, Cartwright H, Pamphlett R, Morris JGL (1995) Ubiquitin-positive achromatic neurons in corticobasal degeneration. Acta Neuropathol 90: 68–75

Hamada K, Fukazawa T, Yanigihara K, Hamada T, Yoshimura N, Tashiro K (1995) Dementia with ALS features and diffuse Pick body-like inclusions (atypical Pick's disease?). Clin Neuropathol 14: 1–6

Handler M, Pahwa R, Hubble J, Koller WC (1995) Parkinsonism associated with neu-
rofibrillary tangles and tufted astrocytes (Abstract). Ann Neurol 38: 301
Hanihara T, Amano N, Takahashi T, Nagatomo H, Yagashita S (1995) Distribution of
tangles and threads in the cerebral cortex in progressive supranuclear palsy.
Neuropathol Appl Neurobiol 21: 319–326
Hansen L, Salmon D, Galasko D, Masliah E, Katzman R, DeTeresa R, Thal L, Pay
RN, Hofstetter R, Klauber M, Rice V, Butters BA, Alford M (1990) The Lewy
body variant of Alzheimer's disease: a clinical and pathologic entity. Neurology 40:
1–8
Hansen LA, Masliah E, Galasko D, Terrry RD (1993) Plaque-only Alzheimer disease is
usually the Lewy body variant and vice versa. J Neuropathol Exp Neurol 52: 648–
654
Harrington CR, Perry RH, Perry EK, Hurt J, McKeith IG, Roth M, Wischik CM (1994a)
Senile dementia of Lewy body type and Alzheimer type are biochemically distinct in
terms of paired helical filaments and hyperphosphorylated tau protein. Dementia 5:
215–228
Harrington GR, Louwagie J, Rossau R, Van Mechelen E, Perry RH, Perry EK, Xuereb
JH, Roth M, Wischik CM (1994b) Influence of apolipoprotein E genotype on senile
dementia of the Alzheimer and Lewy body types: significance for etiological therories
of Alzheimer's disease. Am J Pathol 145: 1472–1484
Hauw JJ, Daniel S, Dickson D, Horoupian DS, Jellinger K, Lantos PL, McKee A,
Tabaton M, Litvan I (1994) Preliminary NINDS neuropathologic criteria for Steele-
Richardson-Olszewski syndrome (progressive supranuclear palsy). Neurology 44:
2015–2019
Hedera P, Lerner AJ, Castellani R, Friedland RP (1995) Concurrence of Alzheimer's
disease, Parkinson's disease, diffuse Lewy body disease, and amyotrophic lateral
sclerosis. J Neurol Sci 128: 219–224
Hedreen JC, Folstein SE (1995) Early loss of neostriatal striosome neurons in
Huntington's disease. J Neuropathol Exp Neurol 54: 105–120
Heinonene O, Soininen H, Sorveri H, Kosunen O, Paljärvi L, Kovisto E, Riekkinen PJ
(1995) Loss of synaptophysin-like immunoreactivity in the hippocampal formation is
an early phenomenon in Alzheimer's disease. Neuroscience 64: 375–384
Heinsen H, Strik M, Bauer M, Luther K, Ulmar G, Gangnus D, Jungkunz G,
Eisenmenger W, Gotz N (1994) Cortical and striatal neurone number in Huntington's
disease. Acta Neuropathol 88: 320–333
Higgins JJ, Vascancelos O, Ide SE, Lavendan C, Goldfarb LG, Polymeropoulos MH
(1996) Mutations in American families with spinocerebellar ataxia (SCA) type 3;
SCA 3 is allelic to Machado-Joseph disease. Neurology 46: 208–213
Hof PR, Bouras C, Perl DP, Morrison H (1994a) Quantitative neuropathologic analysis of
Pick's disease cases: cortical distribution of Pick bodies and coexistance with
Alzheimer's disease. Acta Neuropathol 87: 115–124
Hof PR, Nimchinsky EA, Buée-Scherrer V, Buée L, Nasrallah J, Hottinger AF, Purohit
DP, Loerzel AJ, Steele JC, Delacourte A, Bouras C, Morrison JH, Perl DP (1994b)
Amyotrophic lateral sclerosis/parkinsonsim-dementia complex of Guam: quantita-
tive neuropathology, immunohistochemical analysis of neuronal vulnerability, and
comparison with related neurodegenerative disorders. Acta Neuropathol 88: 397–404
Honer WG, Dickson DW, Gleeson J, Davies P (1992) Regional synaptic pathology in
Alzheimer's disease. Neurobiol Aging 13: 375–382
Hoogendijk WJG, Pall CW, Troost D, Venzweiten E, Swaab DF (1995) Image analysis-
assisted morphometry of the locus ceruleus in Alzheimer's disease, Parkinson's dis-
ease, and amyotrophic lateral sclerosis. Brain 118: 131–143
Horoupian DS, Chuy PL (1994) Unusual case of corticobasal degeneration with tau/
Gallyas-positive neuronal and glial tangles. Acta Neuropathol 88: 592–598
Hughes AJ, Daniel SE, Kilford L, Lees AJ (1992) Accuracy of clinical diagnosis of
idiopathic Parkinson's disease. A clinico-pathological study of 100 cases. J Neurol
Neurosurg Psychiatry 55: 181–184

Hyman BT, Van Hoesen GW, Kromer LJ, Damasio AR (1986) Perforant pathway changes and the memory impairment in Alzheimer disease. Ann Neurol 20: 37–40

Ikeda K, Akiyama H, Kondo H, Haga C (1995) A study of dementia with argyrophilic grains — possible cytoskeletal abnormality in dendrospinal portion of neurons and oligodendroglia. Acta Neuropathol 89: 409–414

Ikeuchi T, Koide R, Tanaka H, Onodera O, et al (1995) Dentatorubral-pallidoluysian atrophy: clinical features are closely related to unstable expansions of trinucleotide (CAG) repeat. Ann Neurol 37: 769–775

Ince PG, Stade J, Chinnery RM, McKenzie J, Royston C, Roberts GVV, Shaw PJ (1995) Quantitative study of synaptophysin immunoreactivity of cerebral cortex and spinal cord in motor neuron disease. J Neuropathol Exp Neurol 54: 673–679

Insausti R, Tunon T, Sobreviela T, Insausti AM, Gonzalo LM (1995) The human entorhinal cortex. A cytoarchitectonic analysis. J Comp Neurol 355: 171–198

Ironside JW (1996) Human prion diseases. J Neural Transm [Suppl] 47: 231–246

Jackson M, Lowe J (1996) The new neuropathology of degenerative frontotemporal dementias. Acta Neuropathol 91: 127–134

Jansen ENH, De Vos RAI, Stam FC, Ravid R, Swaab DF (1994) Lewy bodies, with and without dementia: clinico-pathological correlations in 22 consecutive cases of Parkinson's disease. In: Korczyn AD (ed) Dementia in Parkinson's disease. Monduzzi Ed, Bologna, pp 207–209

Jellinger K (1987) Neuropathological substrates of Alzheimer's and Parkinson's disease. J Neural Transm [Suppl] 24: 109–129

Jellinger KA (1995a) Neurodegenerative disorders with extrapyramidal features. A neuropathological overview. J Neural Transm [Suppl] 46: 33–56

Jellinger KA (1995b) Neuropathological criteria for Pick's disease and frontotemporal lobe dementia. In: Cruz-Sánchez FF (ed) Neuropathological diagnostic criteria for brain banking. IOS Press, Amsterdam Oxford Washington Tokyo, pp 35–54

Jellinger KA (1996) The neuropathological diagnosis of secondary parkinsonian syndromes. Adv Neurol 69: 293–303

Jellinger KA, Bancher C (1994) Classification of dementias based on functional morphology. In: Jellinger KA, Ladurner G, Windisch E (eds) New trends in the diagnosis and treatment of Alzheimer's disease. Springer, Wien New York, pp 9–39

Jellinger KA, Bancher C (1995) Structural basis of mental impairment in Parkinson's disease. Neuropsychiatrie 9: 9–14

Jellinger KA, Bancher C (1996) Dementia with Lewy bodies. Relationship to Parkinson's and Alzheimer's disease. In: Perry E, McKeith LG, et al (eds) Dementia with Lewy bodies. Cambridge University Press, New York (in press)

Jellinger K, Bancher C, Fischer P, Lassmann H (1992) Quantitative histopathologic validation of senile dementia of the Alzheimer type. Eur J Gerontol 3: 146–156

Jellinger KA, Bancher C, Fischer P (1993) Neuropathological correlates of mental dysfunctions in Parkinson's disease. In: Wolters ED, Scheltens P (eds) Mental dysfunction in Parkinson's disease. Vrije Universiteit, Amsterdam, pp 141–161

Jellinger K, Bancher C, Fischer P, Lassmann H (1994) Staging of degenerative dementia. Neurol Croat 43 [Suppl] 2: 39–58

Jellinger KA, Bancher C, Fischer P (1995) Letter to the editor. J Neuropathol Exp Neurol 54: 129–130

Katzman R, Kawan C (1994) The epidemiology of dementia and Alzheimer disease. In: Terry RD, Katzman R, Bick KI (eds) Alzheimer disease. Raven Press, New York, pp 105–122

Kawaguchi Y, Okamoto T, Taniwaki M, Aizawa M, Inoue M, Katayama S, Kawakami H, Nakmura S, Nishimura M, Akiguchi I, Kimura J, Narumiya S, Kakizuka (1994) CAG expansion in a novel gene for Machado-Joseph disease at chromosome 14q32.1. Nature Genet 8: 221–227

Kazee AM, Han LY (1995) Cortical Lewy bodies in Alzheimer's disease. Arch Pathol Lab Med 119: 448–453

Kazee AM, Cox C, Richfield EK (1995) Substantia nigra lesions in Alzheimer disease and normal aging. Alzheimer Dis Assoc Disord 9: 61–67

Kertesz A, Hudson L, Mackenzie JRA, Munoz DG (1994) The pathology and nosology of primary progressive aphasia. Neurology 44: 2065–2072

Khachaturian ZS (1985) Diagnosis of Alzheimer's disease. Arch Neurol 42: 1097–1105

Kim H, Gearing M, Mirra SS (1995) Ubiquitin-positive CA 2(3 neurites in hippocampus coexist with cortical Lewy bodies. Neurology 45: 1766–1770

Kosaka K (1993) Dementia and neuropathology in Lewy body disease. Adv Neurol 60: 456–463

Kosaka K, Yoshimura M, Ikeda K, Budka H (1984) Diffuse type of Lewy body disease: progressive dementia with abundant cortical Lewy bodies and senile changes of various degree — a new disease? Clin Neuropathol 3: 195–192

Kosunen O, Soininen H, Paljärvi L, Heinonen O, Talasniemi S, Riekkinen PJ (1996) Diagnostic accuracy of Alzheimer's disease: a neuropathological study. Acta Neuropathol 91: 185–193

Ksiezak-Reding H, Morgan K, Mattiace LA, Davies P, Liu WK, Yen SH, Weidenheim K, Dickson DW (1994) Ultrastructural and biochemical composition of paired helical filaments in corticobasal degeneration. Am J Pathol 145: 1496–1508

Landwehrmeyer GB, McNeil SMJ, Dure LS, Ge P, et al (1995) Huntington's disease gene: regional and cellular expression in brain of normal and affected individuals. Ann Neurol 37: 218–230

Lang AE, Riley DE, Bergeron C (1994a) Cortico-basal ganglionic degeneration. In: Calne DB (ed) Neurodegenerative diseases. Saunders, Philadelphia, pp 877–894

Lang AE, Rogaeva EA, Tsuda T, Hutterer J, Styeorge-Hyslop P (1994b) Homozygous inheritance of the Machado-Joseph disease gene. Ann Neurol 36: 443–447

Lanska DJ, Currier RD, Cohen M, Gambetti P, et al (1994) Familial progressive subcortical gliosis. Neurology 44: 1633–1643

Lantos PL (1992) Neuropathology of unusual dementias; an overview. In: Baillière's clinical neurology, vol 1. Baillière Tindall, London, pp 485–516

Larner AJ (1995) The cortical neuritic dystrophy of Alzheimer's disease: nature, significance, and possible pathogenesis. Dementia 6: 218–224

Lassmann H, Fischer P, Jellinger K (1993) Synaptic pathology of Alzheimer's disease. Ann NY Acad Sci 695: 59–64

Lassmann H, Weiler R, Fischer P, Bancher C, Jellinger K, Floor E, Danielczyk W, Seitelberger F, Winkler H (1992) Synaptic pathology in Alzheimer's disease: immunological data for markers of synaptic and large dense core vesicles. Neuroscience 46: 1–8

Lippa CF, Smith IW, Swearer JM (1994) Alzheimer's disease and Lewy body disease: a comparative clinicopathological study. Ann Neurol 35: 81–88

Lippa CF, Smith TW, Saunders AM, et al (1995) Apolipoprotein E genotype and Lewy body disease. Neurology 45: 97–103

Litvan I, Hauw JJ, Bartko JJ, Lantos PL, Daniel SE, Horoupian DS, McKee A, Dickson D, Bancher C, Tabaton M, Jellinger K, Anderson DW (1996a) Validity and reliability of the preliminary NINDS neuropathologic criteria for the diagnosis of progressive supranuclear palsy and related disorders. J Neuropathol Exp Neurol 55: 97–105

Litvan I, Hauw JJ, Bartko JJ, Lantos PL, Daniel SE, Horoupian DS, McKee A, Dickson D, Bancher C, Tabaton M, Jellinger K, D'Olhaberriague L, Anderson DW (1996) Reliability and validity of neuropathology in the diagnosis of neurodegenerative disorders with extrapyramidal features. Neurology 46: 922–930

Markowitsch HJ (1994) Anatomical basis of memory disorders. In: Gazzaniga MS (ed) The cognitive neurosciences. MIT Press, Cambridge, MA, pp 765–781

Martinoli MG, Trojanowski JQ, Schmidt ML, Arnold SE, Fujiwara TM, Yee VM-Y, Hurtig, Julein JP, Clarc C (1995) Association of apolipoprotein ε4 allele and neuropathological findings in patients with dementia. Acta Neuropathol 90: 239–243

Masliah E (1995) Mechanisms of synaptic dysfunction in Alzheimer's disease. Histol Histopathol 10: 505–519

Masliah E, Mallory M, Hansen L, DeTeresa R, Alford M, Terrry R (1994) Synaptic and neuritic alterations during the progression of Alzheimer's disease. Neurosci Lett 174: 67–72

McKee AC, Kosik KS, Kowall NW (1992) Neuritic pathology and dementia in Alzheimer's disease. Ann Neurol 30: 156–165

McKeith IG, Galasko D, Kosaka K, Perry EK, et al (1996) Clinical and pathological diagnosis of dementia with Lewy bodies (DLB): report of the COLB International Workshop. Neurology (in press)

McKhann GD, Drachmann DA, Folstein MF, et al (1984) Clinical diagnosis of Alzheimer's disease: report of the NINCDS-ADRDA Work Group under the auspices of the Department of Health and Human Services Task Force on Alzheimer's disease. Neurology 34: 939–944

Mirra SS, Hart N, Terry RD (1993) Making the diagnosis of Alzheimer's disease. A primer for practicing pathologists. Arch Pathol Lab Med 117: 132–144

Mirra SS, Heyman A, McKeef D, Sumi SM, Crain BJ, Brownlee LM, Vogel FS, Hughes JP, Van Belle G, Berg L (1991) The Consortium to Establish a Registry for Alzheimer's Disease (CERAD). II. Standardization of the neuropathologic assessment of Alzheimer's disease. Neurology 41: 479–486

Morris CM, Massey HM, Leake BR, Griffiths BC, Brown LH, Ince GP, et al (1996) Molecular biology of APO E alleles in Alzheimer's and non-Alzheimer's dementias. J Neural Transm [Suppl] 47: 205–218

Morris JC, McKeel DW Jr, Storandt M, Rubin EM, Price JL, Grant EA, Ball MJ, Berg L (1991) Very mild Alzheimer's disease: informant-based clinical, psychometric, and pathological distinction from normal aging. Neurology 41: 469–478

Owen F, Cooper PN, Pickering-Brown S, McAndrew C, Mann DMA, Neary D (1993) The lobar atrophies are non prion encephalopathies. Neurodegeneration 2: 195–199

Papp MI, Lantos PL (1994) The distribution of oligodendroglial inclusions in multiple system atrophy and ist relevance to clinical symptomatology. Brain 117: 235–243

Perry EK, Morris CM, Court JA, Cheng A, Fairbairn AF, McKeith JG, Irving D, Browns A, Perry RH (1995) Alteration in nicotin binding sites in Parkinson's disease, Lewy body dementia and Alzheimer's disease: possible index of early neuropathology. Neuroscience 64: 385–395

Perry EK, Irving D, Kerwin JM, McKeith IG, Thompson P, Collerton D, Fairbairn AP, Ince PG, Morris CM, Cheng AV, Perry RM (1993) Cholinergic transmitter and neurotrophic activities in Lewy body dementia. Similarity to Parkinson's and distinction from Alzheimer disease. Alzheimer Dis Assoc Disord 7: 69–79

Petersen RB, Tabaton M, Monari L, Richardson SL, Lynches T, Manetto V, Lanska DJ, Markesberry WR, Currier RD, Autilio-Gambetti L, Wilhelmsen KC, Gambetti P (1995) Familial progressive subcortical gliosis: presence of prions and linkage to chromosome 17. Neurology 45: 1062–1067

Pillon B, Blin J, Vidalhet M, Deweer B, Sirigu A, Dubois B, Agid Y (1995) The neuropsychological pattern of corticobasal degeneration — comparison with progressive supranuclear palsy and Alzheimer's disease. Neurology 45: 1477–1483

Pillon B, Deweer B, Malapani C, Rogelet P, Agid Y, Dubois B (1994a) Explicit memory disorders of demented parkinsonian patients and underlying neuronal basis. In: Korczyn AD (ed) Dementia in Parkinson's disease. Monduzzi Ed, Bologna, pp 265–271

Pillon B, Michon A, Malapani C, Agid Y, Dubois B (1994b) Are explicit memory disorders of progressive supranuclear palsy related to damage to striatofrontal circuits? Comparison with Alzheimer's, Parkinson's and Huntington's diseases. Neurology 44: 1264–1270

Pollanen MS, Dickson DW, Bergeron C (1993) Pathology and biology of the Lewy body. J Neuropathol Exp Neurol 52: 183–191

Pollanen MS, Weyer L, Bergeron C (1995) Distribution of phosphorylated tau in Pick's disease, corticobasal degeneration, and frontal lobe dementia (Abstract). J Neuropathol Exp Neurol 54: 446

Roman GC, Tatechimi TK, Erkinjuntti T, et al (1993) Vascular dementia: diagnostic criteria for research studies. Report of the NINDS-AIREN International Workshop. Neurology 43: 250–260

Samuel W, Masliah E, Hill LR, Butters N, Terry R (1994a) Hippocampal connectivity and Alzheimer's dementia. Neurology 44: 2081–2088

Samuel W, Terry RD, DeTeresa R, Butters N, Masliah E (1994b) Clinical correlates of cortical and nucleus basalis pathology in Alzheimer dementia. Arch Neurol 51: 772–778

Scheff SW, Price DA (1993) Synapse loss in the temporal lobe in Alzheimer's disease. Ann Neurol 33: 190–199

Schmitt HP, Yang Y, Forstl H (1995) Frontal lobe degeneration of non-Alzheimer type and Picks atrophy — lumping or splitting. Eur Arch Psychiat Clin Neurosci 245: 299–305

Schneider JA, Gearing M, Watts R, Mirra SS (1995) Corticobasal degeneration: a neuropathological, clinical and molecular study (Abstract). J Neuropathol Exp Neurol 54: 446

Schneider JS, Pope-Coleman A (1995) Cognitive deficits precede motor deficits in a slowly progressing model of parkinsonism in the monkey. Neurodegeneration 4: 245–255

Scoones D, Ince PG, Shaw PJ, Perry RH (1995) Neuritic pathology in Huntington's disease is present in the substantia nigra in addition to the cortex: observations in 21 cases, including the rigid variant (Abstract). Neuropathol Appl Neurobiol 21: 445

Sharp AH, Loev SJ, Schilling G, Li SH, et al (1995) Widespread expression of Huntington disease gene (IT15) protein product. Neuron 14: 1065–1074

Skoog I, Nilssen L, Palmertz B, Andreasson LA, Svanborg A (1993) A population-based study of dementia in 85-year olds. N Engl J Med 328: 153–158

Smith MA, Perry G (1994) Is a Lewy body always a Lewy body? In: Korczyn AD (ed) Dementia in Parkinson's disease. Monduzzi Ed, Bologna, pp 187–193

Steele JC, Richardson JC, Olszewski J (1964) Progressive supranuclear palsy. Arch Neurol 10: 333–359

Takauchi S, Yamauchi S, Morimura Y, Ohara K, Morita Y, Hayashi S, Miyoshi K (1995) Coexistance of Pick bodies and atypical Lewy bodies in the locus ceruleus neurons of Pick's disease. Acta Neuropathol 90: 93–100

Talbot PR (1996) Frontal lobe dementia and motor neuron disease. J Neural Transm [Suppl] 47: 125–132

Tatemichi TK, Sacktor N, Mayeux R (1994) Dementia associated with cerebrovascular disease, other degenerative diseases, and metabolic disorders. In: Terry RD, Katzman R, Bick KL (eds) Alzheimer disease. Raven Press, New York, pp 123–166

Terry RD, Masliah E, Hansen LA (1994) Structural basis of the cognitive alterations in Alzheimer's disease. In: Terry RD, Katzman R, Bick KL (eds) Alzheimer disease. Raven Press, New York, pp 179–196

Terry RD, Masliah E, Salomon DP, et al (1991) Physical basis of cognitive alterations in Alzheimer's disease: synapse loss is the major correlate of cognitive impairment. Ann Neurol 30: 572–580

Thompson PD, Day BL, Rothweel JC, Brown P, Britton TC, Marsden CD (1995) The myoclonus in corticobasal degeneration: evidence for two forms of cortical reflex myoclonus. Brain 117;1197–1207

Tierney MC, Fischer H, Lewis AJ, et al (1988) The NINCDS-ADRDA Work Group criteria for the clinical diagnosis of probable Alzheimer's disease: clinicopathological study of 57 cases. Neurology 38: 356–364

Tolnay M, Spillantini M, Goedert M, Probst A (1995) Pick's disease: somatoaxonal distribution of hyperphosphorylated tau protein (Abstract). Neuropathol App Neurobiol 21: 440

Tolosa E, Duvoisin R, Cruz-Sánchez FF (eds) (1994) Progressive supranuclear palsy: diagnosis, pathology, and therapy. J Neural Transm [Suppl 42]

Trojanowski JQ, Shin RW, Schmidt ML, Lee VMY (1995) Relationship between plaques, tangles, and dystrophic processes in Alzheimer's disease. Neurobiol Aging 16: 335–340

Turner RS, Kenyon LC, Trojanowski JQ, Gonatas N, Grossman M (1996) Clinical, neuroimaging, and pathologic features of progressive nonfluent aphasia. Arch Neurol 39: 166–173

Uchihara T, Mitani K, Mori H, Kondo R, Yamada M, Ikeda K (1994) Abnormal cytoskeletal pathology peculiar to corticobasal degeneration is different from that of Alzheimer's disease or progressive supranuclear palsy. Acta Neuropathol 88: 379–383

Uitti RJ, Berry K, Yasuhara O, Eisen A, Feldman H, McGeer PL, Calne DB (1995) Neurodegenerative "overlap" syndrome: clinical and pathological features of Parkinson's disease, motor neuron disease, and Alzheimer's disease. Park Rel Dis 1: 21–34

Uyama E, Kondo I, Uchino M, Fukushima T, Murayama N, Kuwano A, Inokuchi N, Ohtam Y, Ando M (1995) Dentatorubral-pallidoluysian atrophy (DRPLA): clinical, genetic, and neuroradiologic studies in a family. J Neurol Sci 130: 146–153

Vermersch P, Robitaille Y, Bernier L, Wattez A, Gavreau D, Delacourte A (1994) Biochemical mapping of neurofibrillary degeneration in a case of progressive supranuclear palsy: evidence for general cortical involvement. Acta Neuropathol 87: 572–577

Vonsattel JP (1992) Neuropathology of Huntington's disease. In: Joseph AB, Young RR (eds) Movement disorders in neurology and neuropsychiatry. Blackwell Scientific Publications, Oxford London Edinburgh Melbourne Paris Berlin Vienna, pp 186–194

Wakabayashi K, Honer WG, Masliah E (1994) Synapse alterations in the hippocampal-entorhinal formation in Alzheimer's disease with and without Lewy body disease. Brain Res 667: 24–32

Warner TT, Lennox GG, Janota I, Harding AE (1994) Autosomal-dominant dentatorubropallidolysin atrophy in the United Kingdome. Mov Disord 9: 289–296

Warner TT, Williams LD, Walker RWH, Flinter F, Robb SA, Bundey SE, Honavar M, Harding AE (1995) A clinical and molecular genetic study of dentato-rubropallidoluysian atrophy in four european families. Ann Neurol 37: 452–459

Watanabe M, Abe K, Aoki M, Kameya T, Kanako J, et al (1996) Analysis of CAG trinucleotide expansion associated with Machado-Joseph disease. J Neurol Sci 136: 101–107

Wenning GK, Ben-Shlomo Y, Magalhaes M, Daniel SS, Quinn NP (1995) Clinicopathological study of 35 cases of multiple system atrophy. J Neurol Neurosurg Psychiatry 58: 160–166

Wilcock GK, Esiri MM (1982) Plaques, tangles and dementia. A quantitative study. J Neurol Sci 56: 343–356

Williams TL, Shaw PJ, Lowe J, Bates D, Ince PG (1995) Parkinsonism in motor neuron disease: case report and literature review. Acta Neuropathol 89: 275–283

Xuereb JH, Gertz HJ, Huppert F, Brayne C, Wischik CM, Mukaetova-Ladinska E (1995) The application of Braak's staging model of Alzheimer-type pathology to neuropathological diagnosis of dementia (Abstract). Neuropathol Appl Neurobiol 21: 441

Authors' address: Prof. Dr. K. A. Jellinger, L. Boltzmann Institute for Clinical Neurobiology, Lainz Hospital, Wolkersbergenstrasse 1, A-1130 Wien, Austria.

J Neural Transm (1996) [Suppl] 47: 31–46

Cytoskeletal pathology in non-Alzheimer degenerative dementia: new lesions in Diffuse Lewy body disease, Pick's disease, and Corticobasal Degeneration

D. W. Dickson, M. B. Feany, S.-H. Yen, L. A. Mattiace, and **P. Davies**

Departments of Pathology and Neurology, and the Rose F. Kennedy Center for
Research in Mental Retardation and Human Development, Albert Einstein College of
Medicine, Bronx, NY, U.S.A.

Summary. Increasing use of immunocytochemistry for evaluation of dementia disorders has revealed histopathological alterations that were previously unknown, even with sensitive silver techniques. Disorders [Pick's disease (PD), diffuse Lewy body disease (DLBD) and corticobasal degeneration (CBD)] in which immunocytochemistry has revealed occult pathology are discussed. All three disorders have neurofilament (NF) immunoreactive neuronal alterations in the neocortex. In DLBD round, eosinophilic cytoplasmic inclusions referred to as cortical Lewy bodies are neurofilament-positive, while in both PD and CBD neurofilament epitopes are expressed in irregularly swollen neurons and their proximal cell processes, which are referred to as ballooned neurons. Interestingly, the cortical neuronal population that is vulnerable to Lewy bodies is similar to that which is vulnerable to ballooned neurons. Furthermore, Lewy bodies can occasionally be detected within the cytoplasm of ballooned neurons. Besides neurofilament-immunoreactivity, Lewy bodies are immunoreactive for ubiquitin, while ballooned neurons are inconsistently stained with antibodies to ubiquitin. Both Lewy bodies and ballooned neurons can be appreciated with routine histology, but they are much easier to detect with immunocytochemistry. In contrast, a new type of neuritic alteration in the hippocampal CA2/3 region has been recognized in DLBD. These dystrophic neurites cannot be appreciated with routine histology and are only optimally seen with immunocytochemistry for ubiquitin. Their presence is a certain indication of the presence of cortical Lewy bodies.

The microtuble associated protein tau is the major constituent of neurofibrillary tangles in Alzheimer's disease (AD). Biochemical studies have shown that Pick bodies, argyrophilic neuronal inclusions that are highly characteristic of, if not pathognomonic for PD are also composed of abnormal tau protein. Along with Pick bodies, tau has recently been detected in glial cells in PD. Similar so-called "gliofibrillary tangles" are increasingly recognized in progressive supranuclear palsy. Previously, CBD was considered to be free of such lesions, but recent studies have revealed widespread tau-positive neuronal and glial cytoskeletal lesions in CBD. A distinctive type of tau-positive glial lesion in CBD is characterized by annular clusters of grain-like tau immunoreactivity reminiscent of a neuritic plaque in AD, except that the clusters are devoid of amyloid. The tau-positive profiles are consistently located around a central astrocyte cell body. Double labeling studies with glial fibrillary acidic protein, vimentin and CD44, which are markers for reactive astrocytes, demonstrates tau immunoreactivity within astrocytic processes; these "astrocytic plaques" appear to be specific for CBD. Although NF, ubiquitin and tau proteins are present in diverse neuronal and glial inclusions in these disorders, the morphology and distribution of these lesions differentiate non-AD dementias.

Introduction

Although the most common neurodegenerative disorder of mid- to late-adult life is Alzheimer's disease (AD), differentiating AD from non-AD degenerative diseases is a challenge to clinicians and pathologists. Our recent clinicopathological studies have suggested that neurologists are accurate in their clinical diagnosis of AD in about 75% of the cases (Crystal et al., 1993). Postmortem examination remains the only means of confirming the diagnosis. Among centers investigating neurodegenerative disorder, there is variability in the methods of analysis of brain tissue and no universal agreement upon diagnostic criteria. In an effort to improve communication, research criteria for AD and certain non-AD disorders have recently been developed (Gearing et al., 1995; Hauw et al., 1994). For other disorders, especially the rare neurodegenerative diseases, pathological and clinical criteria have not been established.

In the past, staining tissue sections with silver impregnation techniques was the method of choice of neuropathologists to evaluate neurodegenerative disease. A number of silver staining methods have been developed to differentially stain various components of neural tissue. These methods may be very sensitive, but they lack specificity to a varying degree, are sometimes capricious and often dependent upon specific modifications of the procedure that are unique to the individual laboraory. Standardization of silver staining techniques has been difficult to obtain. The problem of lack of specificity and standardization of silver stains can be overcome with methods that make use of the exquisite specificity of immunoglobulins. The relatively unlimited supply of monoclonal antibodies with high specificity also offers the prospect of increased uniformity of results across laboratories. The development of sensitive and simple immunostaining kits has made immunocytochemistry a nearly routine histological procedure in many laboratories.

In addition to the practical issues that widespread application of immunocytochemistry to degenerative diseases raises, immunocytochemistry also offers the prospect of revealing fundamental features that are common to clinically disparate disorders. This brief review will describe select lesions in neurodegenerative disorders that are revealed with immunocytochemistry and discuss implications that these observations have on the pathophysiological relationship of these disorders.

Materials and methods

Case material

Postmortem tissue from degenerative disorders were evaluated by the brain bank at Albert Einstein College of Medicine using a standardized protocol. Multiple tissue sections were routinely examined with H&E and with thioflavin-S fluorescent histochemical methods to document senile changes. Additional tissue sections were stained with silver stains as indicated, but routine with immunocytochemistry as detailed below. The degenerative diseases included in this study and diagnostic considerations are as follows:

Diffuse Lewy body disease (DLBD) was diagnosed as a dementing condition, with or without accompanying extrapyramidal movement disorder or psychiatric complaints, associated with neuronal loss to a varying degree in key monoaminergic and cholinergic nuclei in the brainstem and the basal forebrain, and eosinophilic neuronal cytoplasmic neuronal inclusions, Lewy bodies (LB). Cases had to have widespread LB formation in the neocortex in addition to limbic cortices to be considered to have DLBD (Kosaka et al., 1984).

Pick's disease (PD) was diagnosed as a dementing condition associated with circumscribed atrophy of the frontal and temporal lobes, associated with marked neuronal loss, status spongiosus and specific argyrophilic neuronal inclusions, Pick bodies (PB) (Ball, 1979). Cases lacking PB were not considered to have PD.

Corticobasal degeneration (CBD) (Gibb et al., 1989) was diagnosed as a dementing disorder, with or without dystonic movement disorder or language impairment, associated with atrophy of the frontoparietal convexity, with swollen achromatic neurons in the cortex (Rebeiz et al., 1968), white matter gliosis, and variable gliosis and neuronal loss in the basal ganglia and brainstem monoaminergic nuclei.

Progressive supranuclear palsy (PSP) was diagnosed as a dementing disorder, usually with axial rigidity and vertical eye movement impairment associated with neuronal loss and neurofibrillary degeneration in basal ganglia, thalamus and brainstem nuclei (Steele et al., 1964), according to proposed pathological criteria (Hauw et al., 1994).

Immunocytochemistry

The antibodies used in immunocytochemical studies are listed in Table 1. The immunostaining was performed on paraffin sections (10 μm thick) mounted on glass slides and on free floating vibratome sections (40 μm thick). For paraffin sections the avidin-biotin-peroxidase method was most commonly used, with diaminobenzidine as the chromogen. Ubiquitin staining was optimal on formalin-fixed paraffin sections. For all other antibodies, staining was best on thicker vibratome sections. Before sectioning, tissue was fixed intact in 10% formalin for over 10 days; alternatively, small $1 \times 1 \times 0.5$ cm blocks of tissue were immersion fixed in 4% paraformaldehyde for 12 to 24 hours or in Bouin's solution for 1–2 hours. Fixed tissue blocks were stored at 4°C in 30% sucrose with 0.1% azide before sectioning.

For staining of floating sections, peroxidase-, β-galactosidase- or alkaline phosphatase-conjugated secondary antibodies were used. The secondary antibody was specific to the species and the isotype of the primary antibody. Sections were usually incubated for 16 hours at 4°C. Non-specific antibody binding was usually blocked with 5% normal goat serum or 5% nonfat milk.

Controls included incubations with irrelevant antibodies of the same isotype. For some antibodies assessment of adequacy of staining was possible due to the presence of tissue "internal controls". For example, ubiquitin-positive granular degeneration of myelin is an invariant age-related change. If the white matter lacked this type of staining, the stain quality was considered inadequate and was repeated. For neurofilament antibodies, a similar internal control was staining of axons in white matter. For antibodies that

Table 1. Antibodies used for immunocytochemistry

Antibody	Specificity	Isotype & Dilution	Source
SMI- 31	neurofilament (phosphorylated epitope)	mIgG1 1:5,000	Sternberger-Meyer, Inc.
NP18	neurofilament (phosphorylated epitope)	mIg]M 1:10	Peter Davies, AECOM
Alz-50	tau (nonphosphorylated epitope)	mIgM 1:10	Peter Davies, AECOM
PHF-1	tau (phosphorylated epitope)	mIgG1 1:200	Peter Davies, AECOM
Ab39	NFT (conformational epitope)	mIgG1 1:10	Shu-Hui Yen, AECOM
TG-3	PHF (phosphorylated epitope)	mIgM 1:10	Peter Davies, AECOM
UBQ	ubiquitin (polyclonal antibody)	rIg 1:400	Dennis Dickson, AECOM

recognized pathological structures, staining was done in parallel with a disease control, i.e. AD. For the antibodies used in this study hydrated autoclaving did not produce improved staining (Dickson et al., 1992)

Results

Neurofilament

The most prominent of the pathological structures revealed with neurofilament antibodies is the ballooned neuron (Fig. 1). Ballooned neurons are swollen, achromatic neurons most commonly detected in the deeper cortical layers, especially in the limbic and multimodal association cortices. The soma is swollen and sometimes vacuolated and the proximal apical and basal dendrites are also irregularly expanded. They are most easily detected with phosphorylated neurofilament antibodies (Dickson et al., 1986). Ballooned neurons have a variable degree of immunoreactivity with tau antibodies (Murayama et al., 1990; Feany et al., 1996), but are generally negative with NFT and PHF antibodies (Dickson et al., 1986). They can be distinguished from neurofibrillary tangles by these criteria. Although ballooned neurons are characteristic of PD and CBD, a small number of ballooned neurons can also be detected in the limbic cortices in some aged normal individuals, and those with AD, DLBD and other less common neurodegenerative diseases (Clark et al., 1986). In PD and CBD ballooned neurons are more widespread in the cortex. In CBD they are usually most numerous in the dorsal parietal lobe. Although ballooned neurons can be detected with routine histochemical stains, the differential staining provided by immunocytochemistry permits a

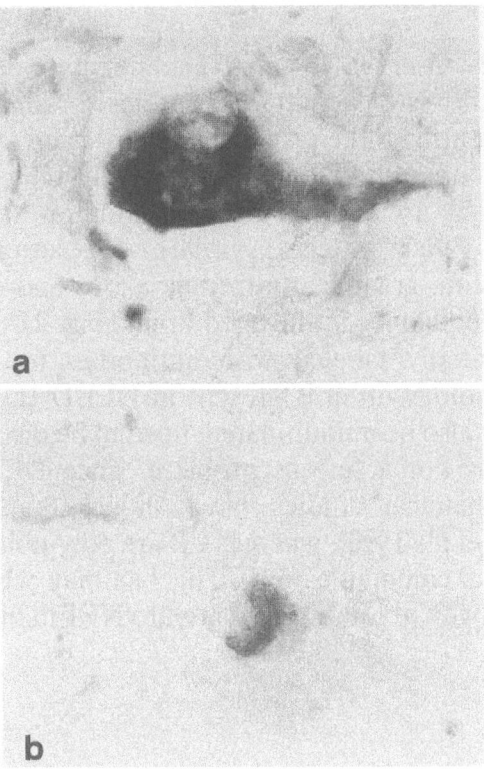

Fig. 1. Neuronal abnormalities in CBD: **a** ballooned neuron immunoreactive for phosphorylated neurofilament; note swelling of cell body and proximal processes; **b** tau-positive neuronal inclusions in CBD are in small non-pyramidal neurons and usually crescent shaped and fibrillar

more accurate assessment of their number and distribution in the aging and diseased brain.

The classic brainstem LB is a compact, hyalin cytoplasmic inclusion that has been recognized for nearly a century in monoaminergic and cholinergic nuclei in the brainstem and basal forebrain. They are the hallmark of idiopathic Parkinson's disease, but are found in a host of neurodegenerative diseases as either an essential or coincidental feature. The biology of LB has been reviewed recently (Pollanen et al., 1993). In contrast, the cortical LB is more indistinct. Cortical LB are less compact, round to slightly irregular, eosinophilic cytoplasmic neuronal inclusions that are difficult to recognize in routine histochemical preparations. They are most abundant in lower cortical layers of the limbic lobe, but also found in the temporal and frontal association cortices in cases of DLBD. Because of their subtle staining properties on routine histological stains, they were greatly underrecognized until the advent of more sensitive and specific staining methods, in particular immunocytochemistry. Although they can detected with antibodies to neurofilament, the most sensitive stain for cortical LB is immunocytochemistry with antibodies to ubiquitin.

Ubiquitin

Ubiquitin is a highly conserved 76 amino acid polypeptide that is involved in non-lysosomal proteolysis of denatured proteins through an energy-dependent mechanism that utilizes the proteosome (reviewed in Dickson and Yen, 1994). Antibodies to ubiquitin label many different types of neuronal inclusions, more of which are filamentous, in addition to age-related non-filamentous lesions (Dickson et al., 1990). The latter include granular degeneration of myelin, granular dystrophic axons and dystrophic neurites associated with senile plaques in the aged brain (Fig. 2).

LB are preferentially labeled with antibodies to ubiquitin (Fig. 2). Alzheimer-type pathology often is present in DLBD (Dickson et al., 1992) and NFT, which may also be ubiquitinated, need to be distinguished from LB. In most cases this is not a serious problem, since NFT are only weakly ubiquitinated. Biochemical studies have shown that NFT are mono-ubiquitinated (Ihara et al., 1990), whereas LB are poly-ubiquitinated (Lee and Trojanowski, personal communication). This fact may account for the differential staining of LB with ubiquitin compared to NFT in brains that have both lesions.

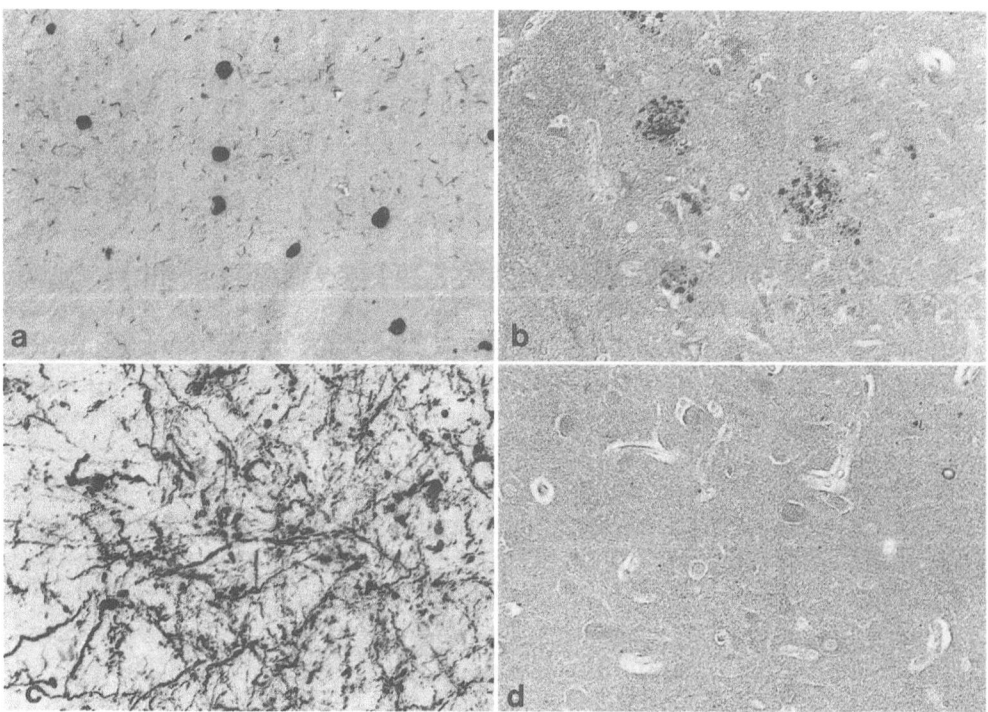

Fig. 2. Ubiquitin positive lesions in DLBD: **a** Cortical Lewy bodies are stained with ubiquitin. **b** Clusters of dystrophic neurites around dense amyloid cores (not shown) are present in senile plaques. **c** A dense plexus of ubiquitin-immunoreactive neurites is present in the CA2/3 region of the hippocampus, but **d** the immediately adjacent CA1 region is devoid of similar structures

In addition to the lesions that are apparent with routine histology, additional pathologic lesions are present in DLBD that are invisible with routine histology and even with most routine silver stains. In particular, dystrophic neurites are often abundant in the medial accessory basal nucleus of the amygdala (Braak et al., 1994) and in the CA2/3 region of the hippocampus (Dickson et al., 1991, 1994). The CA2/3 neurites have a number of staining properties in common with LB, being positive with both neurofilament and ubiquitin (Fig. 2). At the ultrastructural level the neurites contain less organized intact filaments, whereas filaments in LB are more compact and associated with granular amorphous material. These latter observations may in part explain the differential appearance of LB and CA2/3 neurites with histologic methods.

Ballooned neurons share some histological properties with CA2/3 neurites and LB, including immunoreacctivity for neurofilament, but they are inconsistently positive for ubiquitin and more consistently positive for αB crystallin, a small heat shock protein, than either CA2/3 neurites or LB (Lowe et al., 1992) (see Table 2 for summary).

Tau protein

The best means of differentiating cortical LB from NFT is with antibodies to tau protein, since NFT, but not LB, are tau-immunoreactive. Tau protein is a microtubulc-associated phosphoprotein that promotes tubulin polymerization and stabilization. It is inactive in its most highly phosphorylated state. It is present in neurons, preferentially in axons, and until recently was felt to be specific to neurons. More recent immunochemical evidence suggests that tau protein is also present in glial cells. It is the product of a gene that undergoes alternative splicing to generate a family of 3 to 6 proteins (Goedert et al., 1991). It undergoes extensive post-translational modification, including phosphorylation, which controls its functional state. Recently, it has also been shown to be glycated (reviewed in Yen et al., 1995).

Antibodies to tau protein have provided powerful reagents for studying neurodegenerative diseases. Using tau protein on a wide variety of neurodegenerative diseases it is possible to separate disorders associated with extensive tau protein abnormalities from those in which tau protein is not appreciably altered (see Table 3). The variety of tau-positive lesions are discussed with respect to diagnosis.

Table 2. Intermediate filament neuronal inclusions

Structure	Neurofilament	Ubiquitin	αB crystallin
Ballooned neuron	++	±	++
Lewy body	+	++	+
CA2/3 neurite	+	++	±

Table 3. Classification of neurodegenerative disorders based upon presence of abnormal tau

Abnormal tau protein	Neurons	Glia
Alzheimer's disease	NFT & NT & NP	
Progressive supranuclear palsy	NFT & NT	GFT ("tufted astrocytes")
Corticobasal degeneration	"NFT" & NT	GFT (astrocytes and oligodendroglia), astrocytic plaques
Pick's disease	PB	GFT (astrocytes)
Others (see Geddes et al., 1993)		
Guam Parkinson-dementia complex	NFT	
Post-encephalitic parkinsonism	NFT	
Dementia pugilistica	NFT	

No abnormal tau protein
Lewy body disease (including Parkinson's disease and DLBD)
Frontal lobe dementia and other dementias with circumscribed cortical atrophy
Motor neuron disease (ALS)
Multisystem degeneration (olivopontocerebellar degeneration/striatonigral degeneration)

NFT neurofibrillary tangles; *NT* neuropil threads; *NP* neuritic plaques; *GFT* gliofibrillary tangles; *PB* Pick body

Pick's disease

The hallmark of PD is the argyrophilic neuronal inclusion found in small granular neurons and in select pyramidal neurons in the frontal and temporal lobe, but especially the neurons in the hippocampus and the dentate fascia (Ball, 1979). PB contain abnormal tau protein (Yen et al., 1986; Love et al., 1988; Murayama et al., 1990) (Fig. 3). Routine application of tau protein immunocytochemistry reveals additional pathology in PD, in addition to PB.

Not only neurons, but also select glial cells are stained with antibodies to tau protein (Yamazaki et al., 1994) (Fig. 3). Tau-positive glia show cytoplasmic immunoreactivity with extension of immunoreactivity into proximal processes. The labeled cells are more common in gray than white matter and are morphologically consistent with astrocytes. Tau-positive astrocytes have been referred to as gliofibrillary tangles (GFT). Double staining with GFAP, the intermediate filament protein specific to astrocytes, demonstrates that the majority of the GFT in PD are astrocytic. Similar types of GFT have also been consistently detected in progressive supranuclear palsy (PSP) (Fig. 4), where they were first recognized (Yamada et al., 1992; Nishimura et al., 1992; Iwatsubo et al., 1994; Feany et al., 1996). They have been described as "tufted" astrocytes and are highly characteristic of PSP. Tufted astrocytes follow the same general distribution as NFT and are often numerous in the basal ganglia and subthalamic nuclei. The observation of glial tau-positive inclusions was a major breakthrough in understanding these disorders, since it

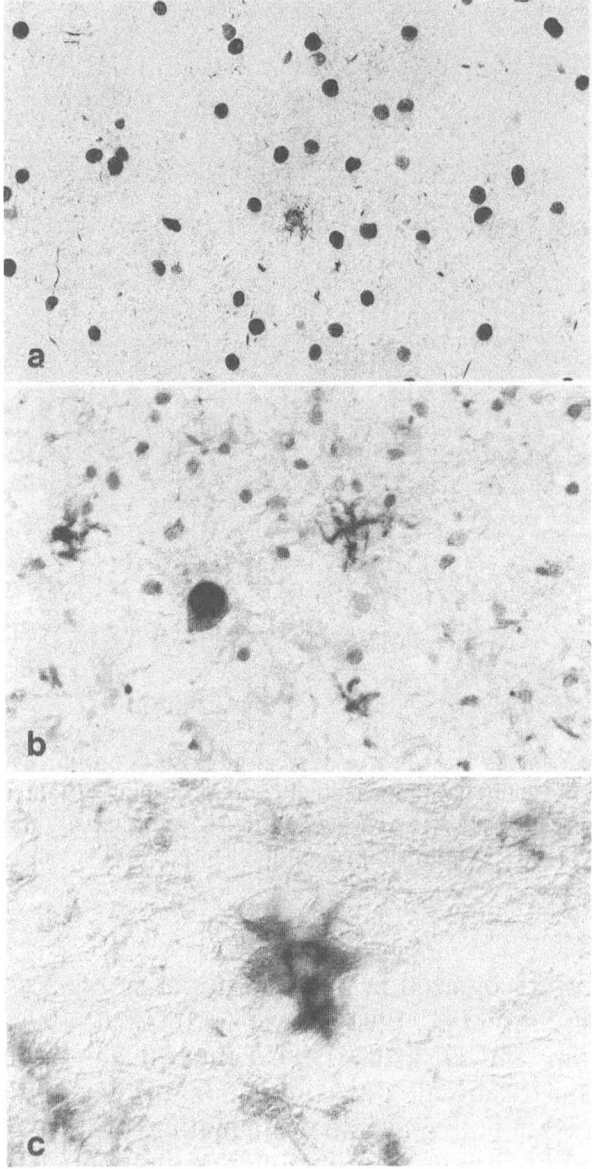

Fig. 3. Tau-positive lesions in PD: **a** Pick bodies and focal astrocytic tau-positive lesions are stained. **b** Higher magnification of several tau-positive astrocytes in PD; **c** another tau-positive astrocyte in the gray matter of PD

implied that the cytoskeletal pathology was more extensive and less neuron-specific than formerly recognized.

Corticobasal degeneration

Although ballooned neurons were the first structural alteration to be noted in CBD, they are by no means as extensive as the tau-positive changes that have

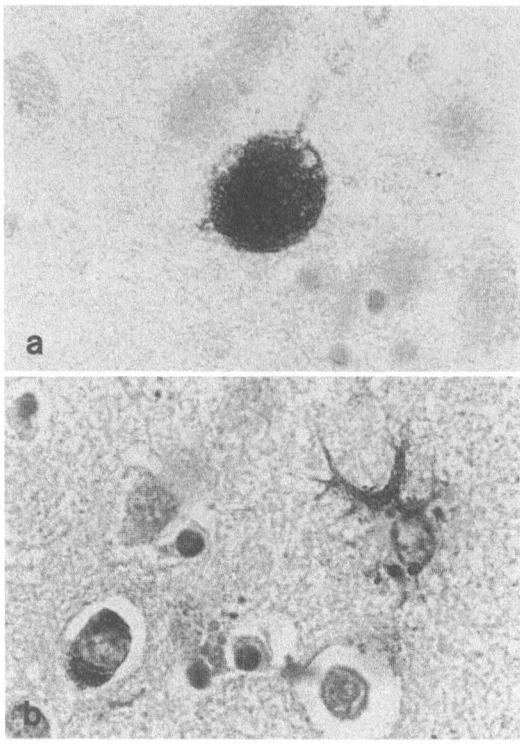

Fig. 4. Tau positive lesions in PSP. **a** A typical globose neurofibrillary tangle from the brainstem shows intense tau immunoreactivity with a fibrillar structure. **b** Astrocytic tau-positive staining (so-called tufted astrocytes); note stellate shaped cell processes, some of which extend to form endfeet of a blood vessel

only recently been recognized in this disorder (Ksiezak-Reding et al., 1994; Ikeda et al., 1994; Mori et al., 1994; Wakabayashi et al., 1994; Horoupian and Chuy, 1994; Feany and Dickson, 1995; Feany et al., 1995). Tau antibody immunocytochemistry reveals widespread immunostaining of glial and neuronal cell processes in both gray and white matter of affected areas of cortex, basal ganglia and brainstem. Tau immunoreactivity in CBD is morphologically diverse and includes both neuronal and glial lesions in both cell soma and processes. Neuronal staining is most often in the form of crescent-shaped cytoplasmic filamentous aggregates similar to NFT (Fig. 1); in CBD tau-positive neurons are often small, nonpyramidal neurons in the upper cortex. In addition, there may be focal tau-positive staining within the cytoplasm of some of the ballooned neurons in CBD, as in PD. In addition to this neuronal perikaryal staining, tau immunostaining is also detected in cellular processes, so-called neuropil threads (Braak et al., 1986). Double staining with neurofilament antibodies proves that at least some of the processes are neuronal and probably axonal, especially in the white matter (Feany and Dickson, 1995). On the other hand, some of the thread-like processes in CBD are glial in origin. In the white matter thread and coil-shaped processes are double stained with Leu-7- and tau and are consistent with oligodendroglial inclusions (Fig. 5). Glial staining is present in astrocytes in addition to oligoden-drocytes, especially in the cortical gray matter, based upon double immunostaining with GFAP (Feany and Dickson, 1995).

Perhaps the most characteristic tau-positive lesion in CBD, particularly in the neocortex, is a cluster of grain-like (Braak and Braak, 1987) processes that is highly suggestive of a neuritic plaque; however, there is no evidence of amyloid in these lesions with histochemical, fluorescent and immunocy-tochemical methods for amyloid. In addition, most of tau immunoreactivity is

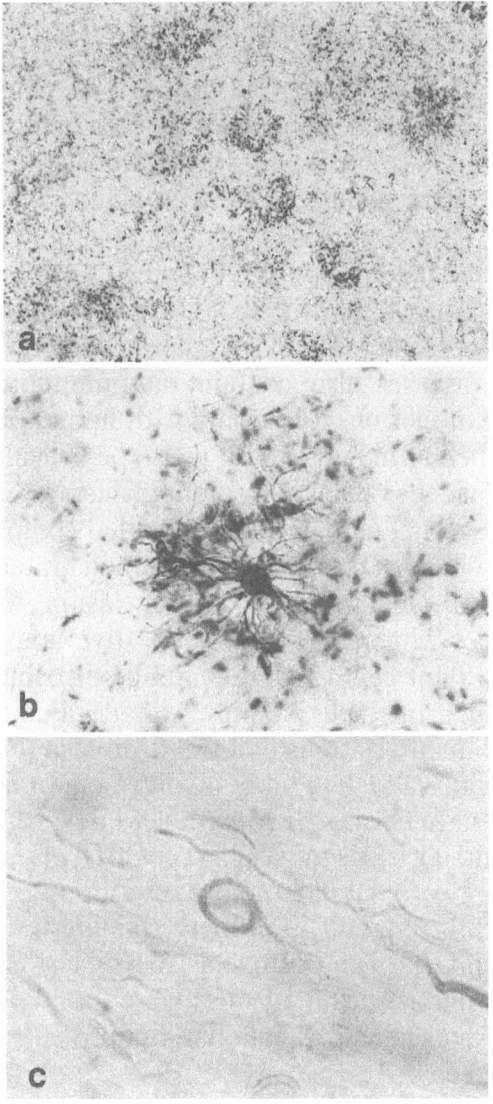

Fig. 5. Tau-positive glial lesions in CBD: **a** Low power image of cortex reveals scattered clusters of grain like cell processes as well as many fine processes in the intervening neuropil. **b** Higher magnification of a section that has been double stained for tau (grain like structures) and vimentin (to detect reactive astrocytes) reveals a central astrocyte in the middle of the grain-like structures. **c** Tau-positive perinuclear filamentous loops and long thread-like processes in the white matter

not within neurons, and thus is not truly "neuritic". Double staining with GFAP, vimentin or CD44, which are all markers with varying degrees of specificity for astrocytes, demonstrates that the tau-positive cell processes in these lesions are derived from astrocytes (Feany and Dickson, 1995) (Fig. 5). We have termed these lesions "astrocytic plaques". To date they have been detected only in CBD. A more extensive survey of additional neurodegenerative disorders is needed to determine if astrocytic plaques are indeed specific for CBD.

Discussion

Biochemical and molecular biological studies have identified microtubule binding protein tau as the predominant component of inclusions in AD (Ihara et al., 1988; Iqbal et al., 1989; Greenberg and Davies, 1990; Lee et al., 1991). The types of tau-positive inclusions in AD include NFT, neuropil threads (Braak et al., 1986; Davis et al., 1992; Tabaton et al., 1989; Kowall and Kosik, 1987) and neuritic elements of senile plaques. All of these structures are neuronal in origin, consistent with the previously held notion that tau is a neuron-specific molecule (Binder et al., 1985). A number of other neurodegenerative diseases also contain tau-immunoreactive lesions, but closer inspection of the lesions, especially with immunoelectron microscopy and with double labeling methods with cell-type-specific markers, has provided unequivocal evidence that tau protein inclusions in neurodegenerative diseases are both neuronal and glial. In a detailed comparison of tau-immunoreactive lesions in PSP, PD and CBD, we demonstrated unexpected pathological similarities in the neuronal and glial inclusions in these diseases, but distinctive differences with respect to the relative abundance of particular types of lesions and their cellular and anatomic distributions that argue for these disorders being distinct, but possibly related, clinicopathological entities rather than variable manifestations of a single disease (Feany et al., 1996). In particular, we found that PSP had more involvement of deep gray matter and PD more involvement of cortical gray matter, while CBD affected both cortical and deep gray matter to a similar degree. CBD was also distinguished by the greater proportion of glial inclusions and tau-positive neuronal and glial processes compared to PSP and PD, where staining was more prominent in cell bodies in PSP and PD. Tau-positive astrocytic lesions were prominent in PSP, CBD and PD, but astrocytic plaques were found only in CBD. Finally, both CBD and PD had far more ballooned neurons than PSP, where they were only rarely detected.

In contrast to PSP, CBD and PD, tau protein abnormalities are not a consistent feature of DLBD, unless there is co-existing AD. On the other hand, DLBD is associated with distinctive lesions that are best demonstrated with ubiquitin antibodies. Among the lesions that are positive with ubiquitin are cortical and brainstem type LB, dystrophic neurites in senile plaques and neurites in the CA2/3 region of the hippocampus and the amygdala. In contrast to LB and dystrophic neurites, CA2/3 and amygdaloid neurites are not visible with routine stains and are only detected with ubiquitin immunocytochemistry. Immunocytochemistry is also the most sensitive means of detecting cortical LB.

Ballooned neurons and cortical LB have a number of similarities in terms of staining properties and distribution, but CBD and PD are different from DLBD in all other respects. Whereas the LB appears to be an essential histopathological hallmark of DLBD, it is not clear that ballooned neurons in CBD and PD carry the same diagnostic significance. Ballooned neurons can be detected in other unrelated disorders, whereas the tau-positive lesions that are the hallmarks of PD (Pick bodies) and CBD (astrocytic plaques) are far more disease-specific.

Ubiquitin-positive glial inclusions are also found in multisystem atrophy (MSA) (Papp et al., 1989; Murayama et al., 1992; Mochizuki et al., 1992; Abe et al., 1992). The current evidence favors an oligodendroglial origin for so-called "glial cytoplasmic inclusions" (GCI) that have come to be recognized as a pathognomonic feature of this disorder. GCI are consistently present in all forms of MSA, including cases with predominantly olivopontocerebellar degeneration or those with predominantly striatonigral degeneration. GCI are positive with ubiquitin antibodies, but not with tau antibodies. They have had variable immunoreactivity for other cytoskeletal markers depending upon the particular study. Identification of GCI as an essential feature of MSA, as with the GFT in PSP, CBG and PD forces one to reconsider the pathobiology of these "neuro"-degenerative diseases and to realize that not only neurons, but also glia are affected, particularly with respect to tau- and ubiquitin-positive cellular inclusions that increasingly contribute to the pathological diagnosis.

Routine use of immunocytochemistry is highly recommended in the evaluation of dementia disorders. In particular, ubiquitin staining should be performed in all cases of suspected DLBD both to adequately document the extent and severity of cortical LB involvement and to reveal supportive lesions in the hippocampus and amygdala. In addition to silver stains, tau immunocytochemistry should be considered an essential tool in evaluation of PD, PSP and CBD. The full extent of cytoskeletal changes in these disorders will be underestimated without such methods. Although ballooned neurons can be detected with routine histological stains, the differential staining provided by neurofilament immunocytochemistry is a useful adjunct for assessing disease severity. Finally, other routine immunocytochemical methods for glial changes and myelin preservation can be applied to illustrate the distribution and severity of reactive glial changes or secondary white matter changes. In contrast to ubiquitin and tau immunostaining, however, the latter methods have yet to prove to be useful in establishing the specificity of any disease process.

Acknowledgement

Supported by grant NIH AG06803.

References

Abe H, Yagishita S, Amano N, Iwabuchi D, Hasegawa K, Kowa K (1992) Argyrophilic glial intracytoplasmic inclusions in multiple system atrophy: immunocytochemical and ultrastructural study. Acta Neuropathol 84: 273–277

Ball MJ (1979) Topography of Pick inclusion bodies in hippocampi of demented patients. A quantiative study. J Neuropathol Exp Neurol 38: 614–620

Binder LI, Frankfurter A, Rebum LI (1985) The distribution of tau in the mammalian central nervous system. J Cell Biol 101: 1371–1378

Braak H, Braak E, Grundke-Iqbal I, Iqbal K (1986) Occurrence of neuropil threads in the senile human brain and in Alzheimer's disease: a third location of paired helical filaments outside of neurofibrillary tangles and neuritic plaques. Neurosci Lett 65: 351–355

Braak H, Braak E (1987) Argyrophilic grains: characteristic pathology of cerebral cortex in cases of adult onset dementia without Alzheimer changes. Neurosci Lett 76: 124–127

Braak H, Braak E, Yilmazer D, de Vos RA, Jansen EN, Bohl J, Jellinger K (1994) Amygdala pathology in Parkinson's disease. Acta Neuropathol 88: 493–500

Clark AW, Manz HJ, White CL 3d, Lehmann J, Miller D, Coyle JT (1986) Cortical degeneration with swollen chromatolytic neurons: its relationship to Pick's disease. J Neuropathol Exp Neurol 45: 268–284

Crystal HA, Dickson DW, Sliwinski M, Lipton R, Grober E, Marks-Nelson H, Antis P (1993) Pathological markers associated with normal aging and dementia in the elderly. Ann Neurol 34: 566–573

Davis DG, Wang HZ, Markesbery WR (1992) Image analysis of neuropil threads in Alzheimer's, Pick's, diffuse Lewy body disease and in progressive supranuclear palsy. J Neuropathol Exp Neurol 51: 594–600

Dickson DW, Wu E, Crystal HA, Mattiace LA, Yen S-HC, Davies P (1992) Alzheimer and age-related pathology in diffuse Lewy body disease. In: Boller F, Forcette F, Khachaturian Z, Poncet M, Christen Y (eds) Heterogeneity of Alzheimer's disease. Springer, Berlin Heidelberg New York Tokyo, pp 168–186

Dickson DW, Yen S-H (1994) Ubiquitin, the cytoskeleton and neurodegenerative disease. In: Mayer RJ, Brown IR (eds) Heat shock or stress proteins and the nervous system. Academic Press, London, pp 235–264

Dickson DW, Ksiezak-Reding H, Liu W-K, Davies P, Crowe A, Yen S-HC (1992) Immunocytochemistry of neurofibrillary tangles (NFT) with antibodies to subregions of tau protein: identification of hidden and cleaved epitopes and a new phosphorylation site. Acta Neuropathol 84: 596–605

Dickson DW, Ruan D, Crystal H, Mark MH, Davies P, Kress Y, Yen S-H (1991) Hippocampal degeneration differentiates diffuse Lewy body disease (DLBD) from Alzheimer's disease: light and electron microscopic immunocytochemistry of CA2–3 neurites specific to DLBD. Neurology 41: 1402–1409

Dickson DW, Schmidt ML, Lee VM-Y, Trojanowski JQ, Yen S-H (1994) Hippocampal neurites in diffuse Lewy body disease: immunocytochemical characterization and local origin Acta Neuropathol 87: 269–276

Dickson DW, Wertkin A, Kress Y, Ksiezak-Reding H, Yen S-H (1990) Ubiquitin-immunoreactive structures in normal brains: distribution and developmental aspects. Lab Invest 63: 87–99

Dickson DW, Yen S-H, Suzuki KI, Davies P, Garcia JH, Hirano A (1986) Ballooned neurons in select neurodegenerative diseases contain phosphorylated neurofilament epitopes. Acta Neuropathol 71: 216–223

Feany MB, Dickson DW (1995) Widespread cytoskeletal pathology characterizes corticobasal degeneration. Am J Pathol 146: 1388–1396

Feany MB, Ksiezak-Reding H, Liu W-K, Vincent I, Yen S-HC, Dickson DW (1995) Epitope expression and hyperphosphorylation of tau protein in corticobasal degeneration: differentiation from progressive supranuclear palsy. Acta Neuropathol 90: 37–43

Feany MB, Mattiace LA, Dickson DW (1996) Neuropathologic overlap of progressive supranuclear palsy, Pick's disease, and corticobasal degeneration. J Neuropathol Exp Neurol 55: 53–67

Gearing M, Mirra SS, Hedreen JC, Sumi SM, Hansen LA, Heyman A (1995) The Consortium to Establish a Registry for Alzheimer's Disease (CERAD), part X. Neuropathology confirmation of the clinical diagnosis of Alzheimer's disease. Neurology 45: 461–466

Geddes JF, Hughes AJ, Lees AJ, Daniel SE (1993) Pathological overlap in cases of parkinsonism associated with neurofibrillary tangles. Brain 116: 281–302

Gibb WRG, Luthert PJ, Marsden CD (1989) Corticobasal degeneration. Brain 112: 1171–1192

Goedert M, Spillantini MG, Crowther RA (1991) Tau proteins and neurofibrillary degeneration. Brain Pathol 1: 279–286

Greenberg SG, Davies P (1990) A preparation of Alzheimer paired helical filaments that displays distinct tau proteins by polyacrylamide gel electrophoresis. Proc Natl Acad Sci USA 87: 5827–5831

Hauw J-J, Daniel SE, Dickson DW, Horoupian DS, Jellinger K, Lantos PL, McKee A, Tabaton M, Litvan I (1994) Preliminary NINDS neuropathologic criteria for Steele-Richardson-Olszewski syndrome (progressive supranuclear palsy). Neurology 44: 2015–2019

Horoupian DS, Chu PL (1994) Unusual case of corticobasal degeneration with tau/Gallyas-positive neuronal and glial tangles. Acta Neuropathol 88: 592–598

Ihara Y, Nukina N, Miura R, Ogawara M (1988) Phosphorylated tau protein is integrated in paired helical filaments in Alzheimer disease. J Biochem 99: 1807–1810

Ikeda K, Akiyama H, Haga C, Kondo H, Arima K, Oda T (1994) Argyrophilic thread-like structure in corticobasal degeneration and supranuclear palsy. Neurosci Lett 174: 157–159

Iqbal K, Grundke-Iqbal I, Smith AJ, George L, Tung Y-C, Zaidi T (1989) Identification and localization of tau peptide to paired helical filaments of Alzheimer disease. Proc Natl Acad Sci USA 86: 5646–5650

Iwatsubo T, Hasegawa M, Ihara Y (1994) Neuronal and glial tau-positive inclusions in diverse neurologic diseases share common phosphorylation characteristics. Acta Neuropathol 88: 129–136

Kosaka K, Yoshimura M, Ikeda K, Budka H (1984) Diffuse type of Lewy body disease: progressive dementia with abundant cortical Lewy bodies and senile changes of varying degree — a new disease? Clin Neuropathol 3: 185–192

Kowall NW, Kosik KS (1987) Axonal disruption and aberrant localization of tau protein characterize the neuropil pathology of Alzheimer's disease. Ann Neurol 22: 639–643

Ksiezak-Reding H, Morgan K, Mattiace LA, Davies P, Liu W-K, Yen S-H, Weidenheim KM, Dickson DW (1994) Ultrastructure and biochemical composition of paired helical filaments in corticobasal degeneration. Am J Pathol 145: 1–14

Lee VM-Y, Balin B, Otvos L Jr, Trojanowski JQ (1991) A68: a major subunit of paired helical filaments and derivatized forms of normal tau. Science 451: 675–678

Love S, Saitoh T, Quijada S, Cole GM, Terry RD (1988) Alz-50, ubiquitin and tau immunoreactivity of neurofibrillary tangles, Pick bodies and Lewy bodies. J Neuropathol Exp Neurol 47: 393–405

Lowe J, Errington DR, Lennox G, Pike I, Spendlove I, Landon M, Mayer RJ (1992) Ballooned neurons in several neurodegenerative diseases and stroke contain alpha B crystallin. Neuropathol Appl Neurobiol 18: 341–350

Mochizuki A, Mizusawa H, Ohkoshi N, Yoshizawa K, Komatsuzaki Y, Inoue K, Kanazawa I (1992) Argentophilic intracytoplasmic inclusions in multiple system atrophy. J Neurol 239: 311–316

Mori H, Nishimura M, Namba Y, Oda M (1994) Corticobasal degeneration: a disease with widespread appearance of abnormal tau and neurofibrillary tangles, and its relation to progressive supranuclear palsy. Acta Neuropathol 88: 113–121

Murayama S, Arima K, Nakazato Y, Satoh J, Oda M, Inose T (1992) Immunocytochemical and ultrastructural studies of neuronal and oligodendroglial cytoplasmic inclusions in multiple system atrophy. 2. Oligodendroglial cytoplasmic inclusions. Acta Neuropathol 84: 32–38

Murayama S, Mori H, Ihara Y, Tomonaga M (1990) Immunocytochemical and ultrastructural studies of Pick's disease. Ann Neurol 27: 394–405

Nishimura M, Namba Y, Ideda K, Oda M (1992) Glial fibrillary tangles with straight tubules in the brains of patients with progressive supranuclear palsy. Neurosci Lett 143: 35–38

Papp MI, Kohn JE, Lantos PL (1989) Glial cytoplasmic inclusions in the CNS of patients with multiple system atrophy and Shy-Drager syndrome. J Neurol Sci 94: 79–100

Pollanen MS, Dickson DW, Bergeron C (1993) Pathology and biology of the Lewy body. J Neuropathol Exp Neurol 52: 183–191

Rebeiz JJ, Kolodny EH, Richardson EP (1968) Corticodentatonigral degeneration with neuronal achromasia. Arch Neurol 18: 20–33

Steele JC, Richardson JC, Olszewski J (1964) Progressive supranuclear palsy: a heterogenous degeneration involving the brain stem, basal ganglia and cerebellum, with vertical gaze and pseudobulbar palsy, nuchal dystonia and dementia. Arch Neurol 10: 333–339

Tabaton M, Mandybur TI, Perry G, Onorato M, Autillo-Gambetti L, Gambetti P (1989) The widespread alteration of neurites in Alzheimer's disease may be unrelated to amyloid deposition. Ann Neurol 26: 771–778

Wakabayashi K, Oyanagi K, Makifuchi T, Ikuta F, Honna A, Honna Y, Horikawa Y, Tokiguchi S (1994) Corticobasal degeneration: etiopathological significance of the cytoskeletal alterations. Acta Neuropathol 87: 545–553

Yamada T, McGeer PL, McGeer EG (1992) Appearance of paired nucleated, tau-positive glia in patients with progressive supranuclear palsy brain tissue. Neurosci Lett 35: 99–102

Yamazaki M, Nakano I, Imazu O, Kaieda R, Terashi A (1994) Astrocytic straight tubules in the brain of a patient with Pick's disease. Acta Neuropathol 88: 587–591

Yen S-H, Dickson DW, Peterson C, Goldman JE (1986) Cytoskeletal abnormalities in neuropathology. In: Zimmerman HM (ed) Progress in neuropathology, vol 6. Raven Press, New York, pp 63–90

Yen S-H, Liu W-K, Hall FL, Yan S-D, Stern D, Dickson DW (1995) Alzheimer neurofibrillary lesions: molecular nature and potential roles of different components. Neurobiol Aging 16: 381–387

Authors' address: D. W. Dickson, M.D., Department of Pathology (Neuropathology), Albert Einstein College of Medicine, 1300 Morris Park Ave., Bronx, NY 10461, U.S.A.

J Neural Transm (1996) [Suppl] 47: 47–59
© Springer-Verlag 1996

The neuropathologic diagnostic criteria of frontal lobe dementia revisited. A study of ten consecutive cases*

J. J. Hauw[1], C. Duyckaerts[1], D. Seilhean[1], S. Camilleri[1], V. Sazdovitch[1], and G. Rancurel[2]

[1]Laboratoire de Neuropathologie R Escourolle, La Salpêtrière Hospital,
Paris VI University and INSERM U 360, Association Claude Bernard, Paris, and
[2]Service de Neurologie, La Salpêtrière Hospital, Paris VI University, France

Summary. Ten successive cases from the Neuropathology Laboratory of La Salpêtrière Hospital in Paris, were selected on the presence of:

— dementia and prominent symptoms and signs of the frontal type;
— a degenerative disease without markers other than Pick cells, Pick bodies or ubiquitin-labelled non argyrophilic inclusions.

We propose the following steps to diagnose the degenerative dementia associated with symptoms and signs of the frontal type:

1. If there is severe frontotemporal atrophy, severe neuronal loss and astrogliosis, many ballooned neurons and characteristic inclusions that are both tau and ubiquitin positive, the diagnosis is Pick disease.
2. If signs of motor involvement (sometimes unnoticed by the clinician) are present with mild cortical atrophy and mild spongiosis of layers II-III, the diagnosis of frontal lobe degeneration associated with motor neuron disease is warranted. Ubiquitin positive inclusions are useful, but non specific, markers.
3. When there are neither Pick inclusions nor motor neuron disease, the diagnosis may be frontal lobe atrophy lacking distinctive histology.

Introduction

The nosology of frontal lobe dementia (FLD) is still a controversial and confusing matter. The central issue is the extension of Pick disease (PD). Those cases with frontal lobe type symptoms and signs, and fronto-temporal lesions: atrophy, neuronal loss and astrogliosis, but without markers such as Pick bodies, Pick cells or a high density of neurofibrillary tangles (NFT), were generally classified as PD, or atypical PD (Escourolle, 1958; Delay and Brion,

---

*This paper has been given at the XIIth International Congress of Neuropathology, Toronto, September 18–23, 1994

1962; Brion et al., 1991; Constantinidis et al., 1974; Tissot et al., 1975), until the term "Frontal lobe degeneration of non-Alzheimer type" was coined by Brun in 1987 (Brun, 1987). Since then, whether cases without markers, together with those of typical PD, form a continuum of disease changes, or represent distinct entities, is debated (Baldwin and Förstl, 1993; Pasquier and Lebert, 1995). An exception is FLD associated with motor neuron disease (MND), which is believed to be a single disease by most neuropathologists, although some (Knopman, 1993) always distinguish a motor neuronopathic form of "Dementia lacking distinctive histology" (DLDH).

Numerous descriptions of FLD without histological markers have been made. The absolute need of the main histological markers for the diagnosis of PD has been progressively emphasized: the presence of swollen cells, also called ballooned, or achromatic, neurons ("Pick cells"), which have been shown to be labelled by antibodies against nonphosphorylated neurofilaments (Dickson et al., 1986), and overall that of argyrophilic neuronal inclusions, which are positive for phosphorylated tau and ubiquitin (Munoz-Garcia and Ludwin, 1984; Love et al., 1988) ("Pick bodies") became mandatory for an increasing number of neuropathologists (Baldwin and Förstl, 1993; Hauw et al., 1994; Jellinger and Bancher, 1994). In the meantime, the umbrella of PD has been progressively left aside: cases with fronto-temporal atrophy associated with severe neuronal loss, and without Pick cells and Pick bodies were gradually included into non-Pick FLD.

Three main papers (Table 1) were dedicated to this topic. Brun and Lund's school first described "Frontal lobe degeneration of non Alzheimer type" in cases with a high familial incidence (Brun, 1987, 1993). There was no or mild gross atrophy of the brain. Histologically, the most striking lesion was microvacuolation ("spongiosis") of layers I to III in the frontal cortex. Neuronal loss and gliosis in the isocortex, hippocampus and amygdala, striatum, substantia nigra, and white matter were mild. These cases contrasted with PD, where marked gross atrophy and neuronal loss, astrogliosis, Pick bodies and Pick cells were found. In 1993, however, Brun (1993) stated that a few cases, although with severe cortical and subcortical lesions, would possibly belong to advanced "Frontal lobe degeneration of non-Alzheimer type".

Knopman et al. (1990) made, three years later, another description that included some cases closer to classic PD. "Cortical variant of DLDH" was also characterized by little (or absent) gross cortical atrophy and by superficial spongiosis in the frontal and temporal neocortex, but prominent neuronal loss and astrogliosis were seen in the cortex, and were not found anymore characteristic for PD. Subcortical nuclei were sometimes affected, especially in a thalamostriate variant, the heterogeneity of which made generalisations about this group difficult. Mild neuronal loss in the cortex and gliosis in the white matter characterized a leukogliotic variant (Knopman et al., 1990; Knopman, 1993).

Mann et al. (1993), summarizing the neuropathological criteria of the Manchester group for frontal type atrophy, included a new set of cases hitherto classified into PD: lobar atrophy and associated severe neuronal loss were not anymore diagnostic for PD. They emphasized the value of microvacuolation

Table 1. Nosology of fronto-temporal lobe degeneration without histological marker

Escourolle (1956) Brion (1962–1993) Constantinidis (1975)	Brun (1987–1993)	Knopman et al. (1990–1993)	Mann (1993)
Pick disease without Pick bodies (Constantinidis C2 type)	*Frontal lobe degeneration of non-Alzheimer type*	*Dementia lacking distinctive histology*	*Dementia of Frontal type Cortical* (subgroup A, and some cases of subgroup B)
Pick disease without Pick bodies with basal ganglia lesions	Advanced FLD (?) with basal ganglia lesions	Thalamostriate variant	DFT + Striato-temporal stereotopy (subgroup C)
Pick disease with motor neuron involvement or ALS and dementia	FLD with ALS	Motor neuronopathic variant	DFT & MND
Pick disease with marked white mater lesions		Leukogliotic variant	

ALS Amyotrophic lateral sclerosis; *DFT* dementia of frontal type; *FLD* Frontal lobe degeneration of non-Alzheimer type; *MND* motor neuron disease

in the cortex in "dementia of frontal type". In this disease, there was severe gross atrophy, severe loss of large cortical neurons with spongiform change of layers II and III, but without, or with minimal, astrocytosis. This was considered different from PD, where there was also a severe loss of large cortical neurons, but where florid astrocytosis occurred without spongiform change. Pick cells and Pick bodies could be missing for the diagnosis of PD. In some cases of both disorders, lesions of basal ganglia could involve caudate and thalamus, together with amygdala and hippocampus. Lastly, one case associated with motor neuron disease had mild atrophy and spongiosis, and neuronal inclusions that were ubiquitin positive, but negative for tau. These inclusions were similar to those already described in the spinal cord of motor neuron disease (Okamoto et al., 1991; Wightman et al., 1992).

The Lund and Manchester groups (1994) formalized their opinions in consensus report on clinical and neuropathological criteria for frontotemporal dementia (FTD).

They emphasized the distinction between the usual slight gross atrophy of the cortex, superficial microvacuolation and mild to moderate astrocytic gliosis with atrophy/loss of neurons of FLD, and the more intense and usually more circumscribed gross atrophy with intense involvement of all cortical layers of PD. Although most cases lacking the histological markers of PD were thought to belong to FLD, some cases with intense astrocytosis were still considered as PD even if they lacked Pick bodies and Pick cells.

This prompted us to study 10 successive cases from the Neuropathology Laboratory of La Salpêtrière Hospital in Paris, selected on two criteria:

— first, patients were demented and exhibited prominent symptoms and signs of the frontal type, sometimes confirmed by hypometabolism in frontal areas;
— second, the disease had been diagnosed as degenerative, and no markers other than Pick cells, Pick bodies or ubiquitin-labelled non argyrophilic inclusions had been found. Cases with tangles above the age-associated density or Lewy bodies (LB), were discarded.

Material and methods

Cases

Inclusion criteria were the following: every FTD of the degenerative type from the files of the Laboratoire de Neuropathologie R Escourolle in La Salpêtrière Hospital, Paris, from 1984 to 1992.

Exclusion criteria were incomplete clinical or pathological data, or the presence of the following changes: infarcts and other vascular disorders, tumours, traumatic lesions, hydrocephalus, encephalitides, AIDS, PrP positive immunohistochemistry, multiple sclerosis and other disorders of the white matter, focal asymmetric cortical atrophy, cortical NFT and neuritic plaques above the age-related density, amyloid deposits in the vessel walls, numerous tangles in the brain stem and basal ganglia, LB and argyrophilic oligodendroglial inclusions.

Ten cases were selected, 6 men and 4 women (Table 2). The mean age at death was 63.2 ± 13.2 years (range: 37–81). The disease duration was 6.3 ± 4.6 years (range: 2–15). No case was known to be familial.

Methods

The brains were formalin-fixed and embedded in celloidin and/or paraffin. Sections from the different cerebral lobes and basal ganglia, cerebellum and three levels of brain stem were stained with haematoxylin-eosin, Bodian impregnation coupled with luxol fast blue for paraffin embedded specimens, hematoxylin-eosin and Loyez stain for celloidin embedded sections. In addition, the Bielschowsky technique modified for paraffin sections, and immunohistochemistry for tau, Aβ peptide, ubiquitin, αB crystallin, and GFAP were performed on sections from the hippocampal formation, the parahippocampal and middle frontal gyri (area 9). PrP immunohistochemistry was performed on cerebellar samples. An immunoblot for PrP was performed in some cases.

The main lesions that were considered included:

1. Symmetrical gross atrophy of fronto-temporal predominance (Fig. 1A,B);
2. Neuronal loss and marked astrogliosis in the frontotemporal cortex (Fig.1E);
3. Spongiosis of layers II-III (Fig. 1C,D);
4. Swollen cells (Fig. 2A);
5. Cytoplasmic inclusions in neurons, either argyrophilic, tau and ubiquitin positive (Fig. 2B), or only ubiquitin positive (Fig. 2C,D).

In addition, neuronal loss, marked astrogliosis and other changes (swollen cells, inclusions) were checked in basal ganglia, brain stem, white matter, cerebellum and peripheral motor neurons.

Table 2. Main data from this series. Under the "Diagnosis" title are listed the diagnoses that can be made following the criteria of Brun (1993), Knopman et al. (1993), Mann (1993) and the Lund and Manchester groups (1994)

Case	Sex	Age at death	Evolution (years)	Distribution of atrophy	Spong	Astrogliosis	Others	Diagnosis			
								Brun	Knopman	Mann	L. & M.
1	M	71	2	Fronto-temp	+ Sup	++	Ball N	FLD	DLDH	FLD	FLD
2	M	71	12	Fronto-temp	—	++	—	FLD	DLDH	Pick	Pick
3	F	64	15	Temp-front ++ Caud	+ Sup	+	Ball N	FLD	DLDH	FLD	FLD
4	M	70	3	Temp-frontal Caud SN	–	+	Ball N	FLD	DLDH	FLD	FLD
5	F	49	6	Temp-front-par ++ Caud Thal SN	– Sup	+	—	FLD	DLDH	FLD	FLD
6	F	81	6	Fronto-temp ++ Caud Thal SN	+	++	—	FLD	DLDH	FLD	FLD
7	M	60	5	Fronto-temp SN	+ Sup	+	MND	MND + dementia	DLDH, Mn	MND + dementia	MND + dementia
8	M	55	10	Fronto-temp ++	+ Sup	++	Ball N Arg Incl	Pick	Pixk	Pick	Pick
9	M	74	2	Frontal	+	+	Ball N Arg Incl	Pick	Pick	Pick	Pick
10	F	37	2	Striatum ++	++	+	—	Prion	Prion	Prion	Prion

Arg Incl Pick body; *Ball N* Ballooned neurons; *Caud* caudate nucleus; *DLDH* dementia lacking distinctive histology, motor neuronopathic variety; *DFT* dementia of the frontal type; *FLD* frontal lobe degeneration; *Front-temp* fronto-temporal lobes (predominantly frontal); *L. & M.* The Lund and Manchester groups criteria; *ND* motor neuron disease; *Prion* Prion disease; *SN* substantia nigra; *Spong* spongiform changes; *Sup* superficial; *Temp-frontal* temporo-frontal lobes (predominantly temporal); *Temp-front-par* temporo-fronto-parietal lobes (predominantly temporal and frontal); *Thal* thalamus

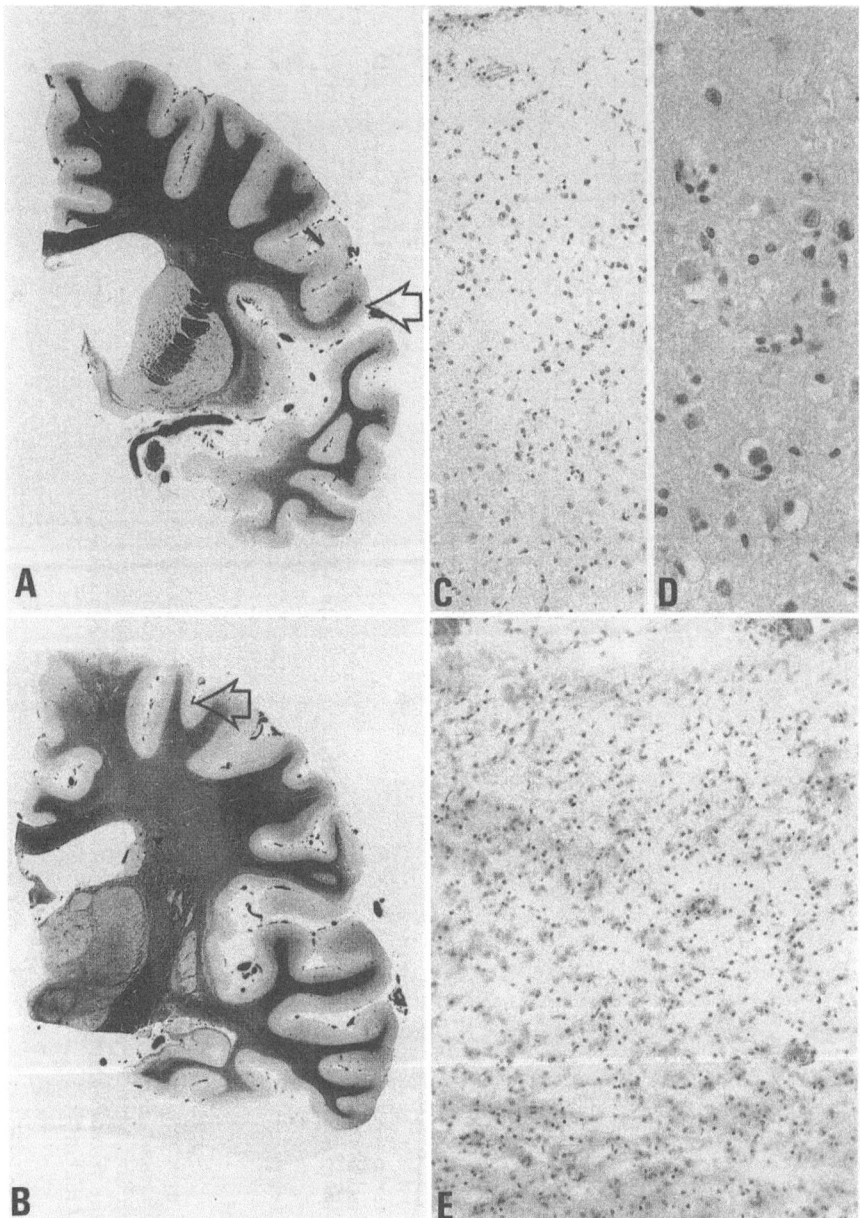

Fig. 1. All the figures are from the same case of Pick disease (N° 8). **A, B** Hemispheric coronal sections showing temporal and frontal atrophy. Arrows point to the lesions seen on adjacent sections stained with haematoxylin and eosin. The white mater and basal ganglia are little or not affected. Celloidin-embedded sections. Loyez stain for myelin. Magnification: 0.8. **C** and **D** Superficial spongiosis seen in the inferior part of area 6. Celloidin-embedded section. Haematoxylin-eosin. (C) ×370; (D) ×680

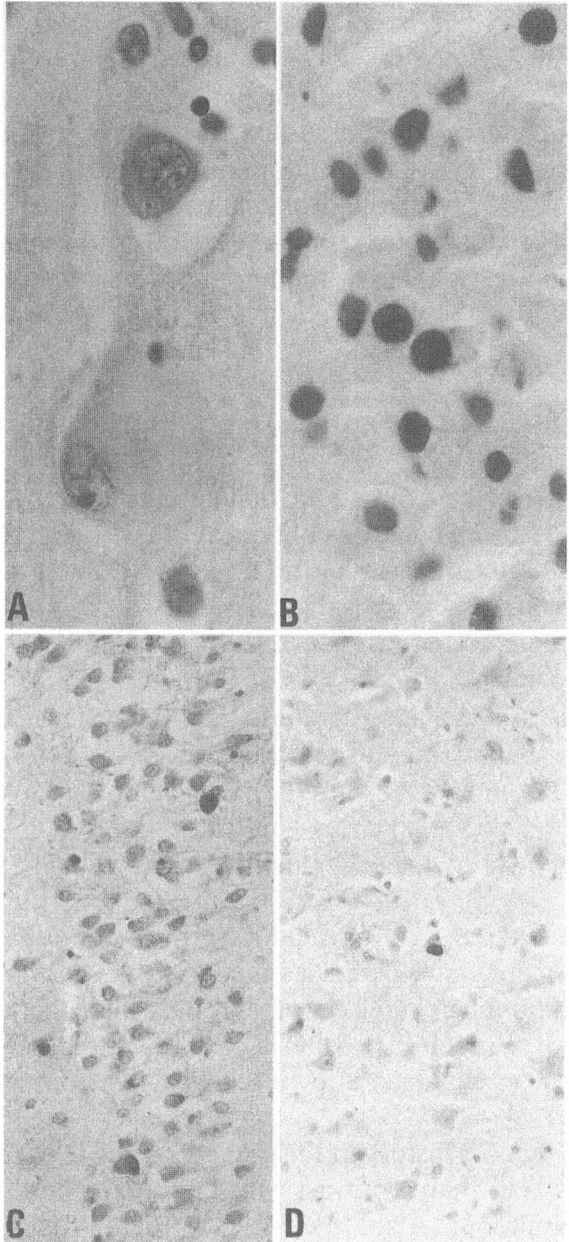

Fig. 2. A Case 8 (Pick disease): Ballooned cell; anterior cingular cortex; area 24. Celloidin-embedded section. Haematoxylin-eosin. ×1,700; **B** Case 8: Pick bodies; dentate gyrus of the hippocampus. Paraffin-embedded section; tau immunohistochemistry. ×1,700. Case 7 (Motor neuron disease and fronto-temporal atrophy): Ubiquitin positive inclusions are seen in the dentate gyrus of the hippocampus (**C**) and in the frontal cortex (**D**) Middle frontal gyrus (area 9). Paraffin-embedded sections; ubiquitin immunohistochemistry. ×680

Results

As shown on Table 2, 9/10 cases could be classified into one of the following categories: PD (2 cases), FLD without pathological marker (7 cases), and FLD + MND characterized by numerous ubiquitin positive inclusions in the neurons of the dentate gyrus, and seldom in the frontal cortex (1 case). One case was peculiar: a 37 year-old woman, with diffuse spongiosis in basal ganglia and in the frontal cortex, some A-β deposits and tau positive cells in the parahippocampus gyrus. PrP immunoblot ascertained the diagnosis of prion disease.

Discussion

In this series of unselected frontal lobe dementias of degenerative type, there was one Prion disease and two cases of typical PD with argyrophilic inclusions and swollen cells. Another case had FLD + MND, with ubiquitin positive inclusions in the brain. Finally, six cases had FLD without pathological marker, four of them being characterized by marked basal ganglia involvement. There were spongiform changes of the superficial layers in the frontal cortex of three cases. The diagnosis would have been different when using the four sets of criteria that we mentioned, however. Every author would agree on the diagnosis of PD in cases 8 and 9, and of Prion disease in case 10. The classification of the seven other cases would have differed. For Knopman et al. (1990) and Knopman (1993), these remaining cases would have been classified as DLDH.

For the other authors, case 7 would have been considered as MND with dementia. Case 2 would have been classified as PD by Mann et al. (1993) and following the Lund and Manchester Groups neuropathological criteria (1994), for there was severe astrogliosis, and the superficial spongiosis that these authors consider characteristic for dementia of frontal type was lacking in the sampled areas.

There was no familial history in the six cases of FLD without pathological markers, and this is in sharp contrast with the data from Sweden, Northern England, and Minnesota. Also, age of 87 at death is unusual. Although the number of cases of this series is low, this likely indicates geographical variations. Five points can be made concerning the diagnostic criteria for FLD:

1. When distinctive markers are lacking, the limits of a classification based only upon the severity and distribution of neuronal loss and astrogliosis are obvious. Different histological aspects may reflect stages in, rather than different forms of, a pathological process. Different distributions may be due to the degeneration of differently connected neuronal systems, or could reflect the different sensitivities of neurons injured together.
2. When unconventional agents are excluded, and this is usually easy (Budka et al., 1995), the significance of spongiosis in the grey matter is obviously

not unique. Spongiform changes, as defined by Masters and Richardson (1978) can be seen in a number of disorders, including Pick and Alzheimer diseases at the latest stages in evolution. When found only in superficial cortical layers, however, spongiosis indicates a subset of tissue degeneration due to the loss of neuronal processes in these layers, associated with a mild isomorphic gliosis. This prevents a shrinkage of the tissue, that is to say a gross atrophy. That such a degeneration would be distinctive for a specific disease is open to discussion, but seems unlikely, as expanded later on.

3. A number of different disorders have in common non-specific lesions in frontal and anterior temporal lobes. Some of them are possible variants of FLD, as emphasized by the Manchester school (Mann et al., 1993; Neary et al., 1993) and by Knopman (1993). The brunt of the pathology is sometimes asymmetrical or involves unusual structures, such as the speech areas in some cases of primary progressive aphasia (Kirshner et al., 1987; Lippa et al., 1991; Snowden et al., 1992; Kertesz et al., 1994), or the limbic system with sparing of the hippocampus (Sima et al., 1994). Other cases involve mainly either the white matter or the basal ganglia. When predominant in the superficial white matter, they are called Neumann's subcortical gliosis, the nosology of which is even more debated than that of PD. In other cases, associated lesions of some basal ganglia or brain stem nuclei are predominant. This is the case for the striatum: type C of frontal lobe atrophy (FLA) (Mann et al., 1993), thalamic atrophies (Martin, 1975; Jellinger, 1994) or mesocorticolimbic dementia (Torack and Morris, 1988) belong to this group. Some of these cases are sporadic, others familial. Familial primary limbic lobe gliosis (Sima et al., 1994) and some cases of familial progressive subcortical gliosis are linked to chromosome 17 (Petersen et al., 1995), the latter being also characterized by the presence of deposits of the protease-resistant PrP isoform.

We propose the following steps to diagnose the degenerative dementia associated with signs and symptoms of the frontal type:

1. If there is severe fronto-temporal atrophy, severe neuronal loss and astrogliosis, many ballooned neurons and characteristic inclusions that are both tau and ubiquitin positive, the diagnosis of PD is made.

2. If signs of motor involvement, sometimes unnoticed by the clinician (Knopman, 1993), are present with mild cortical atrophy and mild spongiosis of layers II-III, the diagnosis of FLD + MND is warranted. Tau negative and ubiquitin positive neuronal inclusions that may be found in peripheral motor neurons, including the nucleus ambiguus, and in cortical neurons, are useful for the diagnosis. However, these inclusions have been reported in a total of 12 cases where no patent peripheral motor neuron involvement has been found (Mann et al., 1993; Jackson et al., 1995). They might thus be the markers of either a special variety of FLA, which would be sometimes associated with MND, or of two different disorders, MND on one hand, and "motor neuron disease inclusion dementia" on the other hand (Jackson et al., 1995). That such inclusions are specific for FLA or for

MND is unlikely because they have been found in a case with pathologi-cally-assessed Joseph disease (Suenaga et al., 1993) and in one non-ALS case: a peripheral lymphoma with chromatolysis of anterior horn cells (Mizutani et al., 1994).

3. When there are neither Pick inclusions nor ubiquitin positive neuronal inclusions and motor neuron disease, the diagnosis may be FLA lacking distinctive histology.

In our opinion, there is no valid reason to make the diagnosis of PD when the characteristic markers are lacking, even if it has been repeatedly argued that Pick bodies, unlike NFT, do not remain unmodified in the nervous tissue after the death of their neuron (Brion et al., 1991; Hulette and Crain, 1992). Their presence in the dentate gyrus of all the cases in the series studied by Hof et al. (1994) tends to indicate that they may persist, at least in some specific areas, until the latest stages of the disease. Neither the involvement of basal ganglia nor even the cortical atrophy are distinctive features. As a matter of fact, the mere presence of Pick's bodies seems diagnostic, whatever the associated pathology. Characteristic histological lesions of PD can be found in the absence of marked brain atrophy, especially when the course of the disease has been short (Delay et al., 1954; Escourolle, 1958). Would the presence of ballooned cells stained by non phosphorylated neurofilaments ("Pick cells") be a sufficient criterion to make the diagnosis of PD in the absence of Pick bodies? We do not think so, since ballooned cells have been described in a variety of disorders which can present with dementia, frontal type symptoms and signs, the lesions of which can be confusing for FLD. These include Creutzfeldt-Jakob disease and other prion diseases (Lantos, 1992), progressive supranuclear palsy (Giaccone et al., 1988; McKee et al., 1993; Higuchi et al., 1995), corticobasal atrophy (Daniel et al., 1994; Lantos, 1992), progressive sub-cortical gliosis (Minagawa and Nagazato, 1973), Alzheimer disease (Higuchi et al., 1995), and even normal aging (Higuchi et al., 1995). This implies that some ballooned cells can be seen in non-Pick frontal atrophy.

4. Is superficial spongiosis such a specific lesion for FLD of non Pick type that it allows to recognise this disease? Certainly not, for it can be observed in other pathological processes, in the first place in PD itself, where isolated superficial spongiosis is often seen in the mildly affected areas. In contrast, marked astrogliosis with neuronal loss, sometimes associated with diffuse status spongiosus, are seen in the most affected areas (Fig. 1). Superficial spongiosis can also be seen in quite different disorders, such as AIDS associated encephalopathy (Seilhean et al., 1993).

In our view, pathologists must rely on the neuropathologic markers, even if imperfect, before more precise diagnostic tools are available. Needless to say, the search for the morphological, biochemical (Vermersch et al., 1995) and, even more, molecular bases of these heterogeneous disorders has not ended, and should be actively pursued. Before a given type of cortical degeneration has been fully identified, on clinical, morphological, biochemical and molecu-lar grounds, we suggest a descriptive approach. The diagnosis of PD would be, for example, beneficially replaced by "fronto-temporal lobe degeneration with superficial spongiosis, few ballooned cells and no specific marker".

Acknowledgments

We thank Profs. Brunet, Derouesné and Laplane for clinical information on some patients. Mrs. Raiton and Mr. Mièle provided expert technical assistance.

References

Baldwin B, Förstl H (1993) "Pick's disease"-101 years on. Still here, but in need of reform. Br J Psychiatry 163: 100–104

Brion S, Plas J, Jeanneau A (1991) Maladie de Pick. Point de vue anatomo-clinique. Rev Neurol (Paris) 147: 693–704

Brun A (1987) Frontal lobe degeneration of non-Alzheimer type. I. Neuropathology. Arch Gerontol Geriatr 6: 193–208

Brun A (1993) Frotal lobe degeneration of non-Alzheimer type revisited. Dementia 4: 126–131

Budka H, Aguzzi A, Brown P, Brucher M, Bugiani O, Collinge J, Diringer H, Gullota F, Haltia M, Hauw JJ, Ironside JW, Kretzschmar HA, Lantos P, Masullo C, Pocchiari M, Schlote W, Tateichi J, Will RG (1995) Tissue handling in suspected Creutzfeldt-Jakob disease (CJD) and other human spongiform encephalopathies (Prion Diseases). Brain Pathol 5: 319–322

Constantinidis J, Richard J, Tissot R (1974) Pick's disease. Histological and clinical correlation. Eur Neurol 11: 208–217

Daniel SE, Geddes F, Revesz T (1994) Clinicopathological overlap between cases of Pick's disease and corticobasal degeneration (Abstract). Brain Pathol 4: 516

Delay J, Brion S (1962) Les démences tardives. Masson, Paris

Delay J, Brion S, Sadoun R (1954) Lésions anatomiques de la maladie de Pick à la phase préatrophique. Rev Neurol (Paris) 91: 81–91

Dickson DW, Yen SH, Suzuki KH, Davies P, Garcia JH, Hirano A (1986) Ballooned neurons in selected neurodegenerative diseases contain phosphorylated neurofilament epitopes. Acta Neuropathol 71: 216–223

Escourolle R (1958) La maladie de Pick. Etude critique d'ensemble et synthèse anatomo-clinique. R Foulon, Paris

Giaccone G, Tagliavini F, Street JS, Ghetti B, Bugiani O (1988) Progressive supranuclear palsy with hypertrophy of the olives: an immunohistochemical study of argyrophilic neurons. Acta Neuropathol 77: 14–20

Hauw J-J, Daniel SE, Dickson D, Horoupian D, Jellinger K, Lantos P, McKee A, Tabaton M, Litvan I (1994) Preliminary NINDS neuropathologic criteria for Steele-Richardson-Olszewski syndrome (Progressive supranuclear palsy). Neurology 44: 2015–2019

Higuchi Y, Iwaki T, Tateishi J (1995) Neurodegeneration in the limbic and paralimbic system in progressive supranuclear palsy. Neuropathol Appl Neurobiol 21: 246–254

Hof PR, Bouras C, Perl DP, Morrison JH (1994) Quantitative neuropathologic analysis of Pick's disease cases: cortical distribution of Pick bodies and coexistence with Alzheimer's disease. Acta Neuropathol 87: 115–124

Hulette CM, Crain BJ (1992) Lobar atrophy without Pick bodies. Clin Neuropathol 11: 151–156

Jackson M, Lennox G, Ward L, Lowe J (1995) Frontal lobe dementia with MND inclusions without clinical ALS: report of eleven cases. Neuropathol Appl Neurobiol 21: 148–149

Jellinger KA (1994) Rare neurodegenerative disorders. In: Calne DB (ed) Neurodegenerative diseases. Saunders, Philadelphia, pp 909–931

Jellinger KA, Bancher C (1994) Classification of dementias based on functional morphology. In: Jellinger KA, Ladurner G, Windisch M (eds) New trends in the diagnosis and therapy of Alzheimer's disease. Springer, Wien New York, pp 9–39

Kertesz A, Hudson L, Mackenzie IRA, Munoz DG (1994) The pathology and nosology of primary progressive aphasia. Neurology 44: 2065–2075

Kirshner HS, Tanridag O, Thurman L, Whetsell WO (1987) Progressive aphasia without dementia: two cases with focal spongiform degeneration. Ann Neurol 22: 527–532

Knopman DS (1993) Overview of dementia lacking distinctive histology: pathological designation of a progressive dementia. Dementia 4: 132–136

Knopman DS, Mastri AR, Frey WHea (1990) Dementia lacking distinctive histological features: a common non-Alzheimer degenerative dementia. Neurology 40: 251–256

Lantos PL (1992) Neuropathology of unusual dementias: an overview. Unusual dementias. Baillière Tindall, London, pp 485–516

Lippa CF, Cohen R, Smith TW, Drachman DA (1991) Primary progressive aphasia with focal neuronal achromasia. Neurology 41: 882–886

Love S, Saitoh T, Quijada S, Cole GM, Terry RD (1989) Alz-50, ubiquitin and Tau immunoreactivity of neurofibrillary tangles, Pick bodies and Lewy bodies. J Neuropathol Exp Neurol 47: 393–405

Mann DMA, South PW, Snowden JS, Neary D (1993) Dementia of frontal lobe type-neuropathology and immunohistochemistry. J Neurol Neurosurg Psychiatry 56: 605–614

Martin JJ (1975) Thalamic degenerations. In: Vinken PJ, Bruyn GW (eds) System disorders and atrophies. Handbook of clinical neurology, vol 21. North Holland, Amsterdam Oxford, pp 587–604

Masters CL, Richardson EP (1978) Subacute spongiform encephalopathy (Creutzfeldt-Jakob disease). The nature and progression of spongiform changes. Brain 101: 333–344

McKee AC, Cole DG, Lee JM, Kowall NW, Growdon JH (1993) Distinctive cortical neuronal degeneration in progressive supranuclear palsy. J Neuropathol Exp Neurol 52: 292

Minagawa M, Nagazato T (1973) A special form of presenile dementia. A case of progressive subcortical gliosis (Neumann). Psychiat Neurol Jpn 75: 36–38

Mizutani T, Kakimi S, Yamaguchi H, Takasu T (1994) Ubiquitin-positive filamentous inclusions in amyotrophic lateral sclerosis (ALS) and other neurological diseases (Abstract). Brain Pathol 4: 528

Munoz-Garcia D, Ludwin SK (1984) Classic and generalized variants of Pick's disease: a clinicopathological, ultrastructural, and immunocytochemical comparative study. Ann Neurol 16: 467–480

Neary D, Snowden JS, Mann DMA (1993) The clinical pathological correlates of lobar atrophy. Dementia 4: 154–159

Okamoto K, Hirai S, Yamazaki Y, Sun X, Nakazato Y (1991) New ubiquitin-positive intraneuronal inclusions in the extra-motor cortices in patients with amyotrophic lateral sclerosis. Neurosci Lett 129: 233–236

Pasquier F, Lebert F (1995) Les démences fronto-temporales. Masson, Paris

Petersen RB, Tabaton M, Chen SG, Monari L, Richardson SL, Lynches T, Manetto V, Lanska DJ, Markesbery WR, Currier RD, Autilio-Gambetti L, Wilhelmsen KC, Gambetti P (1995) Familial progressive subcortical gliosis: presence of prions and linkage to chromosome 17. Neurology 45: 1062–1067

Seilhean D, Duyckaerts C, Vazeux RM, Bolgert F, Brunet P, Katlama C, Gentilini M, Hauw J-J (1993) HIV-1 associated cognitive/motor complex: absence of neuronal loss in the cerebral cortex. Neurology 43: 1492–1499

Sima AAF, D'Amato C, Defendini RF, Jones MZ, Foster NL, Lynch T, Wilhelmsen KC (1994) Primary limbic lobe gliosis. Familial and sporadic cases. Brain Pathol 4: 538

Snowden JS, Neary D, Mann DMA, Goulding PJ, Testa HJ (1992) Progressive language disorder due to lobar atrophy. Ann Neurol 31: 174–183

Suenaga T, Matsushima H, Nakamura S, Akiguchi I, Kimura J (1993) Ubiquitin immunoreactive inclusions in anterior horn cells and hypoglossal neurons in a case with Joseph's disease. Acta Neuropathol (Berlin) 85: 341–344

The Lund and Manchester groups (1994) Clinical and neuropathological criteria for frontotemporal dementia. J Neurol Neurosurg Psychiatry 57: 416–418

Tissot R, Constantinidis J, Richard J (1975) La maladie de Pick. Masson, Paris

Torack RM, Morris JC (1988) The association of ventral tegmental area histopathology with adult dementia. Arch Neurol 45: 497–501

Vermersch P, Bordet R, Ledoze Fea (1995) Mise en èvidence d'un profil particulier de protèines tau pathologiques dans des cas de dèmence fronto-temporale. C R Acad Sci (Paris) 318: 439–445

Wightman J, Anderson VER, Martin J, Swash M, Anderton BH, Neary D, Mann D, Luthert P, Leigh PN (1992) Hippocampal and neocortical ubiquitin-immunoreactive inclusions in amyotrophic lateral sclerosis with dementia. Neurosci Lett 139: 269–274

Authors' address: Prof. J. J. Hauw, Laboratoire de Neuropathologie R Escourolle, Hôpital de la Salpêtrière, 47 Bd. de l'Hôpital, F-75651 Paris Cedex 13, France.

J Neural Transm (1996) [Suppl] 47: 61–71

Cognitive deficits in non-Alzheimer's degenerative diseases

B. Pillon, B. Dubois, and **Y. Agid**

INSERM U-289 and Fédération de Neurologie, Hôpital de la Salpêtrière,
Paris, France

Summary. Although observed in various brain disorders, dementia is particularly frequent in neurodegenerative diseases. Alzheimer's disease is characterized by the association of progressive amnesia with either instrumental (aphasia, apraxia, agnosia) or behavioral (apathy, indifference, anosognosia) disorders, depending upon the location of the underlying neuronal lesions. By contrast, memory, linguistic, praxic, visuo-spatial or comportemental impairments are dissociated in more focal "lobar" atrophies, while planning and retrieval deficits predominate in movement disorders with dementia. Alzheimer's and non-Alzheimer's neurodegenerative diseases can therefore be distinguished insofar as the severity and location of the associated neuronal lesions differ.

Dementia may be observed in various brain diseases, either vascular, metabolic, demyelinating, traumatic, infectious, inflammatory, neoplastic or hydrocephalus (Chui, 1989). It is particularly frequent in neurodegenerative diseases. The recent clinical description of focal lobar atrophies (Weintraub and Mesulam, 1993) and the analysis of cognitive impairment observed in diseases with movement disorders (Cummings and Benson, 1984) have changed the conception of dementia, that may no more be defined as a global deterioration of higher cortical functions. The relative specificity of the cognitive picture of each disease depends on the location of the underlying neuronal lesions. Together with other tools, such as the neurological examination or the functional imagery, the neuropsychological exam may contribute to characterize the clinical picture of a patient with non-Alzheimer's degenerative disease and therefore to determine a clinical diagnosis, that remains probable till the neuropathological confrontation.

Cognitive changes in focal atrophies

Dementia was first conceived as a progressive and parallel deterioration of all cognitive functions (Richards and Constantinidis, 1970). More recent studies, however, have put emphasis on the heterogeneity of neuropsychological deficits even in Alzheimer's disease, in which various pictures have been distinguished according to the predominance of linguistic, visuo-spatial, memory or

62 B. Pillon et al.

behavioral disorders (Martin et al., 1986; Neary et al., 1986); and have been related to the dysfunction of determined brain regions (Celsis et al., 1990; Haxby et al., 1988)

The relationships between the cognitive picture and the location of the associated neuronal lesions is even more evident in focal "lobar" atrophies. Pick's disease, the first described, is characterized by symptoms reflecting the frontal and temporal polar focus of the pathology: 1) personality changes: apathy, desinhibition, roaming and hyperorality; 2) speech disturbances: decreased verbal output, poorly articulated speech, and reiterative speech acts, contrasting with the relative preservation of auditory comprehension and the absence of fluent paraphasic logorrhea often seen in Alzheimer's disease (Mendez et al., 1993). The neuropsychological studies show a marked impairment of executive functions, in relation with the frontal lesions, contrasting with the relative preservation of recent memory, because the hippocampal areas are not disturbed (Knopman et al., 1989).

Atrophy of the frontal and temporal lobes is also found in the pathologically heterogeneous syndrome of dementia of frontal lobe type (Gustafson, 1987; Knopman et al., 1990; Rustan, 1990; Miller et al., 1991; Neary et al., 1988). As in Pick's disease, the clinical picture is characterized by "progressive comportmental dysfunction" with insidious onset of abnormality in attention, motivation, speech initiation, executive functions, judgement and social conducts, but relative preservation of language comprehension and recent memory, at least on recognition (Table 1).

Table 1. Progressive comportmental dysfunction

man, 64 years, 10 years of scolarity
duration of disease: 2 years

correct intellectual efficiency
WAIS-R, verbal scale: IQ = 110
Raven's Progressive Matrices: IQ = 115

correct linguistic functions
naming: 79/80
normal comprehension on the Boston
Diagnostic Aphasia Examination

cognitive slowing and inertia
Wisconsin CST: 3 criteria, 20 perseverations
letter fluency: 10 words beginning with "M", but 4 perseverations
WAIS-R, performance scale: IQ = 80
Rey complex figure (copy): Type IV, 29/36 (organisational difficulties)
frontal behaviors of prehension, imitation and utilisation

impaired free recall but normal cued recall
word list learning
— free recall: 20/48
— cued recall: 48/48

autonomy disturbed only by inertia and environmental dependency

Contrasting with these behavioral abnormalities, language deficits constitute the main detectable impairment in "primary progressive aphasia", in which the fronto-perisylvian regions of the left hemisphere display the most severe pathology (Weintraub and Mesulam, 1993). Metabolic activity in the right cerebral hemisphere can remain normal (Chawluk et al., 1986). The earliest symptom is word-finding difficulty and there may be paraphasic errors in spontaneous speech, both semantic and phonemic. There is no single pattern of language dissolution, and different types of aphasia have been described (Karbe et al., 1993; Snowden et al., 1992).

Although non fluent Broca's or transcortical motor aphasias are particularly frequent (Weintraub and Mesulam, 1993), sensory aphasia may also be observed (Table 2). Daily living activities are limited only by linguistic disorders. These patients demonstrate their remarkable behavioral adaptation by devising their own compensatory strategies and by making use of notebook or alternative signal systems, such as sign language (Weintraub et al., 1990).

Lobar atrophy of the parieto-occipital cortex or "posterior cortical atrophy", also associated with a broad range of pathologies (Weintraub and Mesulam, 1993), may provoke early disorders of ocular fixation, optic ataxia, spatial disorientation, apraxia, acalculia, alexia, visual agnosia and prosopagnosia (Benson et al., 1988; Cogan, 1985; Croisile et al., 1991; De Renzi, 1986; Dick et al., 1989; Tyrell et al., 1990).

Memory, insight and personal conduct are strikingly preserved (Neary, 1990). One of our patients with progressive alexia and simultagnosia was still autonomous in daily life and able to travel alone by train nine years after the beginning of her deficits (Table 3).

Table 2. Primary progressive aphasia

woman, 66 years, 12 years of scolarity
duration of disease: 2 years

correct visuospatial efficiency
Raven's Progressive Matrices: IQ = 118
Rey complex figure (copy): Type I, 32/36

normal verbal memory
list learning of words presented visually
— free recall: 30/48
— cued recall: 48/48

impaired verbal efficiency
WAIS-R, verbal scale: IQ = 102 (Vocabulary: 10; Similarities: 7)
discrete word finding difficulty: 54/60
poor letter fluency: 6 words beginning with "D" in 60 seconds
sensory aphasia with impaired phonemic discrimination and syntactic difficulties but
   correct written comprehension

autonomy mainly disturbed by oral comprehension disorders; evolution toward a global auditory agnosia

bilateral sylvian atrophy on MRI

Table 3. Progressive/ visuospatial dysfunction

---

woman, 72 years, 12 years of scolarity
duration of disease: 9 years

normal executive functions
Wisconsin CST: 6 criteria, no perseveration

normal verbal efficiency
WAIS-R, verbal scale: IQ = 120
oral comprehension: normal on the Boston
Diagnostic Aphasia Examination

correct verbal memory (Wechsler memory scale)
— logical memory: 15
— associate learning: 17

impaired visuospatial functions
WAIS-R, performance scale: IQ = 69
Rey complex figure (copy): 10/36 (simultagnosia)
picture naming: 10/80 (visual agnosia)
disturbed written comprehension (alexia)

autonomy only disturbed by visual disorders

left parieto-occipital atrophy on CT-scan

Table 4. Progressive amnestic dementia

---

man, 68 years, 12 years of scolarity
duration of disease: 5 years

normal intellectual efficiency
WAIS-R, verbal scale: IQ = 109
  performance scale: IQ = 118
  total scale: IQ = 113

normal executive functions
Wisconsin CST: 6 criteria, no perseveration

normal linguistic functions
naming: 80/80
normal comprehension on the
Boston Diagnostic Aphasia Examination

normal visuospatial functions
Rey complex figure (copy): Type I, 36/36

impaired memory
word list learning
— free recall: 1/48
— cued recall: 14/48
— recognition: 2 hits, 17 false positives
Rey complex figure (memory): 2/36

autonomy only disturbed by memory disorders

bitemporal atrophy on MRI

Most of the previous focal atrophies are distinct from Alzheimer's disease by the absence of a true amnesic syndrome. This is not the case for "progressive amnestic dementia", which is characterized by the insidious onset and gradual exacerbation of a primary memory deficit, that accounts for limitations in daily living activities (Weintraub and Mesulam, 1993). Amnesia is related to the atrophy of limbic structures (Tissot et al., 1975; Sulkava et al., 1983). Other cognitive deficits may arise at any time in the course of the disease fitting the definition of probable Alzheimer's disease (McKhann et al., 1984).

Amnesia can also remain isolated for many years raising the question of the underlying pathology. Seven years after the first symptoms of his disease, one of our patients presented only an amnesic syndrome with progressive aggravation, associated with bitemporal atrophy (Table 4). In a similar case, autopsy revealed numerous neurofibrillary tangles in limbic and paralimbic regions but almost no neuritic plaques (Weintraub and Mesulam, 1993).

Even if they are associated with various pathologies, focal atrophies differ, therefore, from the classical picture of Alzheimer's disease by a much more limited cognitive syndrome and a longer preservation of self-governing in daily living activities. Given these features, most of them do not respond to the DSM-IV criteria for dementia (American Psychiatric Association, 1994), at least till an advanced stage of the disease.

Cognitive changes in diseases with movement disorders

Considered as a clinical feature of Huntington's disease (Brandt, 1993) and diffuse Lewy body disease (Gibb et al., 1989), dementia is more debated in Parkinson's disease (Dubois et al., 1991) and progressive supranuclear palsy (Pillon and Dubois, 1992).

Although global cognitive and memory performance is preserved in a great majority of patients with Parkinson's disease, specific impairments appear even at an early stage (Cooper et al., 1991). These basically concern planning (Owen and Robins, 1993) and encoding and retrieval strategies (Taylor et al., 1990). The existence of cognitive slowing and visuospatial deficits is still the subject of debate. Such deficits, when present, may simply result from a frontal lobe dysfunction (Dubois et al., 1991). Dementia occurs mainly in patients with late age at onset of the disease and after several years of evolution (Zetusky et al., 1985). Despite the existence of Alzheimer-like changes in the cerebral cortex (Paulus and Jellinger, 1991), the cognitive syndrome of demented parkinsonian patients differs from that of patients with Alzheimer's disease by the discrete nature of instrumental disorders, the contrast between the severity of retrieval impairment and the absence of storage deficits, and the severity of the dysexecutive syndrome (Litvan et al., 1991; Pillon et al., 1993; Stern et al., 1993). For instance, when testing memory using the same semantic cues (which is the fruit? which is the musical instrument?) at encoding and retrieval (Grober and Buschke, 1987), there is a clear dissociation between impaired free recall and near normal total recall (a good estimation of cued recall), showing that the help of semantic cueing normalizes the performance of these patients, whereas such is not the case in Alzheimer's disease in which cued recall is also severely impaired (Fig. 1). It is therefore possible to distinguish the inefficient planning of memory processes of parkinsonian patients from the genuine amnesic syndrome of patients with Alzheimer's disease. It may be added that, even demented, parkinsonian patients maintain a relative adaptation in daily living activities and are exceptionally institutionalized.

The few studies effected on multiple system atrophy, including the striatonigral degeneration type, display no clear difference from the neuropsychological pattern of Parkinson's disease without dementia (Pillon et al., 1995; Robbins et al., 1992; Testa et al., 1993).

The cognitive profile of cortico-basal degeneration is distinct from that of the previous two, due to the presence of sings suggestive of cortical involvement, particularly gesture disorders that are asymmetric at least at the beginning of the disease (Leiguarda et al., 1994). Manual dexterity, motor

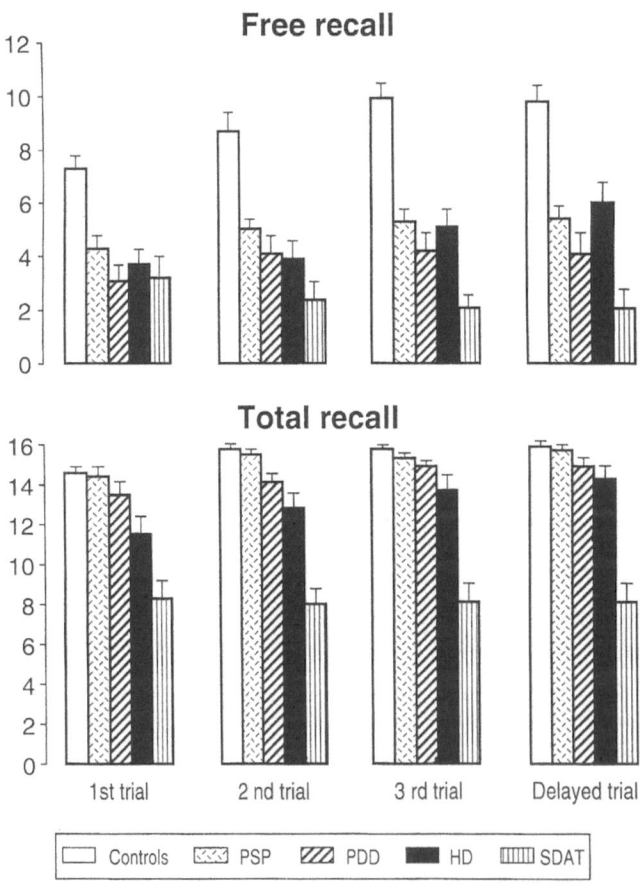

Fig. 1. Grober and Buschke's test. Performance in controls and patients with progressive supranuclear palsy (PSP), Parkinson's disease with dementia (PDD), Huntington's disease (HD) and senile dementia of the Alzheimer's type (SDAT) at the three and delayed trials (from left to right) and in the free and total recall (an estimation of cued recall; from top to bottom). Results are expressed as mean ± SEM

programming, bimanual coordination, posture reproduction, symbolic gesture evocation and imitation, object use and pantomime are precociously disturbed (Pillon et al., 1995).

Although such difficulties do not respond to a strict definition of apraxia, given the underlying severe impairment of manual dexterity, the deficit of voluntary movement goes "beyond that which might be explained by concomitant motor or sensory signs" (Sawle et al., 1991) and raises the question of an underlying apraxic disorder in relation to the parietal involvement. Cortical degeneration may also account for the linguistic perturbations observed in some cases (Riley et al., 1990).

Cognitive and behavioral changes are consistent even in the early stages of progressive supranuclear palsy. They mainly consist in cognitive slowing and severe frontal lobe-like syndrome (Albert et al., 1974; Cambier et al., 1985; Grafman et al., 1990; Maher et al., 1985). Signs of frontal lobe-like dysfunction are generally intense at the time of the diagnosis and more severe than in Parkinson's disease or multiple system atrophy (Pillon et al., 1995).

Patients cannot help imitating the gestures of the examiner, picking up objects placed near their hands and utilizing them without instructions. When asked to clap three times consecutively as quicly as possible, they have a tendency to initiate a series of claps which they are unable to interrupt (Dubois et al., 1995).

Despite a severe free recall deficit, using the Grober and Buschke's test a normal performance is obtained at total recall (Fig. 1) and recognition (Pillon et al., 1994), showing the lack of genuine amnesic syndrome in progressive supranuclear palsy. The cognitive disorders gradually worsen as the disease advances and become severe enough to warrant psychometric criteria of dementia in over 50% of cases.

Dementia is even more frequent in Huntington's disease, being consistently present at end stage. It is dominated by precocious disorders of attention, recall and personality, followed by speech reduction, planning deficits and sometimes psychosis (Brandt, 1991; Cummings, 1993). Even at an early stage, tests of attention, recall and executive functions, allow the disease to be distinguished from other choreiform disorders without the genetic mutation (Durr et al., 1995).

In diffuse Lewy body disease, parkinsonism is associated early with a subacute confusional state, with fluctuations and visual hallucinations, that may be due to severe cell loss in the nucleus basalis of Meynert, and psychotic features, that may reflect limbic involvement (Gibb et al., 1989; Perry et al., 1990). The rapidly progressive dementia is accompanied by aphasia, dyspraxia or spatial disorientation, suggestive of temporo-parietal dysfunction (Burkhardt et al., 1989).

Among the neurodegenerative diseases with movement disorders, diffuse Lewy body disease only shares the association of amnesia and instrumental disorders (aphasia, apraxia, agnosia), characteristic of Alzheimer's disease. However, more rapid onset, cognitive fluctuations and psychosis better predict diffuse Lewy body diseases than Alzheimer's disease. In progressive supranuclear palsy, Huntington's disease and Parkinson's disease with dementia, the predominant striato-frontal dysfunction is so severe that it leads to dramatic planning, monitoring and retrival deficits, evolving toward a dementia. Whereas the possible role of cortical lesions is repeatedly a subject of debate in these so-called "subcortico-frontal dementias" (Jellinger and Bancher, 1992), cognitive disorders generally related to a paralimbic or cortical involvement such as a genuine amnesic syndrome, an aphasia, an apraxia or an agnosia, do not usually occur in these diseases. In Parkinson's disease without dementia, multiple system atrophy and corticobasal degeneration, only specific cognitive impairments are found.

Conclusion

Alzheimer's disease is characterized by the association of a progressive amnesia with either instrumental or behavioral disorders, depending upon the underlying neuronal lesions (Hauw and Delaère, 1991). Such an association of cognitive and comportmental impairments may be observed in diffuse Lewy body disease, in which the same extended cortical areas may be disturbed, whereas in the more limited "lobar" atrophies, memory, linguistic, praxic, visuo-spatial or behavioral disorders are dissociated. The nature of these deficits is modified in predominantly subcortical degenerative diseases, in which the cortical programs may be preserved but insufficiently activated (Agid et al., 1987). Alzheimer's and non-Alzheimer's degenerative diseases can therefore the distinguished insofar as the severity and location of the underlying neuronal lesions differ. By contrast, the nature of histologic changes seems less determinant for the cognitive and behavioral profile than the location of lesions or dysfunction of the neuronal networks, since the same clinical syndrome may apparently be associated with different pathologies (Olichney et al., 1995).

References

Albert ML, Feldman RG, Willis AL (1974) The subcortical dementia of progressive supranuclear palsy. J Neurol Neurosurg Psychiatry 37: 121–130

Agid Y, Ruberg M, Dubois B, Pillon B (1987) Anatomo-clinical and biochemical concepts of subcortical dementia. In: Stahl SM, Iversen SD, Goodman EC (eds) Cognitive neurochemistry. Oxford University Press, New York Oxford, pp 248–271

American Psychiatric Association (1994) Diagnostic and statistical manual of mental disorders, 4th edn. DSM-IV™. American Psychiatric Association, Washington, DC

Benson DF, Davis RJ, Snyder BD (1988) Posterior cortical atrophy. Arch Neurol 45: 789–793

Brandt J (1991) Cognitive impairments in Huntington's disease: insights into the neuropsychology of the striatum. In: Boller F, Grafman J (eds) Handbook of neuropsychology, vol 5. Elsevier Sciences Publishers BV, Amsterdam, pp 241–264

Burkhardt CR, Filley CM, Kleinschmidt-DeMasters BK, De La Monte S, Norenberg MD, Schneck SA (1988) Diffuse Lewy body disease and progressive dementia. Neurology 38; 1520–1528

Byrne EJ, Lennox G, Lowe J, Godwin-Austen RB (1989) Diffuse Lewy body disease: clinical features in 15 cases. J Neurol Neurosurg Psychiatry 52: 709–717

Cambier J, Masson M, Viader F, Limodin J, Strube A (1895) Le syndrome frontal de la paralysie supranucléaire progressive. Rev Neurol 141: 528–536

Celsis P, Agniel A, Puel M, Le Tinnier A, Viallard G, Démonet JF, Rascol A, Marc-Vergnes JP (1990) Lateral asymmetries in primary degenerative dementia of the Alzheimer type. A correlative study of cognitive, haemodynamic and EEG data, in relation with severity, age of onset and sex. Cortex 26: 585–596

Chawluk JB, Mesulam MM, Hurtig H, Kushner M, Weintraub S, Saykin A, Rubin N, Alavi A, Reivitch M (1986) Slowly progressive aphasia without generalized dementia: studies with positron emission tomography. Ann Neurol 19: 68–74

Chui HC (1989) Dementia. A review emphasizing clinico-pathologic correlation and brain-behavior relationship. Arch Neurol 46: 806–814

Cogan DG (1985) Visual disturbances with focal progressive dementing disease. Am J Ophthalmol 100: 68–72

Cooper JA, Sagar HJ, Jordan N, Harvey NS, Sullivan EV (1991) Cognitive impairment in early untreated Parkinson's disease and its relationship to motor disability. Brain 114: 2095–2122.

Croisile B, Trillet M, Hibert O, Cinotti L, Le Bars D, Mauguière F, Aimard G (1991) Désordres visuo-constructifs et alexie-agraphie associés à une atrophie corticale postérieure. Rev Neurol 147: 138–143

Cummings JL (1993) Psychosis in basal ganglia disorders. In: Wolters E, Scheltens P (eds) Mental dysfunction in Parkinson's disease. Vrije Universiteit, Amsterdam, pp 257–268

Cummings JL, Benson DF (1984) Subcortical dementia. Review of an emerging concept. Arch Neurol 41: 874–879

De Renzi E (1986) Slowly progressive visual agnosia or apraxia without dementia. Cortex 22: 171–180

Dick JP, Snowden J, Northern B, Goulding PJ, Neary D (1989) Slowly progressive apraxia. Behav Neurol 2: 101–114

Dubois B, Boller F, Pillon B, Agid Y (1991) Cognitive deficits in Parkinson's disease. In: Boller F, Grafman J (eds) Handbook of neuropsychology, vol 5. Elsevier Sciences Publishers BV, Amsterdam, pp 195–240

Dubois B, Défontaines B, Deweer B, Malapani C, Pillon B (1995) Cognitive and behavioral changes in patients with focal lesions of the basal ganglia. Adv Neurol 65: 29–41

Durr A, Dodé C, Hahn V, Pêcheux C, Pillon B, Feingold J, Kaplan JC, Agid Y, Brice A (1995) Diagnosis of "sporadic" Huntington's disease. J Neurol Sci 129: 51–55

Gibb WR, Luthert PJ, Janota I, Lantos PL (1989) Cortical Lewy body dementia: clinical features and classification. J Neurol Neurosurg Psychiatry 52: 185–192

Gibb WRG, Luthert PJ, Marsden CD (1989) Corticobasal degeneration. Brain 112: 1171–1192

Grafman J, Litvan I, Gomez C, Chase T (1990) Frontal lobe function in progressive supranuclear palsy. Arch Neurol 47: 553–558

Grober E, Buschke H (1987) Genuine memory deficits in dementia. Dev Neuropsychol 3: 13–36

Gustafson L (1987) Frontal lobe degeneration of non-Alzheimer type. II. Clinical picture and differential diagnosis. Arch Gerontol Geriatr 6: 209–223

Hauw JJ, Delaère P (1991) Topographie des lésions. In: Signoret JL, Hauw JJ (eds) Maladie d'Alzheimer et autres démences. Flammarion Médecine-Sciences, Paris, pp 22–38

Haxby JV, Grady CL, Koss E, Horwitz B, Schapiro M, Friedland RP, Rapoport SI (1988) Heterogeneous anterior-posterior metabolic patterns in dementia of the Alzheimer type. Neurology 38: 1853–1863

Jellinger KA, Bancher C (1992) Neuropathology. In: Litvan I, Agid Y (eds) Progressive supranuclear palsy: clinical and research approaches. Oxford University Press, New York Oxford, pp 44–88

Karbe H, Kertesz A, Polk M (1993) Profiles of language impairment in primary progressive aphasia. Arch Neurol 50: 193–201

Knopman DS, Christensen KJ, Schut LJ, Harbaugh RE, Reeder T, Ngo T, Frey W (1989) The spectrum of imaging and neuropsychological findings in Pick's disease. Neurology 39: 362–368

Knopman DS, Mastric AR, Frey WH, Sung JH, Rustan T (1990) Dementia lacking distinctive histologic features: a common non-Alzheimer degenerative dementia. Neurology 40: 251–256

Leiguarda R, Lees AJ, Merello M, Starkstein S, Marsden CD (1994) The nature of apraxia in corticobasal degeneration. J Neurol Neurosurg Psychiatry 57: 455–459

Litvan I, Mohr E, Williams J, Gomez C, Chase TN (1991) Differential memory and executive functions in demented patients with Parkinson's and Alzheimer's disease. J Neurol Neurosurg Psychiatry 54: 25–29

Maher ER, Smith EM, Lees AJ (1985) Cognitive deficits in the Steele-Richardson-Olszewski syndrome (progressive supranuclear palsy). J Neurol Neurosurg Psychiatry 48: 1234–1239

McKhann G, Drachman D, Folstein M, Katzman R, Price D, Stadlan EM (1984) Clinical diagnosis of Alzheimer's disease: report of the NINCDS-ADRDA work group under the auspices of Department of Health and Human Servicies task force on Alzheimer's disease. Neurology 34: 939–944

Mendez MF, Selwood A, Mastri AR, Frey WH (1993) Pick's disease versus Alzheimer's disease: a comparison of clinical characteristics. Neurology 43: 289–292

Miller BL, Cummings JL, Villanueva-Meyer J, Boone K, Mehringer CM, Lesser IM, Mena I (1991) Frontal lobe degeneration: clinical, neuropsychological and SPECT characteristics. Neurology 41: 1374–1382

Neary D (1990) Non Alzheimer's disease form of cerebral atrophy. J Neurol Neurosurg Psychiatry 53: 929–931

Neary D, Snowden JS, Northen B, Goulding P (1988) Dementia of frontal lobe type. J Neurol Neurosurg Psychiatry 51: 353–361

Olichney JM, Galasko D, Corey-Bloom J, Thal LJ (1995) The spectrum of diseases with diffuse Lewy bodies. Adv Neurol 65: 159–170

Owen AM, Robbins TW (1993) Comparative neuropsychology of Parkinsonian syndromes. In: Wolters EC, Scheltens P (eds) Mental dysfunction in Parkinson's disease. Vrije Universiteit, Amsterdam, pp 221–241

Paulus W, Jellinger K (1991) The neuropathologic basis of different clinical subgroups of Parkinson's disease. J Neuropathol Exp Neurol 50: 473–755

Perry RH, Irving D, Blessed G, Fairbairn A, Perry EK (1990) Senile dementia of Lewy body type. A clinically and neuropathologically distinct form of Lewy body dementia in the elderly. J Neurol Sci 95: 119–139

Pillon B, Blin J, Vidailhet M, Deweer B, Sirigu A, Dubois B, Agid Y (1995) The neuropsychological pattern of corticobasal degeneration. Comparison with progressive supranuclear palsy and Alzheimer's disease. Neurology 45: 1477–1483

Pillon B, Deweer B, Agid Y, Dubois B (1993) Explicit memory in Alzheimer's, Huntington's, and Parkinson's diseases. Arch Neurol 50: 374–379

Pillon B, Deweer B, Michon A, Malapani C, Agid Y, Dubois B (1994) Are explicit memory disorders of progressive supranuclear palsy related to damage to striatofrontal circuits? Comparison with Alzheimer's, Parkinson's, and Huntington's diseases. Neurology 44: 1254–1270

Pillon B, Dubois B (1992) Cognitive and behavioral impairments. In: Litvan I, Agid Y (eds) Progressive supranuclear palsy; clinical and research approaches. Oxford University Press, New York Oxford, pp 223–239

Pillon B, Gouider-Khouja N, Deweer B, Vidhailhet M, Malapani C, Dubois B, Agid Y (1995) Neuropsychological pattern of striatonigral degeneration: comparison with Parkinson's disease and progressive supranuclear palsy. J Neurol Neurosurg Psychiatry 58: 174–179

Richard J, Constantinidis J (1970) Les démences de la vieillesse; notions acquises et problèmes cliniques actuels. Confront Psychiat 3: 39–61

Riley DE, Lang AE, Lewis A, Resch L, Ashby P, Hornykiewicz O, Black S (1990) Corticobasal ganglionic degeneration. Neurology 40: 1203–1212

Robbins TW, James M, Lange KW, Owen AM, Quinn NP, Marsden CD (1992) Cognitive performance in multiple System Atrophy. Brain 115: 271–291

Sawle GV, Brooks DJ, Marsden CD, Frackoviack RJ (1991) Corticobasal degeneration. A unique pattern of regional cortical oxygen hypometabolism and striatal fluorodopa uptake demonstrated by positron emission tomography. Brain 114: 541–556

Snowden JS, Neary D, Mann DW, Goulding PJ, Testa HJ (1992) Progressive language disorder due to lobar atrophy. Ann Neurol 31: 174–183

Stern Y, Richards M, Sano M, Mayeux R (1993) Comparison of cognitive changes in patients with Alzheimer's and Parkinson's disease. Arch Neurol 50: 1040–1045

Sulkava R, Haltia M, Paetau A, Wilkstrom J, Palo J (1983) Accuracy of clinical diagnosis in primary degenerative dementia: correlation with neuropathological findings. J Neurol Neurosurg Psychiatry 46: 9–13

Taylor AE, Saint-Cyr JA, Lang AE (1990) Memory and learning in early Parkinson's disease: evidence for a "frontal lobe syndrome". Brain Cogn 13: 211–232

Testa D, Fetoni V, Soliveri P, Musicco M, Palazzini E, Girotti F (1993) Cognitive and motor performance in multiple system atrophy and Parkinson's disease compared. Neuropsychologia 31: 207–210

Tissot R, Constantinidis J, Richard J (1975) La maladie de Pick. Masson, Paris

Tyrell PJ, Warrington EK, Frackowiak RS, Rossor MN (1990) Progressive degeneration of the right temporal lobe studied with positron emission tomography. J Neurol Neurosurg Psychiatry 53: 1046–1050

Weintraub S, Mesulam MM (1993) Four neuropsychological profiles in dementia. In: Boller F, Grafman J (eds) Handbook of neuropsychology, vol 8. Elsevier, Amsterdam, pp 253–282

Weintraub S, Rubin N, Mesulam M (1990) Primary progressive aphasia: longitudinal course, neuropsychological profile and language features. Arch Neurol 47: 1329–1335

Zetusky WJ, Jankovic J, Pirozzolo FJ (1985) The heterogeneity of Parkinson's disease; clinical and prognostic implications. Neurology 35: 522–526

Authors' address: Dr. B. Pillon, INSERM U-289 and Fédération de Neurologie, Hôpital de la Salpêtrière, 47 Bd de l'Hôpital, F-75651 Paris Cedex 13, France.

J Neural Transm (1996) [Suppl] 47: 73–101

The neurochemistry of Alzheimer type, vascular type and mixed type dementias compared

W. Gsell, I. Strein, and **P. Riederer**

Clinical Neurochemistry, Department of Psychiatry, University of Würzburg,
Würzburg, Federal Republic of Germany

Summary. We present the results of a meta-analysis of neurochemical changes in human post mortem brains of Alzheimer type (AD), vascular type (VD) and mixed type (MF) dementias, and matched controls based on 275 articles published between January 1980 and February 1994.

Severity of degeneration between the different neurochemical systems is as follows, although ranking is difficult with regard to limited numbers of investigations in some neurochemical systems: Cholinergic system > serotonergic system > excitatory amino acids > GABAergic system > energy metabolsim > NA > oxidative stress parameters > neuropeptides > DA. But, within a neurochemical system, degeneration is not evenly distributed. Spared parameters, e.g. muscarinic receptors and MAO-B, allow to make some suggestions for future therapeutic strategies.

Aims

We present the results of a meta-analysis of neurochemical changes in human post mortem brains of Alzheimer type (AD), vascular type (VD) and mixed type (MF) dementias and matched controls based on 275 papers published between January 1980 and February 1994. Data research has been done by using Medline. All articles used are original publications. Our data pool includes 9,535 patient records.

The aim of our study was to demonstrate unequivocal pathologic findings, separate them from precarious findings due to reduced numbers of investigations and patients, and to point at patches, either regions or neurochemical parameters, where and which post mortem investigations should be done in the near future. A second goal was to get assistance for future therapeutic strategies.

Terminology

The term Alzheimer type dementia (AD) is used in this paper to cover presenile as well as the senile, severe and mild dementias, dementia of Lewy body type and familial Alzheimer's disease. We did not separate between presenile versus senile, mild versus severe, or familial versus sporadic dementias, because missing characterization in many publications will limit number of studies and patients. The term vascular dementia (VD) mainly covers multiinfarct dementias and Binswanger's disease. Classification of patients was made mainly by DSM-III-R and/or ICD 9.

Methods

To avoid problems caused by different units of measurement, all data were transformed to percent of controls. Data of different authors on one parameter in a specific region were weighted by the number of cases. As many parameters were measured in different regions of one patient, the number of single records is given instead of the number of patients. An overall mean and standard deviation has been calculated from the mean of each publication with respect to the region and neurochemical parameter. The overall mean is shown in a symbolic way (+, −, 0; see Table 1: legend to the tables) for cortical regions (CO), limbic structures (LIM) and regions of the motor loop (MO) in this order for the cholinergic system, biogenic amines (serotonin, dopamine and noradrenaline), the GABAergic system, excitatory amino acids, neuropeptides, second messengers, energy metabolism and oxidative stress. The number of single records is shown symbolically (n < 10: +, −, 0 (small size); n < 50: +, −, 0 (middle size); n > 50: +, −, 0 (large size); Table 1). Within each neurochemical system parameters are arranged in the following way: precursors, synthesizing enzymes, neurotransmitter, metabolizing enzymes, older receptor studies, where subtypes have not been separated, and newer receptor analyses with differentiation of different receptors subtypes and their respective B_{max} and K_D.

Results

Cholinergic system (Table 2)

Within the cholinergic system choline acetyltransferase (ChAT) is the most thoroughly examined parameter as shown by 8,848 single records for ChAT in AD. ChAT activity generally declines to 48% (CO), 51% (LIM) and 78% (MO) of control values, while changes in VD (260 single records) are not as prominent with 85% (CO), 64% (LIM) and 87% (MO). For MF (167 single records) corresponding data are 55% (CO) and 49% (LIM). Acetylcholinest-

Table 1. Legend to Tables 2 to 9

Deviation from control values	Number of cases
− − − : <60% of controls	−, +, 0 (small size): up to 10 cases
− − : <80% of controls	−, +, 0 (middle size): up to 50 cases
− : between 80% and <100% of controls	−, +, 0 (large size): >50 cases
0 : 100% of controls	
+ : up to 120% of controls	
+ + : up to 150% of controls	
+ + + : >150% of controls	

Table 2. Cholinergic system

	Choline			ChAT			Acetylcholine			AChE			Cholinesterase			Phosphoesterase		
	AD	VD	MF	AD	VD	MF	AD	VD	MF	AD	VD	MF	AD	VD	MF	AD	VD	MF
Cortex																		
undifferentiated				- -														
frontal	- -		-	- -	-	-			- -	-			-					
parietal				- -	-				-	-			-					
temporal	- -			- -	-	-	-		- -	- - -	-		- -			-	-	
occipital				-	-					- -	-					-		
limbic structures	- - -			- - -	- -	-			- -	- -			- -					
motor loop	+ +			- -	-		-			- -			-					

	Muscarinic rec.			Muscarine Bmax			Muscarine KD			M1 Receptor			M1 Rec. Bmax			M1 Rec. KD		
	AD	VD	MF	AD	VD	MF	AD	VD	MF	AD	VD	MF	AD	VD	MF	AD	VD	MF
Cortex																		
undifferentiated	+									-								
frontal	-	-		- -	-		-			+						+		
parietal	+									+								
temporal	+				-		+			-			+ +			-	-	
occipital	+ +									-			- -			-	-	
limbic structures	+	-	- -	- -	-		-			+			+ +			+		
motor loop	-	-	-	-			-			+ +			+ + +			+		

	M2 Receptor			M2 Rec. Bmax			M2 Rec. KD			Nicotinic rec.			Nicotine Bmax			Nicotine KD		
	AD	VD	MF	AD	VD	MF	AD	VD	MF	AD	VD	MF	AD	VD	MF	AD	VD	MF
Cortex																		
undifferentiated	- -									-						+ + +		
frontal	- -						0			- -	-		- - -			-		
parietal	- -						+			- -						+		
temporal	- -			- -			-	-		- -			- - -			+ +		
occipital	- -						+			- -	+					+ +		
limbic structures	-			- -			+			-						-		
motor loop	-						-			- -						+ +		

erase (AChE) activity in AD (294 single records) declines to 59% (CO), 38% (LIM) and 69% (MO). Again changes in VD (10 single records) are smaller with 75% (CO) and 70% (MO). No data exist for MF. Within the cholinergic receptor subtypes focus on muscarinic receptors is more frequent than on nicotinic receptors. In most cases unspecified muscarinic receptor binding in AD (2,937 single records) has been performed. For CO, LIM and MO corresponding data are 108%, 109% and 100%. KD values (188 single records) are 96%, 85% and 78% respectively, while Bmax values (31 single records) have been determined in CO (74%) only. Muscarinic M1 receptor binding (286 single records) shows a decrease to 96% (CO), and increases of 117% (LIM) and 141% (MO) with KD values (203 single records) of 105%, 128% and 109%. Bmax values (94 single records) show increases to 98%, 139% and 159%. M2 receptor binding studies (168 single records) show a decrease to 83%, 80% and 89%. M2 KD (196 single records) have been determined to 94%, 112% and 105%, while Bmax values (46 single records) decrease to 57%, 44% and 95%. In VD 128 single records have been reported regarding muscarinic binding studies. Data show a decrease to 86%, 86% and 84%. In MF 113 single records show a decrease to 77%, 81% and 90% respectively.

Unspecified nicotinic binding studies (NICOTINE) were performed in 1,328 (AD) and 81 (VD) single records. Nicotinic binding decreases in AD (1,079 single records) with 60%, 75% and 74%. KD values in AD (218 single records) slightly change to 101% (CO) and increase to 123% (MO) while they decrease to 74% in limbic structures. Bmax values only exist for AD (31 single records) in cortical regions and show a decline to 40%. Data in VD (81 single mesurements) are 45% (CO) and 106% (LIM). No data have been reported for MF.

Biogenic amines

Within the serotonergic system (Table 3) serotonin in AD (1,190 single records) decreases to 63%, 64% and 61%. Changes in VD (101 single records) are not as prominent with 79%, 78% and 82%. 5-HIAA in AD (1297 single records) is reduced to 75%, 74% and 82%. In VD 5-HIAA (101 single records) shows a decrease to 81%, 68% and 69%. No data exist for MF. Unspecified serotonin receptor binding studies were performed on AD patients (1188 single records) and MF patients (36 single records). In AD (221 single records) it is reduced to 78%, 47% and 55%. In MF (36 single records) there is an increase to 128% (CO) but a decrease to 83% (MO). No data exist for VD. Serotonergic HT-2 receptor binding studies (940 single records) have only be reported for AD. There is a significant reduction to 66%, 61% and 84%, while KD values (27 single records) are 100% (CO) and 112% (LIM).

Within the dopaminergic system (Table 4) concentrations for dopamine in AD (1,283 single records) show a decrease to 91%, 75% and 87%. In VD (137 single records) concentrations are 121%, 103% and 99%. No analyses have been reported for MF. In AD MAO-A activities (311 single records) increases

Table 3. Serotonergic system

	Tryptophan			5-HT			5-HT uptake			5-HT upt. Bmax			5-HT upt. KD			5-HIAA		
	AD	VD	MF	AD	VD	MF	AD	VD	MF	AD	VD	MF	AD	VD	MF	AD	VD	MF
Cortex																		
undifferentiated																		
frontal				- -						- -			-			- -		
parietal				- - -												- -		
temporal	+			- -	-		-									- -	-	
occipital				-												- -		
limbic structures	+			- -	-											-	- -	
motor loop	- -			- -	-											-	- -	

	5-HT Receptor			5-HT 2 Receptor			5-HT 2 Rec. KD		
	AD	VD	MF	AD	VD	MF	AD	VD	MF
Cortex									
undifferentiated									
frontal	- -		+	- -					
parietal	- -		+ +	- - -					
temporal	-		+ + +	- -			0		
occipital				- -					
limbic structures	- - -			- -			+		
motor loop	- -		-	-					

Table 4. Dopaminergic system

	Phenylalanine			Tyrosine			Tyrosine hydroxylase			Dopamine			Dopamine ß hydroxylase			MAO-A		
	AD	VD	MF	AD	VD	MF	AD	VD	MF	AD	VD	MF	AD	VD	MF	AD	VD	MF
Cortex																		
undifferentiated										–				–		+++		
frontal										–	–		– –	–		+		
parietal										–	+					++		
temporal	– –			–						–	–		– – –			–		
occipital																++		
limbic structures	+			++						–	+		–	–		+		
motor loop	– –			– –			– – –	– –		–	–		– –	–		+		+++

	MAO-B			MAO-undiff.			DOPAC			HVA			3-Methoxytyramine			Dopamine receptor		
	AD	VD	MF	AD	VD	MF	AD	VD	MF	AD	VD	MF	AD	VD	MF	AD	VD	MF
Cortex																		
undifferentiated	+++			+						++								
frontal	++						– –			++								
parietal	+++						–			++								
temporal	+++						–			–	–							
occipital	+++									+++								
limbic structures	+			+			–			+	–							
motor loop	+			–			+	– –		–	–		– –	–		– – –		+++

	D1 Receptor			D1 Rec. Bmax			D1 Rec. KD			D2 Receptor			D2 Rec. Bmax			D2 Rec. KD		
	AD	VD	MF	AD	VD	MF	AD	VD	MF	AD	VD	MF	AD	VD	MF	AD	VD	MF
Cortex																		
undifferentiated																		
frontal										– –								
parietal																		
temporal																		
occipital																		
limbic structures	– –	–		– –			–			–	+++			+++				
motor loop	–	–	+	–		–				–	++	–		++	–	+++		

to 139%, 106% and 106%. MAO-B in AD (722 single records) are even higher with 155%, 127% and 113%. DOPAC in AD (509 single records) decreases to 99%, 80% and shows only a very mild change in the motor loop with 101%. Data for VD (5 single records) show a decline within the motor loop to 57%. No data are reported for MF. HVA concentrations in AD (1,166 single records) are 110%, 99% and show a decrease to 76% in the motor loop. HVA in VD (56 single records) decreases to 80%, 91% and 92%. No data exist for MF. Dopamine receptor studies were performed on AD (236 measurements), VD (77 measurements) and MF (84 measurements) patients. Data for unspecified dopamine receptor measured on AD (7 measurements) and MF (6 measurements) patients rise up to 116% (MO) in AD and 220% (MO) in MF. More specific dopamine D1 receptor binding in AD (81 measurements) shows 64% (LIM), 88% (MO) of control values. In VD (43 measurements) a mild decrease to 85% (LIM) and 92% (MO) has been foud while change has been reported in MF (52 measurements) to 99% (LIM) and 103% (MO). Bmax values in AD (6 measurements) decline to 65% (LIM) with KD values (6 measurements only) of 97%. Data for unspecified dopamine D2 receptor binding studies in AD (115 measurements) are 71%, 86% and 98%. Data for VD (34 measurements) are 158% (LIM) and 142% (MO). Bmax values in AD (6 measurements) decline to 38% (MO) with KD's as high as 188% (MO). Data for MF (26 measurements) are 95% (LIM) and 90% (MO).

Within the noradrenergic system (Table 5) in AD concentrations for noradrenaline (1,518 measurements) decline to 64%, 75% and 83%. In VD (132 measurements) data change to 120% in cortical regions, but decrease to 87% (LIM) and 81% (MO). No data are available for MF. MHPG concentrations only are reported for AD (732 measurements) and show an increase to 105%, 112% and 138%. In general, adrenergic receptor binding studies were performed on AD- (1092 measurements), VD- (80 measurements) and MF- (40 measurements) patients. Unspecified adrenergic B receptor show mild changes to 105%, 114% and 95% in AD (306 measurements). In VD (30 measurements) there is an increase to 139% (CO) and in MF (21 measurements) to 118% (CO) and 98% (LIM). Adrenergic A1 receptor binding in AD (126 measurements) changes to 104% (CO) and 93% (LIM). In MF (19 measurements) respective data for CO are 142% (CO) while there is a decrease to 71% (LIM). Data for VD (30 measurements) have only be reported for MO (127%). Bmax values decrease in AD (54 measurements) to 80% (CO), 69% (LIM) and 76% (MO). In addition, KD values (54 measurements) in AD also decline to 77%, 65% and 75%. Adrenergic A2 receptor binding data in AD (188 measurements) change to 92%, 102% and 62%. Data for VD (20 measurements) are 128% (CO). Bmax values only exist for AD (54 measurements) and show changes to 83%, 72% and 92%. Respective KD values (54 measurements) for AD decline to 75%, 76% and 91%. Adrenergic B1 receptor binding data only exist for AD (128 measurement) and show 102%, 125% and 85% of control values. However, adrenergic B2 receptor binding shows an increase in AD (128 measurements) to 122%, 165% and 137%.

Table 5. Noradrenergic system

	Noradrenaline			PNMT			MHPG			ADR. B Receptor			ADR. B Rec. KD			A1 Receptor		
	AD	VD	MF	AD	VD	MF	AD	VD	MF	AD	VD	MF	AD	VD	MF	AD	VD	MF
Cortex																		
undifferentiated										+ +	+ +					+	+ +	+ +
frontal	- -	-		+ + +			+			-		+	- -			+		+ + +
parietal	- -			- -			+ +			+		+ +				- -		+
temporal	- -	+ +					+			+		+ +				+		
occipital	-	0					-			-						+		
limbic structures	- -	-		- - -			+			+		-				-		- -
motor loop	-	-		+ + +			+			+								

	A1 Rec. Bmax			A1 Rec. KD			A2 Recptor			A2 Rec. Bmax			A2 Rec. KD			B1 Receptor		
	AD	VD	MF	AD	VD	MF	AD	VD	MF	AD	VD	MF	AD	VD	MF	AD	VD	MF
Cortex																		
undifferentiated							-			- -			- -			-		
frontal	-			-			+	+ +		- -			- -			-		
parietal																		
temporal	- -			- -			-			-			- -			+ + +		
occipital							-											
limbic structures	- -			- -			+			- -			- -			+ +		
motor loop	- -			- -			- -						-			-		

	B2 Receptor		
	AD	VD	MF
Cortex			
undifferentiated	+ + +		
frontal	+ +		
parietal			
temporal	-		
occipital			
limbic structures	+ + +		
motor loop	+ +		

Table 6. GABAergic system

	Glutamate decarboxyl.			GABA			GABA-Transaminase			GABA uptake			GABA binding			GABA binding Bmax		
	AD	VD	MF	AD	VD	MF	AD	VD	MF	AD	VD	MF	AD	VD	MF	AD	VD	MF
Cortex undifferentiated																		
frontal	- -			-	- -		+			- -			- -			- -		
parietal	-			-			- -			- -			- -					
temporal	- -			- -			- -			- - -			-					
occipital				-	+		+ + +			- -			-					
limbic structures	- -			-			-			-			- -					
motor loop	+ +			+						- -								

	GABA binding KD			Benzodiazepine rec.			Benzo. Rec. KD		
	AD	VD	MF	AD	VD	MF	AD	VD	MF
Cortex undifferentiated				-					
frontal	-			+ +	- -				
parietal	-			+ + +					
temporal	-			+	-				
occipital				+ + +					
limbic structures	- -			-			- - -		
motor loop	+ +			-					

GABAergic system (Table 6)

Within the GABAergic system GABA concentration in AD (861 measurements) shows a decrease to 78% (CO), 80% (LIM) and a slight increase in MO with 105%. In VD only few patients (8 measurements) have been examined. Data show 76% (CO) and 108% (LIM). No data exist for MF. GABA uptake in AD (97 measurements) shows a general reduction to 40%, 77% and 71%. No data have been reported for VD and MF. GABA binding studies also only exist for AD (138 measurements) with an overall reduction to 89%, 64% and 56%. Bmax values for this unspecified GABA receptor (16 measurements) show a decline to 58% (CO). KD values (40 measurements) change slightly in cortical regions with 108% and show a decrease to 61% in LIM. Benzodiazepine receptor binding studies in AD (365 measurements) show an increase to 145% (CO) and a slight decrease to 91% (LIM) and 97% (MO), while it decreaes to 81% (CO) in VD (35 measurements). KD values (24 measurements) decrease to 57% (CO) in AD.

Excitatory amino acids (EAA) (Table 7)

For EAA's no data have been reported for MF. Glutamate and aspartate in AD show the most striking changes. In AD glutamate concentrations (647 single records) are generally reduced to 86%, 81% and 84%. In VD only 4 patients were examined with concentrations being 121% (CO) and 99% (LIM). Glutamate uptake in AD (39 single records) shows a significant reduction to 37%, 34% and 72%. No data have been reported for VD. In AD aspartate concentrations (435 measurements) are also generally reduced to 89%, 85% and 83%. In VD only 4 patients were examined and show an increase to 208% (CO) and a decrease to 80% of contol values (LIM). Asparate uptake in AD (118 records) is significantly reduced to 34%, 34% and 69%. No data exist for VD. EAA-transporter studies were done in 390 single records only in AD and there is a decrease to 76% (CO) and 92% (LIM). Unspecified glutamate receptor densities in AD (744 single records) show a decrease to 84%, 76% and a slight increase to 115% (MO). Bmax values (11 single records) show a decline to 74% (CO), while KD values (35 patients) change to 137%, 105% and 107%. NMDA receptor studies performed in 338 single records in AD patients and only show slight changes to 102% (CO) and 95% (LIM), while KD values (30 single records) change to 97%, 131% and 88%. No data on receptor studies exist for VD.

Second messenger systems (Table 9)

Hardly any data exist for DA-sensitive adenylatecyclase (10 measurements in AD patients). Such data show a reduction to 54% of control values (CO).

Table 7. Excitatory amino acids

	Glutamate			Glutamate uptake			Aspartate			Aspartate uptake			Asparagine			EAA-Tranporter		
	AD	VD	MF	AD	VD	MF	AD	VD	MF	AD	VD	MF	AD	VD	MF	AD	VD	MF
Cortex																		
undifferentiated	- -																	
frontal	-	+ +		- -			-	+ + +		- -			+			-		
parietal	-			- -			-			- -			+			- -		
temporal	- -			- -			-			- -			+			- -		
occipital	-			- -			- -			- -						- -		
limbic structures	- -	-		- -			-			- -			+			-		
motor loop	-			- -			-	-		- -						-		

	g-Glutamyl transaminase			Glutamate receptor			Glut. Rec. Bmax			Glut. Rec. KD			NMDA-Receptor			NMDA Rec. KD		
	AD	VD	MF	AD	VD	MF	AD	VD	MF	AD	VD	MF	AD	VD	MF	AD	VD	MF
Cortex																		
undifferentiated	0			- -						+ + +			+ +					
frontal	-			- -						+			+ +					
parietal	+			-						+ +			-			-		
temporal	+			-						,			-			+		
occipital	-												-					
limbic structures				-						+			-			+ +		
motor loop				+						+			-					

	Quisqualate receptor			Quisqu. Rec. Bmax			Quisqu. Rec. KD			Phencyclidine Rec.			PHEN REZ. Bmax			PHEN. REZ. KD		
	AD	VD	MF	AD	VD	MF	AD	VD	MF	AD	VD	MF	AD	VD	MF	AD	VD	MF
Cortex																		
undifferentiated																		
frontal																		
parietal																		
temporal							+											
occipital																		
limbic structures	- -									- -			- -			-		
motor loop																		

Table 8. Neuropeptides

	alpha-MSH			CCK			Corticotropin-RH			CRH-Rec.			CRH-Rec. KD			Galanine		
	AD	VD	MF	AD	VD	MF	AD	VD	MF	AD	VD	MF	AD	VD	MF	AD	VD	MF
Cortex																		
undifferentiated				0														
frontal	-			-			- -			+ +			+			+		
parietal	-			-			-											
temporal	-			-			-			+ +			-			+		
occipital	- -			+			- - -			+ + +			-			- -		
limbic structures	+			-												+		
motor loop	- -			+			+ +											

	Metencephaline			Neuropeptide Y			Neurotensine			Opiate Rec.			Oxytocine			Somatostatin		
	AD	VD	MF	AD	VD	MF	AD	VD	MF	AD	VD	MF	AD	VD	MF	AD	VD	MF
Cortex																		
undifferentiated																		
frontal	+ +			- -			0						+ +			- -		
parietal	+			0			0						+ +			- -		
temporal	+			-			- -			+			+ +			- -		
occipital				- -									-			- -		
limbic structures	-			-			+			- -			-			-		
motor loop				-			+ +			+ +			-			-		

	Somatostatin Rec.			Somato. Rec. Bmax			Somato. Rec. KD			Substance P			VIP			Vasopressine		
	AD	VD	MF	AD	VD	MF	AD	VD	MF	AD	VD	MF	AD	VD	MF	AD	VD	MF
Cortex																		
undifferentiated																		
frontal	+			- -			- -			-			+			+ +		
parietal	- - -						- -			-		- -	-			+		
temporal	- -			- - -			- -			-		- -	-			+ +		
occipital										- -			-			-		
limbic structures	- - -									-			+			-		
motor loop										+	-	+	-			-		

Chromogranine A measured in only 5 AD patients shows an increase to 227% (CO). Signal transduction measurements in AD (162 single records) show a mild change to 98% (CO). In VD (2 patients only) data decline to 47% (CO). No other regions have been examined so far. No data exist for MF.

Neuropeptides (Table 8)

Within the various neuropeptide studies most data exist on somatostatin and show the most severe changes in cortical regions. Cholecystokinin (CCK) in AD (426 single records) is hardly changed to 102%, 93% and 106%. Neuropeptide Y (NPY) in AD (395 single records) is decreased to 80%, 87% and 82%. Somatostatin (SOM) in AD (2091 single records) declines to 60%, 93% and 87%. Somatostatin receptor (SOM-R) studies were performed in 204 single measurements in AD patients. SOM-R binding in AD patients shows a significant decline to 80% (CO) and 48% (LIM). Bmax values (68 single records) decline to 59% (CO) while the respective KD values (68 single measurements) decline to 64% (CO). Substance P (SP) concentrations in AD (762 single records) decrease to 79%, 88% and slightly increase to 104% (MO). In VD only 4 patients were examined and data show a general reduction to 66%, 70% and 82%. In MF (20 single records) data show 73%, 68% and 101%. SP generally declines in all three types of dementia in cortical and limbic regions. Vasopressine in AD (411 single measurements) changes to 115%, 94% and 78%. No data exist for VD and MF.

Energy metabolism (Table 9)

In AD pyruvate dehydrogenase activity (82 single records) declines to 65% (CO) and 87% (MO). No data exist for VD and MF. ATP-citrate lyase activity in AD (36 single measurements) significantly declines to 64%, 49% and 78%. No data exist for VD and MF. Phosphoactivated glutaminase activity in AD (85 single records) severely declines to 22% (CO) and 31% (MO). For unspecified glutamate dehydrognease activity only very few data are available. In AD 14 patients were examined and the activities show a significant reduction to 42% (CO). In AD NAD+ linked glutamate dehydrogenase activity (7 patients) shows hardly any change to 103% (CO). No other regions were examined. Lactate concentrations measured in AD patients (41 single measurements) change to 113% (CO) and 93% (MO). Acetyl-CoA synthase activity in AD (36 single records) declines to 65%, 87% and 80%. No data exist for MF.

Oxidative stress (Table 9)

Still little data are available on oxidative stress. Data only exist on 36 AD patients and show a general increase in oxidative parameters. Glu-

Table 9. Second messengers, energy metabolism, oxidative stress

	Adenylate cyclase			Chromogranine A			Guanylate cyclase			Signal transduction			Pyruvate dehydrogenase			Acetyl-CoA synthase		
	AD	VD	MF	AD	VD	MF	AD	VD	MF	AD	VD	MF	AD	VD	MF	AD	VD	MF
Cortex																		
undifferentiated										−	− − −							
frontal				+ + +			−						−					
parietal							−						−			− −		
temporal													−			− −		
occipital													− − −					
limbic structures	− − −						+									,		
motor loop							−			+			−			,		

	Lactate			Citrate synthase			ATP Citrate lyase			Succinate dehydrogen.			Fumarase			Glutamate dehydrogen.		
	AD	VD	MF	AD	VD	MF	AD	VD	MF	AD	VD	MF	AD	VD	MF	AD	VD	MF
Cortex																		
undifferentiated																		
frontal	+									−			−			− − −		
parietal				−			− −											
temporal							− −											
occipital																		
limbic structures				−			− −											
motor loop	−			−			− −			+								

	Glut. DH NAD+ linked			Glutaminase			Glutathione			Glutathione transferase			SOD		
	AD	VD	MF	AD	VD	MF	AD	VD	MF	AD	VD	MF	AD	VD	MF
Cortex															
undifferentiated															
frontal	−			− − −			+			+ +					
parietal				− − −											
temporal				− − −											
occipital							+ +								
limbic structures	,						+ +			+			+		
motor loop				− − −			+			+			+		

tathione concentration in AD (37 single records) rises to 117%, 127% and 107%. Glutathione transferase activity in AD (43 single measurements) increases to 128%, 111% and 105%. Superoxide dismutase activity (SOD) in 14 AD patients (224 single records) shows an increase to 104% (LIM) and 106% (MO). No other regions were examined.

Discussion

Most data are available to characterize parameters of the cholinergic system which shows the most prominent degeneration in all types of dementias investigated. ChAT activity which is reduced in all three types of dementias shows the most striking reduction in AD, with significant deficits in all regions except the occipital cortex. Within the receptor sites, nicotinic receptors seem to be more affected by degeneration than muscarinic receptors. Precise distinction between M1 and M2 receptors shows even less prominent changes than older studies did. However, muscarinic receptor density seems to increase in dementia, due to transmitter deficits.

Within the serotonergic system, 5-HT concentrations and 5-HT receptor binding, especially 5-HT-2 receptor, are significantly reduced in all regions examined. Although 5-HIAA is generally reduced, it shows a significant increase within the motor loop. Compared to other transmitter systems there are little data available on dopaminergic receptor binding studies. Existing data show no significant changes in AD. The EAA system seems to be generally reduced. Within the peptides somatostatin shows significant reduction in cortical regions. Few data exist on second messengers. Data on oxidative stress show an overall increase in antioxidant activity and oxidative damage. Newer data, which had not been included in this study, confirm this by findings on increased thiobarbituric acid reactive substances, iron and changes in the mitochondrial electron transport system. Data on energy metabolism which only exist for AD show significant reduction.

In general, degeneration in AD seems to be more severe than in VD. For MF the number of studies must be increased. Large amounts of data existing on neurotransmitter systems, especially the cholinergic system, definitely allow further conclusions, e.g. for therapy. Data dealing with etiological hypothesis, e.g. EAA, energy metabolism, oxidative stress, calcium and NO, however, must be increased to ascertain any conclusion.

Concerning therapy, the following conclusions can be drawn and strategies can be suggested. With respect to the cholinergic system, besides the well-known AChE inhibitors, muscarinic antagonists and/or nicotinic agonists should be beneficial. For the treatment of the biogenic amine systems, inhibitors of the degradation process, like monoamine oxidase inhibitors, especially against MAO-B, will be worthy. All other neurochemical systems preclude any considerations at the moment due to insufficient number of investigations.

References

Adem A (1987) Characterization of muscarinic and nicotinic receptors in neural and non-neural tissue: changes in Alzheimer's disease. Acta Universitas Uppsaliensis: Comprehensive summaries of Uppsala Dissertations from the Faculty of Pharmacy, vol 32: 4–61

Adolfsson R, Gottfries CG, Oreland L, Wiberg A, Winblad B (1980) Increased activity of brain and platelet monoamine oxidase in dementia of Alzheimer type. Life Sci 27: 1029–1034

Allard P, Alafuzoff I, Carlsson A, Eriksson K, Ericson E, et al (1990) Loss of dopamine uptake sites labeled with ^{3H}GBR-12935 in Alzheimer's disease. Eur Neurol 30: 181–185

Antuono P, Sorbi S, Bracco L, Fusco T, Amaducci L (1980) A discrete sampling technique in senile dementia of the Alzheimer type and alcoholic dementia: study of the cholinergic system. In: Amaducci L, et al (eds) Aging of the brain and dementia. Raven Press, New York, pp 151–158

Aoyagi T, Wada T, Nagai M, Kojima F, Harada S, et al (1990) Increased gamma-aminobutyrate aminotransferase activity in brain of patients with Alzheimer's disease. Chem Pharm Bull 38: 1748–1749

Arai H, Moroji T, Kosaka K (1984) Somatostatin and vasoactive intestinal polypeptide in postmortem brains from patients with Alzheimer-type dementia. Neurosci Lett 52: 73–78

Arai H, Kobayashi K, Ichimiya Y, Kosaka K, Iizuka R (1984) A preliminary study of free amino acids in the postmortem temporal cortex from Alzheimer-type dementia patients. Neurobiol Aging 5: 319–321

Arai H, Kosaka K, Iizuka R (1984) Changes of biogenic amines and their metabolites in postmortem brains from patients with Alzheimer-type dementia. J Neurochem 43: 388–393

Arai H, Takashi M, Kosaka K, Iizuka R (1986) Extrahypophyseal distribution of alpha-melanocyte stimulating hormone (alpha-MSH)-like immunoreactivity in postmortem brains from normal subjects and Alzheimer-type dementia patients. Brain Res 377: 305–310

Araujo DM, Lapchak PA, Robitaille Y, Gauthier S, Quirion R (1988) Differential alteration of cholinergic markers in cortical and subcortical regions of human brain in Alzheimer's disease. J Neurochem 50: 1914–1923

Arregui A, Perry EK, Rossor M, Tomlinson BE (1982) Angiotensin converting enzyme in Alzheimer's disease: increased activity in caudate nucleus and cortical areas. J Neurochem 38: 1490–1492

Atack JR, Perry EK, Bonham JR, Perry RH, Tomlinson BE, et al (1983) Molecular forms of acetylcholinesterase in senile dementia of Alzheimer type: selective loss of the intermediate (10S) form. Neurosci Lett 40: 199–204

Aubert I, Araujo DM, Cecyre D, Robitaille Y, Gauthier S, et al (1992) Comparative alterations of nicotinic and muscarinic binding sites in Alzheimer's and Parkinson's disease. J Neurochem: 529–541

Baker GB, Reynolds GP (1989) Biogenic amines and their metabolites in Alzheimer's disease: noradrenaline, 5-hydroxytryptamine and 5-hydroxyindol-3-acetic acid depleted in hippocampus but not in substantia innominata. Neurosci Lett 100: 335–339

Beal MF, Mazurek M, Tran VT, Chattha G, Bird E, et al (1985) Reduced numbers of somatostatin receptors in the cerebral cortex in Alzheimer's disease. Science 229: 289–291

Beal MF, Mazurek MF, Chatta G, Bird ED, Martin JB (1985) Neuropeptide Y immunoreactivity is reduced in Alzheimer's disease cerebral cortex. Soc Neurosci Abstr 11: 1119

Beal MF, Mazurek MF, Svendsen CN, Martin JB, Chatta GK, et al (1986) Neuropeptide Y immunoreactivity is reduced in cerebral cortex in Alzheimer's disease. Ann Neurol 20: 282–288

Beal MF, Mazurek MF, Svendsen CN, Bird ED, Martin JB, et al (1986) Widespread reduction of somatostatin-like immunoreactivity in the cerebral cortex in Alzheimer's disease. Ann Neurol 20: 489–495

Beal MF, Clevens R, Chattha GK, MacGarvey UM, Mazurek MF, et al (1988) Galanin-like immunoreactivity is unchanged in Alzheimer's disease and Parkinson's disease dementia cerebral cortex. J Neurochem 51: 1935–1941

Biggins JA, Perry EK, McDermott JR, Smith AI, Perry RH, et al (1983) Post mortem levels of thyrotropin-releasing hormone and neurotensin in the amygdala in Alzheimer's disease, schizophrenia and depression. J Neurol Sci 58: 117–122

Bird TD, Stranahan S, Sumi SM, Raskind M (1983) Alzheimer's disease: choline acetyltransferase activity in brain tissue from clinical and pathological subgroups. Ann Neurol 14: 284–293

Blusztajn JK, Gonzalez-Coviella IL, Logue M, Growdon JH, Wurtman RJ (1990) Levels of phospholipid catabolic intermediates, glycerophosphocholine and glycerophosphoethanolamine, are elevated in brains of Alzheimer's disease but not of Down's syndrome patients. Brain Res 536: 240–244

Bowen DM (1981) Alzheimer's disease. In: Davison AN, Thompson RHS (eds) The molecular basis of neuropathology. Igaku-Shoin, NY Tokyo, pp 649–661

Bowen DM (1983) Biochemical assessment of neurotransmitter and metabolic dysfunction and cerebral atrophy in Alzheimer's disease. In: Biological aspects of Alzheimer's disease. Banbury Report No 15, Cold Spring Harbor Lab NY, pp 219–230

Bowen DM, Davison AN (1980) Biochemical changes in the cholinergic system of the aging brain and in senile dementia. Psychol Med 10: 315–319

Bowen DM, Allen SJ, Benton JS, Goodhardt MJ, Haan EA, et al (1983) Biochemical assessment of serotonergic and cholinergic dysfunction and cerebral atrophy in Alzheimer's disease. J Neurochem 41: 266–272

Bowen DM, Davison AN, Francis PT, Palmer AM, Pearce BR, et al (1985) Neurotransmitter and metabolic dysfunction in Alzheimer's dementia: relationship to histopathological features. Interdisc Topics Geront 19: 156–174

Bowen DM, Najlerahim A, Procter AW, Francis PT (1989) Circumscribed changes of the cerebral cortex in neuro- psychiatric disorders of later life. Proc Natl Acad Sci USA 86: 9504–9508

Burke WJ, Chung HD, Nakra BRS, Grossberg GT (1987) Phenylethanolamine N-methyl transferase activity is decreased in Alzheimer's disease brains. Ann Neurol 22: 278–280

Burke WJ, Chung HD, Strong R, Marshall GL, Davies JW, et al (1987) Phenylethanolamine N-methyltransferase in normal and Alzheimer's disease brains. In: Wood WG, Strong R (eds) Geriatric clinical pharmacology. Raven Press, New York, pp 47–69

Butterworth J, Tennant M, Yates CM (1988) Brain enzymes in agonal state and dementia. Biochem Soc Trans 17: 208–209

Candy JM, Perry RH, Perry EK, Irving D, Blessed G, et al (1983) Pathological changes in the nucleus of Meynert in Alzheimer's and Parkinson's disease. J Neurol Sci 54: 277–289

Candy JM, Gascoigne AD, Biggins JA, Smith AI, Perry RH, et al (1985) Somatostatin immunoreactivity in cortical and some subcortical regions in Alzheimer's disease. J Neurol Sci 71: 315–323

Candy JM, Perry EK, Perry RH, Court JA, Oakley AE, et al (1986) The current status of the cortical cholinergic system in Alzheimer's disease and Parkinson's disease. Progr Brain Res 70: 105–132

Carlsson A (1986) Brain neurotransmitters in normal and pathological aging. Biol Subst Alz Dis 193–203

Carlsson A (1987) Brain neurotransmitters in aging and dementia: similar changes across diagnostic dementia groups. Gerontology 33: 159–167

Carlsson A, Adolfsson R, Aquilonius S, Gottfries C, Oreland L, et al (1980) Biogenic amines in human brain in normal aging, senile dementia and chronic alcoholism. In: Goldstein M, et al (eds) Ergot compounds and brain function: neuroendocrine and neuropsychiatric aspects. Raven Press, New York, pp 295–304

Carlsson A, Gottfries CG, Svennerholm L, Adolfsson R, Oreland L, et al (1980) Neurotransmitters in human brain analyzed post mortem: changes in normal aging, senile dementia and chronic alcoholism. In: Rinne UK, Klinger M, Stamm G (eds) Parkinson's disease — current progress, problems and management. Elsevier Biomedical Press, Amsterdam, pp 121–133

Carlsson A, Gottfries CG, Eckernäs SA, Alafuzoff I, Winblad B (1988) Neurotransmitter changes in dementia: failure to demonstrate relation to histopathologic lesions or multiple infarctions. Biogen Amines 5: 199–204

Caulsfield MP, Straughan DW, Cross AJ, Crow T, Bridsall NJM (1982) Cortical muscarinic receptor subtypes and Alzheimer's disease. Lancet 4: 1277

Chu DCM, Penney JB, Young AB (1987) Cortical GABA-B and GABA-A receptors in Alzheimer's disease: a quantitative autoradiographic study. Neurology 37: 1454–1459

Clevens RA, Beal MF (1989) Substance P-like immunoreactivity in brains with pathological features of Parkinson's and Alzheimer's disease. Brain Res 486: 387–390

Cole G, Dobkins KR, Hansen LA, Terry RD, Saitoh T (1988) Decreased levels of protein kinase C in Alzheimer brain. Brain Res 452: 165–174

Cortes R, Probst A, Tobler HJ, Palacios JM (1986) Muscarinic cholinergic receptor subtypes in the human brain. II. Quantitative autoradiographic studies. Brain Res 362: 239–253

Cowburn RF, Barton AJL, Hardy JA, Wester P, Winblad B (1987) Region-specific defects in glutamate and gamma-aminobutyric acid innervation in Alzheimer's disease. Biochem Soc Trans 15: 505–506

Cowburn R, Hardy J, Roberts P, Briggs R (1988) Regional distribution of pre- and postsynatic glutamatergic function in Alzheimer's disease. Brain Res 452: 403–407

Cowburn RF, Hardy JA, Briggs RS, Roberts P (1989) Characterisation, density, and distribution of kainate receptors in normal and Alzheimer's diseased human brain. J Neurochem 52: 140–147

Cowburn RF, Fowler CJ, Garlind A, Alafuzoff I, Nilsson L, et al (1991) Somatostatin receptors and the modulation of adenylyl cyclase activity in Alzheimer's disease. J Neurol Neurosurg Psychiatry 54: 748–749

Cowburn RF, O'Neill C, Ravid R, Alafuzoff I, Winblad B, et al (1992) Adenylyl cyclase activity in postmortem human brain: evidence of altered G protein mediation in Alzheimer's disease. J Neurochem 58: 1409–1419

Crino PB, Ullman MD, Vogt BA, Bird ED, Volicer L (1989) Brain gangliosides in dementia of the Alzheimer type. Arch Neurol 46: 398–401

Cross A, Crow TJ, Perry E, Perry R, Blessed G, et al (1981) Reduced dopamine-beta-hydroxylase activity in Alzheimer's disease. Br Med J 282: 93–94

Cross AJ, Crow TJ, Johnson JA, Joseph MH, Perry EK, et al (1983) Monoamine metabolism in senile dementia of Alzheimer type. J Neurol Sci 60: 383–392

Cross A, Crow TJ, Johnson JA, Perry EK, Perry RH, et al (1984) Studies on neurotransmitter receptor systems in neocortex and hippocampus in senile dementia of the Alzheimer-type. J Neurol Sci 64: 109–117

Cross AJ, Ferrier IN, Crow TJ, Johnson JA, Markakis D (1984) Striatal dopamine receptors in Alzheimer-type dementia. Neurosci Lett 52: 1–6

Cross AJ, Crow TJ, Ferrier IN, Johnson JA, Bloom SR, et al (1984) Serotonin receptor changes in dementia of the Alzheimer type. J Neurochem 43: 1574–1581

Cross AJ, Crow TJ, Ferrier IN, Johnson JA (1986) The selectivity of the reduction of serotonin S2 receptors in Alzheimer-type dementia. Neurobiol Aging 7: 3–7

Cross AJ, Slater P, Simpson M, Royston C, Deakin JFW, et al (1987) Sodium dependent D-3H-aspartate binding in cerebral cortex in patients with Alzheimer's and Parkinson's disease. Neurosci Lett 79: 213–217

Cross AJ, Slater P, Candy JM, Perry EK, Perry RH (1987) Glutamate deficits in Alzheimer's disease. J Neurol Neurosurg Psychiatry 50: 357–358

Crow TJ, Cross AJ, Cooper SJ, Deakin JFW, Ferrier IN, et al (1984) Neurotransmitter receptors and monoamine metabolites in the brains of patients with Alzheimer-type dementia and depression, and suicides. Neuropharmacology 23: 1561–1569

Crystal HA, Davies P (1982) Cortical substance P-like immunoreactivity in cases of Alzheimer's disease and senile dementia of the Alzheimer type. J Neurochem 38: 1781–1784

D'Amato RJ, Zweig RM, Whitehouse RJ, Wenk GL, Singer HS, et al (1987) Aminergic systems in Alzheimer's disease and Parkinson's disease. Ann Neurol 22: 229–236

Danielsson E, Eckernäs SA, Westlind-Danielsson A, Nordström ò, Bartfai T, et al (1986) VIP-sensitive adenylate cyclase, guanylate cyclase, muscarinic receptors, choline acetylteransferase and acetylcholinesterase, in brain tissue afflicted by Alzheimer's disease/SDAT. In: Muscarinic receptors and cGMP synthesis: studies on human and rat tissue. Thesis, Stockholm Universitet, Sweden

Danielsson E, Eckernäs SA, Westlind-Danielsson A, Nordström ò, Bartfai T, et al (1988) VIP-sensitive adenylate cyclase, guanylate cyclase, muscarinic receptors, choline acetyltransferase and acetylcholinesterase, in brain tissue afflicted by Alzheimer's disease/SDAT. Neurobiol Aging 9: 153–162

Davies P, Terry R (1981) Cortical Somatostatin-Like immunoreactivity in cases of Alzheimer's disease and senile dementia of the Alzheimer type. Neurobiol Aging 2: 9–14

Davies P, Katzman R, Terry RD (1980) Reduced somatostatin-like immunoreactivity in cerebral cortex from cases of Alzheimer disease and Alzheimer senile dementia. Nature 288: 279–280

Davies P, Katz DA, Crystal HA (1982) Choline acetyltransferase, somatostatin, and substance P in selected cases of Alzheimer's disease. In: Corkin S, et al (eds) Alzheimer's disease: a report of progress. Raven Press, New York, pp 9–14

Dawbarn D, Rossor MN, Mountjoy CQ, Roth M, Emson PC (1986) Decreased somatostatin immunoreactivity but not neuropeptide Y immunoreactivity in cerebral cortex in senile dementia of Alzheimer type. Neurosci Lett 70: 154–159

Dewar D, Horsburgh K, Graham DI, Brooks DN, McCulloch J (1990) Selective alterations of high affinity 3H-forskolin binding sites in Alzheimer's disease: a quantitative autoradiographic study. Brain Res 511: 241–248

Dziedzic JD, Wisniewski HM, Iqbal K (1981) Monoamine oxidase activity in normal and Alzheimer brains. Ann Neurol 9: 618–619

Ebinger G, Bruyland M, Martin JJ, Herregodts P, Cras P, et al (1987) Distribution of biogenic amines and their catabolites in brains from patients with Alzheimer's disease. J Neurol Sci 77: 267–283

Ellison DW, Beal MF, Mazurek MF, Bird ED, Martin JB, et al (1986) A postmortem study of amino acid neurotransmitters in Alzheimer's disease. Ann Neurol 20: 616–621

Ellison DW, Beal MF, Martin JB (1987) Phosphoethanolamin and ethanolamin are decreased in Alzheimer's disease and Huntington's disease. Brain Res 417: 389–392

Etienne P, Robitaille Y, Wood P, Gauthier S, Nair NPV, et al (1986) Nucleus basalis neuronal loss, neuritic plaques and choline acetyltransferase activity in advanced Alzheimer's disease. Neuroscience 19: 1279–1291

Farooqui AA, Liss L, Horrocks LA (1989) Lipolytic enzyme activities in different brain regions in Alzheimer's disease. In: Bazan NG, Horrocks LA, Toffano G (eds) Phospholipids in the nervous system: biochemical and molecular pathology. Liviana Press, Padova (Fidia Research Series, vol 17)

Ferrier IN, Cross AJ, Johnson JA, Roberts GW, Crow TJ, et al (1983) Neuropeptides in Alzheimer type dementia. J Neurol Sci 62: 159–170

Fishman EB, Siek GC, MacCallum RD, Bird ED, Volicer L, et al (1986) Distribution of the molecular forms of acetylcholinesterase in human brain: alterations in dementia of the Alzheimer type. Ann Neurol 19: 246–252

Flynn DD, Mash DC (1986) Characterization of L-³H-nicotine binding in human cerebral cortex: comparison between Alzheimer's disease and the normal. J Neurochem 47: 1948–1954

Foster NL, Tamminga CA, O'Donohue TL, Tanimoto K, Bird ED, et al (1986) Brain choline acetyltransferase activity and neuropeptide Y concentrations in Alzheimer's disease. Neurosci Lett 63: 71–75

Fowler CJ, Wiberg A, Oreland L, Marcusson J, Winblad B (1980) The effect of age on the activity and molecular properties of human brain monoamine oxidase. J Neural Transm 49: 1–20

Francis PT, Palmer AM, Sims NR, Bowen DM, Davison AN, et al (1985) Neurochemical studies of early-onset Alzheimer's disease. Possible influence on treatment. N Engl J Med 313: 7–11

Fujiyoshi K, Suga H, Okamoto K, Nakamura S, Kameyama M (1987) Reduction of arginin-vasopressin in the cerebral cortex in Alzheimer type senile dementia. J Neurol Neurosurg Psychiatry 50: 929–932

Geddes JW, Chang-Chui H, Cooper SM, Lott IT, Cotman CW (1986) Density and distribution of NMDA receptors in the human hippocampus in Alzheimer's disease. Brain Res 399: 156–161

Geola FL, Yamada T, Warwick RJ, Tourtelotte WW, Hershman JM (1981) Regional distribution of somatostatin-like immunoreactivity in the human brain. Brain Res 229: 35–42

Giacobini E, DeSarno P, McIlhany M, Clark B (1988) The cholinergic receptor system in the frontal lobe of Alzheimer patients. In: Clementi F, Gotti C (eds) Nicotinic acetylcholine receptors in the nervous system. Springer, Berlin Heidelberg New York Tokyo, pp 367–378

Gilbert JJ, Kish SJ, Chang LJ, Morito C, Shannak K, et al (1988) Dementia, parkinsonism, and motor neuron disease: neurochemical and neuropathological correlates. Ann Neurol 24: 688–691

Gottfries CG (1980) Amine metabolism in normal aging and in dementia disorders. In: Roberts PJ (ed) Biochemistry of dementia. Wiley and Sons, Chichester, pp 213–234

Gottfries CG, Adolfsson R, Aquilonius SM, Carlsson A, Eckernäs SA, et al (1983) Biochemical changes in dementia disorders of Alzheimer type (AD/SDAT). Neurobiol Aging 4: 261–271

Gottfries CG, Bartfai T, Carlsson A, Eckernäs S, Svennerholm L (1986) Multiple biochemical deficits in gray and white matter of Alzheimer brains. Prog Neuropsychopharmacol Biol Psychiatry 10: 405–413

Gramsbergen JBP, Mountjoy CQ, Rossor MN, Reynolds GP, Roth M, et al (1987) A correlative study on hippocampal cation shifts and amino acids and clinicopathological data in Alzheimer's disease. Neurobiol Aging 8: 487–494

Greenamyre JT, Penney JB, Young AB, D'Amato CJ, Hicks SP (1985) Alterations in L-glutamate binding in Alzheimer's and Huntington's disease. Science 227: 1496–1499

Greenamyre JT, Penney JB, D'Amato CJ, Young AB (1987) Dementia of the Alzheimer's type: changes in hippocampal L-³H-glutamate binding. J Neurochem 48: 543–551

Gulya K, Watson M, Vickroy TW, Roeske WR, Perry R, et al (1986) Examination of cholinergic and neuropeptide receptor alterations in senile dementia of the Alzheimer's type (SDAT). In: Alzheimer's and Parkinson's disease. Strategies for research and development, vol 29. Plenum Press, New York, pp 109–116

Hammond P, Brimijoin S (1988) Acetylcholinesterase in Huntington's and Alzheimer's diseases: simultaneous enzyme assay and immunoassay of multiple brain regions. J Neurochem 50: 1111–1116

Hansen LA, De Teresa R, Davies P, Terry R (1988) Neocortical morphometry, lesion counts, and choline acetyltransferase levels in the age spectrum of Alzheimer's disease. Neurology 38: 48–54

Hardy J, Cowburn R, Barton A, Reynolds G, Lofdahl E, et al (1986) Glutamate deficits in Alzheimer's disease. J Neurol Neurosurg Psychiatry 50: 356–357

Hardy J, Cowburn R, Barton A, Reynolds G, Lofdahl E, et al (1987) Region-specific loss of glutamate innervation in Alzheimer's disease. Neurosci Lett 73: 77–80

Hays S, Paul SM (1982) CCK receptors and human neurological disease. Life Sci 31: 319–322

Herregodts P, Bruyland M, Keyser J, Solheid C, Michotte Y, et al (1989) Monoaminergic neurotransmitters in Alzheimer's disease. J Neurol Sci 92: 101–116

Horoupian DS, Thal L, Katzmann R, Terry RD, Davies P, et al (1984) Dementia and motor neuron disease: morphometric, biochemical, and Golgi studies. Ann Neurol 16: 305–313

Hyman BT, Van Hoesen GW, Damasio AR (1987) Alzheimer's disease: glutamate depletion in the hippocampal perforant pathway zone. Ann Neurol 22: 37–40

Ichimiya Y, Arai H, Kosaka K, Iizuka R (1986) Morphological and biochemical changes in the cholinergic and monoaminergic systems in Alzheimer-type dementia. Acta Neuropathol 70: 112–116

Iimoto DS, Masliah E, DeTeresa R, Terry R, Saitoh T (1989) Aberrant casein kinase II in Alzheimer's disease. Brain Res 507: 273–280

Inada M, Toyoshima M, Kameyama M (1982) Cobalamin contents of the brain in some clinical and pathological states. Int J Vit Nutr Res 52: 423–429

Iversen LL, Rossor MN, Reynolds GP, Hills R, Roth M, et al (1983) Loss of pigmented dopamine-β-hydroxylase positive cells from locus coeruleus in senile dementia of Alzheimer's type. Neurosci Lett 39: 95–100

Iwamoto N, Kobayashi K, Kosaka K (1989) The formation of prostaglandins in the postmortem cerebral cortex of Alzheimer-type dementia patients. J Neurol 236: 80–84

Jagust W, Davies P, Tiller-Borcich J, Reed B (1990) Focal Alzheimer's disease. Neurology 40: 14–19

Jansen KLR, Faull RLM, Dragunow M, Synek BL (1990) Alzheimer's disease: changes in hippocampal N-methyl-D-aspartate, quisqualate, neurotensin, adenosin, benzodiazepin, serotonin and opioid receptors in an autoradiographic study. Neuroscience 39: 613–627

Jellinger K, Riederer P (1984) Dementia in Parkinson's disease and (pre) senile dementia of Alzheimer type: morphological aspects and changes in the intracerebral MAO activity. Adv Neurol 40: 199–210

Jenni-Eiermann S, Hahn von HP, Honegger CG, Ulrich J (1984) Studies on neurotransmitter binding in senile dementia. Gerontol 30: 350–358

Kalaria RN, Andorn AC, Tabaton M, Whitehouse PJ, Harik SI, et al (1989) Adrenergic receptors in aging and Alzheimer's disease: increased a2-receptors in prefrontal cortex and hippocampus. J Neurochem 53: 1772–1781

Kanazawa I, Kwak S, Sasaki H, Muramoto O, Mitzutani T, et al (1988) Studies on neurotransmitter markers of the basal ganglia in Pick's disease, with special references to dopamine reduction. J Neurol Sci 83: 63–74

Kanfer JN, McCartney DG (1986) Reduced phosphorylcholine hydrolysis by homogenates of temporal regions of Alzheimer's brain. Biochem Biophys Res Comm 139: 315–319

Kanfer JN, Pettegrew JW, Moossy J, McCartney DG (1993) Alterations of selected enzymes of phospholipid metabolism in Alzheimer's disease brain tissue as compared to Non-Alzheimer's demented controls. Neurochem Res 18: 331–334

Katzman R, Terry R, DeTeresa R, Brown T, Davies P, et al (1988) Clinical, pathological, and neurochemical changes in dementia: a subgroup with preserved mental status and numerous neocortical plaques. Ann Neurol 23: 138–144

Kellar KJ, Whitehouse PJ, Martino-Barrows AM, Marcus K, Price DL (1987) Muscarinic and nicotinic cholinergic binding sites in Alzheimer's disease cerebral cortex. Brain Res 436: 62–68

Kerwin JM, Morris CM, Perry RH, Perry EK (1992) Hippocampal nerve growth factor receptor immunoreactivity in patients with Alzheimer's and Parkinson's disease. Neurosci Lett 143: 101–104

Kish SJ, Robitaille Y, EI-Awar M, Deck JHN, Simmons J, et al (1989) Non-Alzheimer-type pattern of brain cholineacetyltransferase reduction in dominantly inherited olivopontocerebellar atrophy. Ann Neurol 26: 362–367

Kosaka K, Iizuka R, Mizutani Y, Kondo T, Nagatsu T (1981) Striatonigral degeneration combined with Alzheimer's disease. Acta Neuropathol 54: 253–256

Koshimura K, Kato T, Tohyama I, Nakamura S, Kameyama M (1986) Qualitative abnormalities of choline acetyltransferase in Alzheimer type dementia. J Neurol Sci 76: 143–150

Krantic S, Robitaille Y, Quirion R (1992) Deficits in the somatostatin SS1 receptor subtype in frontal and temporal cortices in Alzheimer's disease. Brain Res 573: 299–304

Lang W, Henke H (1983) Cholinergic receptor binding and autoradiography in brains of non-neurological and senile dementia of Alzheimer-type patients. Brain Res 267: 271–280

Leake A, Perry EK, Perry RH, Fairbairn AF, Ferrier IN (1990) Cortical concentrations of corticotropin-releasing hormone and its receptor in Alzheimer type dementia and major depression. Biol Psychiatry 28: 603–608

Leake A, Perry EK, Perry R, Jabeen S, Fairbairn AF, et al (1991) Neocortical concentrations of neuropeptides in senile dementia of the Alzheimer and Lewy Body Type: comparison with Parkinson's disease and severity correlations. Biol Psychiatry 29: 357–364

Lemmer B, Langer L, Ohm T, Bohl J (1993) Beta-adrenoceptor density and subtype distribution in cerebellum and hippocampus from patients with Alzheimer's disease. Naunyn Schmiedebergs Arch Pharmacol 347: 214–219

London ED, Ball MJ, Waller SB (1989) Nicotinic binding sites in cerebral cortex and hippocampus in Alzheimer's dementia. Neurochem Res 14: 745–750

Lowe SL, Francis PT, Procter AW, Palmer AM, Davison AN, et al (1988) Gamma-aminobutyric acid concentration in brain tissue at two stages of Alzheimer's disease. Brain 111: 785–799

Mann DMA, Lincoln J, Yates PO, Stamp JE, Toper S (1980) Changes in the monoamine containing neurones of the human CNS in senile dementia. Br J Psychiatry 136: 533–541

Mann DMA, Yates PO, Hawkes J (1982) The noradrenergic system in Alzheimer and multiinfarct dementias. J Neurol 45: 113–119

Mantle D, Lauffart B, Perry EK, Perry RH (1989) Comparison of major cortical aminopeptidase activity in normal brain and brain from patients with Alzheimer's disease. J Neurol Sci 89: 227–234

Marcusson JO, Alafuzoff I, Bäckström IT, Ericson E, Gottfries CG, et al (1987) 5-Hydroxytryptamine-sensitive ^{3}H-imipramine binding of protein nature in the human brain. II. Effect of normal aging and dementia disorders. Brain Res 425: 137–145

Marklund SL, Adolfsson R, Gottfries CG, Winblad B (1985) Superoxid dismutase isoenzymes in normal brains and in brains from patients with dementia of Alzheimer type. J Neurol Sci 67: 319–325

Mazurek MF, Beal MF, Bird ED, Martin JB (1986) Vasopressin in Alzheimer's disease: a study of postmortem brain concentrations. Ann Neurol 20: 665–670

Mazurek M, Beal MF, Bird E, Martin J (1987) Oxytocin in Alzheimer's disease: postmortem brain levels. Neurology 3: 1001–1003

McGeer EG, Singh E, McGeer PL (1987) Sodium-dependent glutamate binding in senile dementia. Neurobiol Aging: 219–223

McGeer EG, Singh EA, McGeer PL (1987) Gamma-glutamyltransferase: normal cortical levels in Alzheimer disease. Alzheimer Dis Assoc Disord 1: 38–42

McGeer PL, Itagaki S, Boyes BE, McGeer EG (1988) Reactive microglia are positive for HLA-DR in the substantia nigra of Parkinson's and Alzheimer's disease brains. Neurology 38: 1285–1291

McGeer E, Singh EA, McGeer P (1988) Peripheral-type benzodiazepine binding in Alzheimer disease. Alzheimer Dis Assoc Disord 2: 331–336

Meana JJ, Barturen F, Garro MA, Garcia-Sevilla JA (1992) Decreased density of presynaptic alpha-2-adrenoceptors in postmortem brains of patients with Alzheimer's disease. J Neurochem 58: 1896–1904

Middlemiss DN, Palmer AM, Edel N, Bowen DM (1986) Binding of the novel serotonin agonist 8-hydroxy-2-(di-n-propylamino) tetralin in normal and Alzheimer brain. J Neurochem 46: 993–996

Moroni F, Lombardi G, Robitaille Y, Etienne P (1986) Senile dementia and Alzheimer's disease: lack of changes of the cortical content of quinolinic acid. Neurobiol Aging 7: 249–253

Mouradian MM, Contreras PC, Monahan JB, Chase TN (1988) ^{3}H-MK-801 binding in Alzheimer's disease. Neurosci Lett 93: 225–230

Nazarali AJ, Reynolds GP (1992) Monoamine neurotransmitters and their metabolites in brain regions in Alzheimer's disease: a postmortem study. Cell Mol Neurobiol 12: 581–587

Nemeroff CB, Kizer JS, Reynolds GP, Bissette G (1989) Neuropeptides in Alzheimer's disease: a postmortem study. Regul Pept 25: 123–130

Nordberg A, Winblad B (1981) Cholinergic receptors in human hippocampus — regional distribution and variance with age. Life Sci 29: 1937–1944

Nordberg A, Winblad B (1986) Brain nicotinic and muscarinic receptors in normal aging and dementia. In: Winblad B (ed) Alzheimer's and Parkinson's disease. Strategies for research and development, vol 29. Plenum Press, New York, pp 95–108

Nordberg A, Winblad B (1986) Reduced number of ^{3}H-nicotine and ^{3}H-acetylcholine binding sites in the frontal cortex of Alzheimer brains. Neurosci Lett 72: 115–119

Nordberg A, Adolfsson R, Marcusson J, Winblad B (1982) Cholinergic receptors in the hippocampus in normal aging and dementia of Alzheimer type. In: Giacobini E, et al (ed) The aging brain: cellular and molecular mechanisms of aging in the nervous system. Raven Press, New York, pp 231–245

Nordberg A, Larsson C, Adolfsson R, Alafuzoff I, Winblad B (1983) Muscarinic receptor compensation in hippocampus of Alzheimer patients. J Neural Transm 56: 13–19

Nordberg A, Alafuzoff I, Winblad B (1986) Muscarinic receptor subtypes in hippocampus in Alzheimer's disease and mixed dementia type. Neurosci Lett 70: 160–164

Nordberg A, Adem A, Hardy J, Winblad B (1988) Change in nicotinic receptor subtypes in temporal cortex of Alzheimer brains. Neurosci Lett 86: 317–321

Nordberg A, Alafuzoff I, Winblad B (1992) Nicotinic and muscarinic subtypes in the human brain: changes with aging and dementia. J Neurosci Res 31: 103–111

Nyberg P, Adolfsson R, Hardy JA, Nordberg A, Wester P, et al (1985) Catecholamine topochemistry in human basal ganglia. Comparison between normal and Alzheimer brains. Brain Res 333: 139–142

O'Neill C, Fowler CJ, Winblad B (1989) Alpha 1-adrenergic receptor binding sites in post-mortal human cerebral microvessel preparations: preservation in multi-infarct dementia and dementia of Alzheimer type. J Neural Transm [P-DSect] 1: 303–310

Ogane N, Giacobini E, Struble R (1992) Differential inhibition of acetylcholinesterase molecular forms in normal and Alzheimer disease brain. Brain Res 589: 307–312

Ohm T, Bohl J, Lemmer B (1989) Reduced cAMP-signal transduction in postmortem hippocampus of demented old people. Alzheimer Dis Related Disord 0: 501–509

Ohm TG, Bohl J, Lemmer B (1991) Reduced basal and stimulated (isoprenaline, Gpp(NH)p, forskolin) adenylate cyclase activity in Alzheimer's disease correlated with histopathological changes. Brain Res 540: 229–236

Oreland L, Gottfries CG (1986) Brain and brain monoamine oxidase in aging and in dementia of Alzheimer's type. Prog Neuropsychopharmacol Biol Psychiatry 10: 533–540

Oreland L, Adolfsson R, Fowler CJ, Gottfries CG, Wiberg A, et al (1981) Increased activity of monoamine oxidase in dementia of Alzheimer type. In: Perris C, Struwe G, Jansson B (eds) Biological psychiatry. Elsevier/North Holland Biochemical Press, Amsterdam, pp 973–976

Palmer AM, Bowen DM (1984) 5-Hydroxyindoleacetic acid and homovanillic acid in the cerebrospinal fluid and caudate nucleus of histologically verified examples of Alzheimer's disease. Biochem Soc Trans 13: 167–168

Palmer AM, Francis PT, Bowen DM (1986) The stability of 5-hydroxyindolacetic acid and noradrenaline in normal and Alzheimer postmortem brain. Biochem Soc Trans 14: 608–6090

Palmer AM, Procter AW, Stratmann GC, Bowen DM (1986) Excitatory amino acid-releasing and cholinergic neurones in Alzheimer's disease. Neurosci Lett 66: 199–204

Palmer AM, Wilcock GK, Esiri MM, Francis PT, Bowen DM (1987) Monoaminergic innervation of the frontal and temporal lobes in Alzheimer's disease. Brain Res 401: 231–238

Parks KM, Sugar JE, Haroutunian V, Bierer L, Perl D, et al (1991) Reduced in vitro phosphorylation of synapsin I (site 1) in Alzheimer's disease postmortem tissues. Mol Brain Res 9: 125–134

Pearce BR, Bowen DM (1984) ^{3}H-Kainic acid binding and choline acetyltransferase activity in Alzheimer's dementia. Brain Res 310: 376–378

Pearce BR, Palmer AM, Bowen DM, Wilcock GK, Esiri MM, et al (1984) Neurotransmitter dysfunction and atrophy of the caudate nucleus in Alzheimer's disease. Neurochem Pathol 2: 221–232

Perdahl E, Adolfsson R, Alafuzoff I, Albert KA, Nestler EJ, et al (1984) Synapsin I (Protein I) in different brain regions in senile dementia of Alzheimer type and in multiinfarct dementia. J Neural Transm 60: 133–141

Perry E, Perry R (1980) The cholinergic system in Alzheimer's disease. Biochem Dementia 0: 135–183

Perry E, Perry R, Tomlinson BE, Blessed G, Gibson P (1980) Coenzyme A-acetylating enzymes in Alzheimer's disease: possible cholinergic compartment of pyruvate dehydrogenase. Neurosci Lett 18: 105–110

Perry E, Tomlinson BE, Blessed G, Perry RH, Cross AJ, et al (1981) Noradrenergic and cholinergic systems in senile dementia of Alzheimer type. Lancet: 149

Perry E, Marshall E, Perry R, Irving D, Smith CJ, et al (1990) Cholinergic and dopaminergic activities in senile dementia of Lewy Body Type. Alzheimer Dis Assoc Disord 4: 87–95

Perry E, Marshall E, Kerwin J, Smith C, Jabeen S, et al (1990) Evidence of a monoaminergic-cholinergic imbalance related to visual hallucinations in Lewy Body Dementia. J Neurochem 55: 1454–1456

Perry E, Irving D, Perry RH (1991) Cholinergic controversies. Letters to the editor. Trends Neurosci 14: 483

Perry EK, Blessed G, Tomlinson BE, Perry RH, Crow TJ, et al (1981) Neurochemical activities in human temporal lobe related to aging and Alzheimer-type changes. Neurobiol Aging 2: 251–256

Perry EK, Tomlinson BE, Blessed G, Perry RH, Cross AJ, et al (1981) Neuropathological and biochemical observations on the noradrenergic system in Alzheimer's disease. J Neurol Sci 51: 279–287

Perry EK, Perry RH, Candy JM, Fairbairn AF, Blessed G, et al (1984) Cortical serotonin-

S2 receptor binding abnormalities in patients with Alzheimer's disease: comparisons with Parkinson's disease. Neurosci Lett 51: 353–357

Perry EK, Perry RH, Smith CJ, Dick DJ, Candy JM, et al (1987) Nicotinic receptor abnormalities in Alzheimer's and Parkinson's diseases. J Neurol Neurosurg Psychiatry 50: 806–809

Perry EK, Smith CJ, Court JA, Perry RH (1990) Cholinergic nicotinic and muscarinic receptors in dementia of Alzheimer, Parkinson and Lewy body types. J Neural Transm [PD-Sect] 2: 149–158

Perry RH, Dockray GJ, Dimaline R, Perry EK, Blessed G, et al (1981) Neuropeptides in Alzheimer's disease, depression and schizophrenia. J Neurol Sci 51: 465–472

Perry TL, Yong VW, Bergeron C, Hansen S, Jones K (1987) Amino acids, glutathione, and glutathione transferase activity in the brains of patients with Alzheimer's disease. Ann Neurol 21: 331–336

Procter AW, Palmer AM, Bowen DM, Murphy E, Neary D (1987) Glutamatergic denervation in Alzheimer's disease — A cautionary note. J Neurol Neurosurg Psychiatry 50: 825

Procter AW, Lowe SL, Palmer AM, Francis PT, Esiri M, et al (1988) Topographical distribution of neurochemical changes in Alzheimer's disease. J Neurol Sci 84: 125–140

Procter AW, Palmer AM, Francis PT, Lowe SL, Neary D, et al (1988) Evidence of glutamatergic denervation and possible abnormal metabolism in Alzheimer's disease. J Neurochem 50: 790–802

Procter AW, Stirling JM, Stratmann GC, Cross AJ, Bowen DM (1989) Loss of glycine-dependent radioligand binding to the N-methyl-#NAME? Alzheimer's disease. Neurosci Lett 10: 62–66

Procter AW, Wong EHF, Stratmann GC, Lowe SL, Bowen DM (1989) Reduced glycine stimulation of (^{3}H)-MK-801 binding in Alzheimer's disease. J Neurochem 53: 698–704

Quirion R, Martel JC, Robitaille Y, Etienne P (1986) Neurotransmitter and receptor deficits in senile dementia of the Alzheimer type. Can J Neurol Sci 13: 503–510

Quirion R, Aubert I, Lapchak P, Schaum R, Teolis S, et al (1989) Muscarinic receptor subtypes in human neurodegenerative disorders: focus on Alzheimer's disease. Trends Pharmacol Sci 0: 80–84

Reinikainen KJ, Riekkinen PJ, Jolkkonen J, Kosma VM, Soininen H (1987) Decreased somatostatin-like immunoreactivity in cerebral cortex and cerebrospinal fluid in Alzheimer's disease. Brain Res 402: 103–108

Reinikainen KJ, Riekkinen PJ, Halonen T, Laakso M (1987) Decreased muscarinic receptor binding in cerebral cortex and hippocampus in Alzheimer's disease. Life Sci 41: 453–461

Reinikainen KJ, Paljärvi L, Halonen T, Malminen O, Kosma VM, et al (1988) Dopaminergic system and monoamine oxidase-B activity in Alzheimer's disease. Neurobiol Aging 9: 245–252

Reinikainen KJ, Riekkinen PJ, Paljärvi L, Soininen H, Hekala EL, et al (1988) Cholinergic deficit in Alzheimer's disease: a study based on CSF and autopsy data. Neurochem Res 13: 135–146

Reinikainen KJ, Paljärvi L, Huuskonen M, Soininen H, Laakso M, et al (1988) A postmortem study of noradrenergic, serotonergic and GABAergic neurons in Alzheimer's disease. J Neurol Sci 84: 101–116

Reisine TD, Pedigo NW, Meiners B, Iqbal K, Yamamura HI (1980) Alzheimer's disease: studies on neurochemical alterations in the brain. In: Amaducci L, et al (eds) Aging of the brain and dementia. Raven Press, New York, pp 147–150

Reynolds GP, Arnold L, Rossor MN, Iversen LL, Mountjoy CQ, et al (1983) Reduced binding of (^{3}H) Ketaserin to 5-HT$_2$ receptors in senile dementia of the Alzheimer type. Neurosci Lett 44: 47–51

Richter J, Perry E, Tomlinson B (1980) Acetylcholine and choline levels in postmortem human brain tissue: preliminary observations in Alzheimer's disease. Life Sci 26: 1683–1689

Riederer P, Jellinger K (1982) Morphological and biochemical changes in the aging brain: pathophysiological and possible therapeutic consequences. Exp Brain Res [Suppl] 5: 158–166

Riekkinen PJ, Soininen H, Sirviö J, Reinikainen K, Helkala EL, et al (1987) Dementia without cholinergic deficit. Gerontol 33: 268–272

Rinne JO (1987) Muscarinic and dopaminergic receptors in the aging human brain. Brain Res 404: 162–168

Rinne JO, Rinne JK, Laakso K, Paljärvi L, Rinne UK (1984) Reduction in muscarinic receptor binding in limbic areas of Alzheimer brain. J Neurol Neurosurg Psychiatry 47: 651–653

Rinne JO, Laakso K, Lönnberg P, Mölsö P, Paljörvi L, et al (1985) Brain muscarinic receptors in senile dementia. Brain Res 336: 19–25

Rinne JO, Säkö E, Paljärvi L, Mölsö PK, Rinne UK (1986) Brain dopamine D-2 receptor in senile dementia. J Neural Transm 65: 51–62

Rinne JO, Säkö E, Paljärvi L, Mölsö PK, Rinne UK (1986) Brain dopamine D-1 receptors in senile dementia. J Neurol Sci 73: 219–230

Rinne JO, Säkö E, Paljärvi L, Mölsö PK, Rinne UK (1987) A comparison of brain choline acetyltransferase activity in Alzheimer's disease, multiinfarct dementia, and combined dementia. J Neural Transm 73: 121–128

Rinne JO, Lönneberg P, Marjamäki P, Rinne UK (1989) Brain muscarinic receptor subtypes are differently affected in Alzheimer's disease and Parkinson's disease. Brain Res 483: 402–406

Rinne JO, Myllykylä T, Lönnberg P, Marjamäki P (1991) A postmortem study of brain nicotinic receptors in Parkinson's and Alzheimer's disease. Brain Res 547: 167–170

Rossor MN, Emson PC, Mountjoy CQ, Roth M, Iversen LL (1980) Reduced amounts of immunoreactive somatostatin in the temporal cortex in senile dementia of Alzheimer type. Neurosci Lett 20: 373–377

Rossor M, Fahrenkrug J, Emson P, Mountjoy C, Iverson L, et al (1980) Reduced cortical choline acetyltransferase activity in senile dementia of Alzheimer type is not accompanied by change in vasoactive intestinal polypeptide. Brain Res 201: 249–253

Rossor MN, Iversen LL, Mountjoy CQ, Roth M, et al (1980) Arginine vasopressin and choline acetyltransferase in brains of patients with Alzheimer type senile dementia. Lancet: 1367–1368

Rossor MN, Rehfeld JF, Emson PC, Mountjoy CQ, Roth M, et al (1981) Normal cortical concentration of cholecystokinin-like immunoreactivity with reduced choline acetyltransferase activity in senile dementia of Alzheimer type. Life Sci 29: 405–410

Rossor MN, Svendsen C, Hunt SP, Mountjoy CQ, Roth M, et al (1982) The substantia innominata in Alzheimer's disease: an histochemical and biochemical study of cholineregic marker enzymes. Neurosci Lett 28: 217–222

Rossor MN, Emson PC, Mountjoy CQ, Roth M, Iversen LL (1982) Neurotransmitters of the cerebral cortex in senile dementia of Alzheimer type. Exp Brain Res 5: 153–157

Rossor MN, Garrett NJ, Johnson AL, Mountjoy CQ, Roth M, et al (1982) A postmortem study of the cholinergic and GABA systems in senile dementia. Brain 105: 313–330

Rossor MN, Emson PC, Iversen LL, Mountjoy CQ, Roth M, et al (1982) Neuropeptides and neurotransmitters in cerebral cortex in Alzheimer's disease. In: Corkin S, et al (eds) Alzheimer's disease: a report of progress. Raven Press, New York, pp 15–24 (Aging, vol 19)

Rossor MN, Iversen LL, Reynolds GP, Mountjoy CQ, Roth M (1984) Neurochemical characteristics of early and late onset types of Alzheimer's disease. Br Med J 288: 961–964

Rossor MN, Emson PC, Iversen LL (1984) Patterns of neuropeptide deficits in Alzheimer's disease. In: Wurtman RJ (ed) Alzheimer's disease: advances in basic research and therapies. Raven Press, New York, pp 29–38

Rylett RJ, Ball MJ, Colhoun EH (1983) Evidence for high affinity transport in synaptosomes prepared from hippocampus and neocortex of patients with Alzheimer's disease. Brain Res 289: 169–175

Sakurada T, Alafuzoff I, Winblad B, Nordberg A (1990) Substance P-like immunoractivity, choline acetyltransferase activity and cholinergic muscarinic receptors in Alzheimer's disease and multi-infarct dementia. Brain Res 521: 329–332

Sanders DJ, Zahedi-Asl S, Marr AP (1982) Glucagon and CCK in human brain: controls and patients with senile dementia of Alzheimer type. Prog Brain Res 55: 465–471

Sasaki H, Muramoto O, Kanazawa I, Arai H (1986) Regional distribution of amino acid transmitters in postmortem brains of presenile and senile dementia of Alzheimer type. Ann Neurol 19: 263–269

Sawada M, Hirata Y, Arai H, Iizuka R, Nagatsu T (1987) Tyrosine hydroxylase, trytophan hydroxylase, biopterin, and neopterin in brains of normal controls and patients with senile dementia of the Alzheimer type. J Neurochem 4: 760–764

Schegg K, Nielsen S, Zweig R, Peacock J (1989) Decrease in membrane-bound G4 form of acetylcholinesterase in postmortem Alzheimer brain. In: Alzheimer's disease and related disorders. Alan R Liss, New York, pp 437–452

Schotte A, Maloteaux JM, Laduron PM (1983) Characterization and regional distribution of serotonin S2 receptors in human brain. Brain Res 276: 231–235

Schwarcz R, Whetsell WO (1982) Post-mortem high affinity glutamate uptake in human brain. Neuroscience 7: 1771–1778

Severson JA, Marcusson J, Winblad B, Finch CE (1982) Age-related loss of dopaminergic binding sites in human basal ganglia. J Neurosci 39: 1623–1631

Sherif F, Gottfries CG, Alafuzoff I, Oreland L (1992) Brain gamma-aminobutyrate aminotransferase (GABA-T) and monoamine oxidase (MAO) in patients with Alzheimer's disease. J Neural Transm [PD-Sect] 4: 227–240

Sheu KFR, Kim YT, Blass JP, Weksler ME (1985) An immunochemical study of the pyruvate dehydrogenase deficit in Alzheimer's disease brain. Ann Neurol 17: 444–449

Shimohama S, Taniguchi T, Fujiwara M, Kameyama M (1986) Biochemical characterization of alpha-adrenergic receptors in human brain and changes in Alzheimer-type dementia. J Neurochem 47: 1294–1301

Shimohama S, Taniguchi T, Fujiwara M, Kameyama M (1986) Changes in nicotinic and muscarinic cholinergic receptors in Alzheimer-type dementia. J Neurochem 46: 288–293

Shimohama S, Taniguchi T, Fujiwara M, Kameyama M (1987) Changes in β-adrenergic receptor subtypes in Alzheimer-type dementia. J Neurochem 48: 1215–1221

Shimohama S, Taniguchi T, Fujiwara M, Kameyama M (1988) Changes in benzodiazepine receptors in Alzheimer-type dementia. Ann Neurol 23: 404–406

Simpson MDC, Royston MC, Cross AJ, Slater P, Mann DMA, et al (1987) Brain regional ^{3}H-D-aspartate and ^{3}H-TCP binding in Alzheimer's disease and Down's syndrome. Br J Pharmacol [Suppl] 92: 609

Simpson MDC, Cross AJ, Slater P, Deakin JFW (1988) Loss of cortical GABA uptake sites in Alzheimer's disease. J Neural Transm 71: 219–226

Simpson MDC, Royston MC, Deakin JFW, Cross AJ, Mann DMA, et al (1988) Regional changes in ^{3}H-D-aspartate and ^{3}H-TCP binding sites in Alzheimer's disease brains. Brain Res 462: 76–82

Smith CJ, Perry EK, Perry RH, Fairbairn AF, Birdsall NJM (1987) Guanine nucleotide

modulation of muscarinic cholinergic receptor binding in postmortem human brain
— a preliminary study in Alzheimer's disease. Neurosci Lett 82: 227–232

Smith CJ, Perry EK, Perry RH, Candy JM, Johnson M, et al (1988) Muscarinic cholinergic
receptor subtypes in hippocampus in human cognitive disorders. J Neurochem 50:
847–856

Sofic E, Halket J, Przyborowska A, Riederer P, Beckmann H, et al (1989) Brain
quinolinic acid in Alzheimer's dementia. Eur Arch Psychiatr Neurol Sci 239: 177–
179

Sorbi S, Antuono P, Amaducci L (1980) Choline acetyltransferase and acetylcholinesterase abnormalities in senile dementia: importance of biochemical measurements in
human post-mortem brain specimens. Ital J Neurol Sci 2: 75–83

Sorbi S, Bird ED, Blass JP (1983) Decreased pyruvate dehydrogenase complex activity in
Huntington and Alzheimer brain. Ann Neurol 13: 72–78

Sparks DL, Slevin JT (1985) Determination of tyrosine, tryptophan and their
metabolic derivitives by HPLC-electrochemical detection: application to
postmortem samples from patients with Parkinson's and Alzheimer's disease. Life Sci
36: 449–457

Stokes CE, Hawthorne JN (1987) Reduced phosphoinositide concentrations in anterior
temporal cortex of Alzheimer-diseased brains. J Neurochem 48: 1018–1021

Sugaya K, Giacobini E, Chiappinelli VA (1990) Nicotine acetylcholine receptor
subtypes in human frontal cortex: changes in Alzheimer's disease. J Neurosci Res 27:
349–359

Tamminga CA, Foster NL, Chase TN (1985) Reduced brain somatostatin levels in
Alzheimer's disease. N Engl J Med 313: 1294–1295

Tamminga CA, Foster NL, Fedio P, Bird ED, Chase TN (1987) Alzheimer's disease: low
cerebral somatostatin levels correlate with impaired cognitive function and cortical
metabolism. Neurology 37: 161–165

Tarbit I, Perry EK, Perry RH, Blessed G, Tomlinson BE (1980) Hippocampal free amino
acids in Alzheimer's disease. J Neurochem 35: 1246–1249

Trocewicz J, Oka K, Nagatsu T, Nagastsu I, Iizuka R, et al (1982) Phenylethanolamine N-
methyltransferase activity in human brains. Biochem Med 27: 317–324

Unden A, Meyerson B, Winblad B, Sachs C, Bartfai T (1983) Postmortem changes in
binding to the muscarinic receptor from human cerebral cortex. J Neurochem 41:
102–106

Vanderheyden P, Ebinger G, Dierckx R, Vauquelin G (1987) Muscarinic cholinergic
receptor subtypes in normal human brain and Alzheimer's presenile dementia. J
Neurol Sci 82: 257–269

Waller S, Ball M, Reynolds M, London E (1986) Muscarinic binding and choline
scetyltransferase in postmortem brains of demented patients. Can J Neurol Sci 13:
528–532

Wallin A, Alafuzoff I, Carlsson A, Eckernäs SA, Gottfries CG, et al (1989) Neurotransmitter deficits in a non-multi-infarct category of vascular dementia. Acta Neurol
Scand 79: 397–406

Wang JX, Roeske WR, Mei L, Wang W, Perry E, et al (1987) Nicotinic and muscarinic M2
receptor alteration in the cerebral cortex of patients with senile dementia of the
Alzheimer type (SDAT). In: Rand MJ, Raper C (eds) Excerpta Medica 750 Pharmacology. Elsevier Science Publ, Amsterdam, pp 83–86

Weber S, Louis RB, Trombley L, Bissette G, Davies P, et al (1992) Metabolic half-life of
somatostatin and peptidase activities are altered in Alzheimer's disease. J Gerontol
47: 18–25

Weiler R, Lassmann H, Fischer P, Jellinger K, Winkler H (1990) A high ratio of
chromogranin A to synaptin/synaptophysin is a common feature of brains in
Alzheimer and Pick disease. FEBS Lett 263: 337–339

Whitehouse PJ, Martino AM, Antuono PG, Lowenstein PR, Coyle JT, et al (1986)
Nicotinic acetylcholine binding in Alzheimer's disease. Brain Res 371: 146–151

Whitehouse PJ, Vale WW, Zweig RM, Singer HS, Mayeux R, et al (1987) Reductions in corticotropin releasing factor-like immunoreactivity in cerebral cortex in Alzheimer's disease, Parkinson's disease, and progressive supranuclear palsy. Neurology 37: 905–909

Whitehouse PJ, Martino AM, Wagster MV, Price DL, Mayeux R, et al (1988) Reductions in ^{3}H-nicotinic acetylcholine binding in Alzheimer's disease and Parkinson's disease. An autoradiographic study. Neurology 38: 720–723

Whitford C, Candy J, Edwardson J, Perry R (1988) Cortical somatostatinrgic system not affected in Alzheimer's and Parkinson's diseases. J Neurol Sci 86: 13–18

Wilcock GK (1983) The temporal lobe in dementia of Alzheimer's type. Gerontology 29: 320–324

Wilcock GK, Esiri MM, Bowen DM, Smith CCT (1982) Alzheimer's disease. Correlation of cortical choline acetyltransferase activity with the severity of dementia and histological abnormalities. J Neurol Sci 57: 407–417

Wilcock GK, Esiri MM, Bowen DM, Smith CCT (1983) The nucleus basalis in Alzheimer's disease: cell counts and cortical biochemistry. Neuropathol Appl Neurobiol 9: 175–179

Winblad B, Adolfsson R, Carlsson A, Gottfries CG, Oreland L (1981) Brain biogenic amines in dementia of Alzheimer type. In: Peris C, Struwe G, Jansson B (eds) Biol psychiatry. Elsevier/North Holland Biochemical Press, Amsterdam, pp 965–968

Winblad B, Adolfsson R, Carlsson A, Gottfries CG (1982) Biogenic amines in brains of patients with Alzheimer's disease. Alz Dis A Report Prog 19: 25–33

Wolfe LS, Ng Ying Kin NMK, Palo J, Haltia M (1982) Raised levels of cerebral cortex dolichols in Alzheimer's disease. Lancet 10: 99

Wood PL, Etienne P, Lal S, Nair NPV, Finlayson MH, et al (1983) A postmortem comparison of the cortical cholinergic system in Alzheimer's disease and Pick's disease. J Neurol Sci 62: 211–217

Yates CM, Simpson J, Maloney AFJ, Gordon A, Reid AH (1980) Alzheimer-like cholinergic deficiency in Down syndrome. Lancet 979

Yates CM, Ritchie IM, Simpson J, et al (1981) Noradrenaline in Alzheimer-type dementia and Down syndrome. Lancet: 39–40

Yates CM, Harmar AJ, Rosie R, Sheward J, et al (1983) Thyreotropin-releasing hormone, luteinizing hormone-releasing hormone and substance P immunoreactivity in post-mortem brain from cases of Alzheimer-type dementia and Down's syndrome. Brain Res 258: 45–52

Yates CM, Simpson J, Gordon A, Maloney AFJ, Allison Y, et al (1983) Catecholamines and cholinergic enzymes in presenile and senile Alzheimer-type dementia and Down's syndrome. Brain Res 280: 119–126

Yates CM, Simpson J, Gordon A (1986) Regional brain 5-hydroxytryptamine levels are reduced in senile Down's syndrome as in Alzheimer's disease. Neurosci Lett 65: 189–192

Yates CM, Butterworth J, Gordon A (1989) Gamma-glutamyl transpeptidase in dementia. Neurobiol Aging 10: 107–108

Yates CM, Simpson J, Gordon A, Christie JE (1989) Cholinergic enzymes in the spinal cord in Alzheimer-type dementia. J Neural Transm [PD-Sect] 1: 311–315

Yates CM, Butterworth J, Tennant MC, Gordon A (1990) Enzyme activities in relation to pH and lactate in postmortem brain in Alzheimer-type and other dementias. J Neurochem 5: 1624–1630

Younkin SG, Goodridge B, Locket G, Katz J, Nafziger D, et al (1986) Molecular forms of acetylcholinesterases in Alzheimer's disease. Fed Proc 45: 2982–2988

Authors' address: Dr. W. Gsell, Clinical Neurochemistry, Department of Psychiatry, University of Würzburg, Füchsleinstrasse 15, D-97080 Würzburg, Federal Republic of Germany.

J Neural Transm (1996) [Suppl] 47: 103–123

Clinical features of frontal lobe dementia in comparison to Alzheimer's disease

C. A. Gregory[1] and **J. R. Hodges**[2]

[1] Psychiatry Services for Adults, Fulbourn Hospital, and [2] University Neurology Unit,
University of Cambridge, United Kingdom

Summary. Over the past decade it has become evident that a substantial minority of patients with primary dementing diseases, particularly those presenting in the presenium, have dementia of frontal lobe type (DFT) due to non-Alzheimer's pathology. Although post-mortem remains the only method of definitive diagnosis, DFT and Alzheimer's disease (AD) can, we would claim, be separated with a high degree of certainty based on a combination of informant history, neuropsychology and neuroimaging.

In DFT, changes in personality, motivation, social interaction and organisational abilities, in the presence of well preserved memory and visuo-spatial abilities, are characteristic. The lack of insight emphasises the need for independent information particularly as patients may perform normally on bedside (and more sophisticated) tests of cognition. Psychiatric features especially mood disturbance appear to be common, but their prevalence remains to be established. In contrast, AD is a progressive amnestic disorder with episodic and semantic memory deficits, followed by breakdown in other attentional, perceptual and visuo-spatial abilities, which reflects the major locus of pathology in AD, namely the medial temporal lobe. These features are illustrated by reference to a longitudinal study of 52 patients with minimal to moderate AD. In addition, we shall describe the results of retrospective and prospective neuropsychiatric studies of a group of DFT patients.

Introduction

Although all authorities agree that Alzheimer's disease (AD) remains the commonest case of dementia, accounting for some 60–80% of cases (Cooper, 1991; Jorm et al., 1987), it is now clear that a substantial proportion of patients who would previously have received a diagnosis of Alzheimer's disease have, instead, other clinico-pathological syndromes which are characterised by non-Alzheimer's forms of pathology (Brun, 1987; Knopman et al., 1990; Miller et al., 1991; Neary et al., 1986). Among these are the so-called focal lobar atrophies which, as the term suggests, manifest with features of progressive frontal and/or temporal lobe degeneration (Brun et al., 1994; Gregory and

Hodges, 1993; Neary et al., 1993). This paper concerns the clinical and neuropsychological features of the commonest form of focal lobar atrophy, dementia of frontal type (DFT) which are contrasted with those found in AD.

The cognitive deficit of early AD

The most pervasive feature of AD is undoubtedly a failure of memory. When patients present in the early stages of the disease, complaints of memory difficulty are by far the commonest symptom noticed by the patient, and more particularly by their spouse. In patients who are seen for the first time at a more advanced stage of deterioration, a retrospective history of insidiously progressive memory failure can almost invariably be elicited from the carer. As will be discussed below, there are growing number of case reports documenting atypical presentations of AD (aphasia, apraxia, visual agnosia etc.), but our own experience suggests that these represent only a tiny minority of cases. Moreover, in the context of this paper, a predominately frontal presentation of AD seems to be exceptional.

Our own experience of dementia derives from a Memory and Cognitive Disorders Clinic run jointly by the University Departments of Neurology, Psychiatry and Neuropsychology in Cambridge in which over 400 patients have been assessed. In 1991, we enrolled into an MRC-funded project a consecutive series of 52 patients (chosen simply on the basis of their willingness to participate in an intensive longitudinal study) with probable AD, according to the NINCDS-ADRDA (McKhann et al., 1984) criteria. The aims of this study were to document the pattern of cognitive deficits in patients with minimal and mild AD, both cross-sectionally and over time. We defined "minimal" cases as those scoring 24 or greater on the Mini-Mental State Examination (MMSE); mild cases were in the range of 18–23. In order to obtain "pseudo-longitudinal" information, we included within the cohort some cases with more established disease (labelled as moderate AD; MMSE 6–17). Most of the patients in this latter category have, predictably, dropped out of the study but we are still following up the majority of cases in the minimal and mild categories. The basic demographic data on our cohort is shown in Table 1.

The focus of the project has been on aspects of memory and language which have been investigated using a combination of standard (e.g., subtests from the Wechsler Memory Scale-Revised, Warrington's Recognition Memory Test, the National Adult Reading Test, the Token Test, the Cookie theft picture description task from the Boston Diagnostic Aphasia Examination etc.) and experimental tasks (e.g., the Hodges semantic memory battery, the Pyramids and Palm Trees Test, tests of reading and writing ability which manipulate word frequency and the regularity of spelling-to-sound correspondence etc.). We have also included tests of global intellectual ability (the MMSE, Mattis' Dementia Rating Scale) as well as tests of visuo-perceptual and -spatial function (Rey Complex Figure Test, Judgement of Line Orientation, Unusual Views Matching Test). A full description of the methodology of

Table 1. Basic demographic data of the AD patient group and controls in the Cambridge AD study

| | Controls | AD subgroups | | |
		Minimal	Mild	Moderate
n	24	17	17	18
Age				
mean (SD)	69.7 (7.8)	72.2 (7.2)	67.0 (8.3)	63.4 (8.8)
Educ'n in yrs				
mean (SD)	10.7 (2.2)	11.2 (2.8)	11.4 (3.6)	10.9 (2.5)
MMSE				
mean (SD)	29.1 (1.0)	25.6 (1.8)	20.9 (1.7)	10.0 (4.6)
range	27–30	24–30	18–23	6–17
DRS				
mean (SD)	140 (2.4)	123.8 (8.8)	111.6 (10.1)	72.7 (20.2)
range	135–144	103–137	97–132	32–102

the project and the tests employed is published elsewhere (Hodges and Patterson, 1995; Patterson et al., 1994).

A decade of intensive neuropsychological research into the nature of the memory deficit has established that not all aspects of memory are affected equally in early AD. The major impairment is in the domain of anterograde episodic memory (e.g., Grady et al., 1988; Heindel et al., 1993; Hodges and Patterson, 1995; Welsh et al., 1991, 1992). The term "episodic" refers to memory for temporally-specific events in a person's own experience. Our work has confirmed that the ability to retain new information after a period (delayed recall) is the most sensitive measure of AD and that memory for both verbal and visual material is affected in the majority of cases (Greene et al., 1995; Hodges and Patterson, 1995), as illustrated in Fig. 1. This profound deficit in episodic memory has been attributed principally to defective encoding and storage of new information, whereas an accelerated rate of forgetting appears to make only a minor contribution to the patients' memory failure (Brandt and Rich, 1994; Greene et al., in press; Kopelman, 1985). In other words, patients are unable to learn new information, but the little they learn is retained reasonably well.

It is also apparent that patients with AD show progressive disruption of semantic memory. The term semantic memory is applied to the component of long-term memory containing knowledge of objects, facts and concepts as well as words and their meaning (Tulving, 1987). In contrast to episodic memory, semantic memory is culturally shared rather than personal and is not temporally specific. Tasks dependent on semantic memory include object naming, generation of definitions for spoken words, word-picture and picture-picture matching and the generation of exemplars on category fluency tests (e.g., animals, vegetables etc.). Patients with AD are characteristically impaired on these tests, although they are of differential sensitivity. Category fluency is a sensitive measure and early in the course of AD there is dispropor-

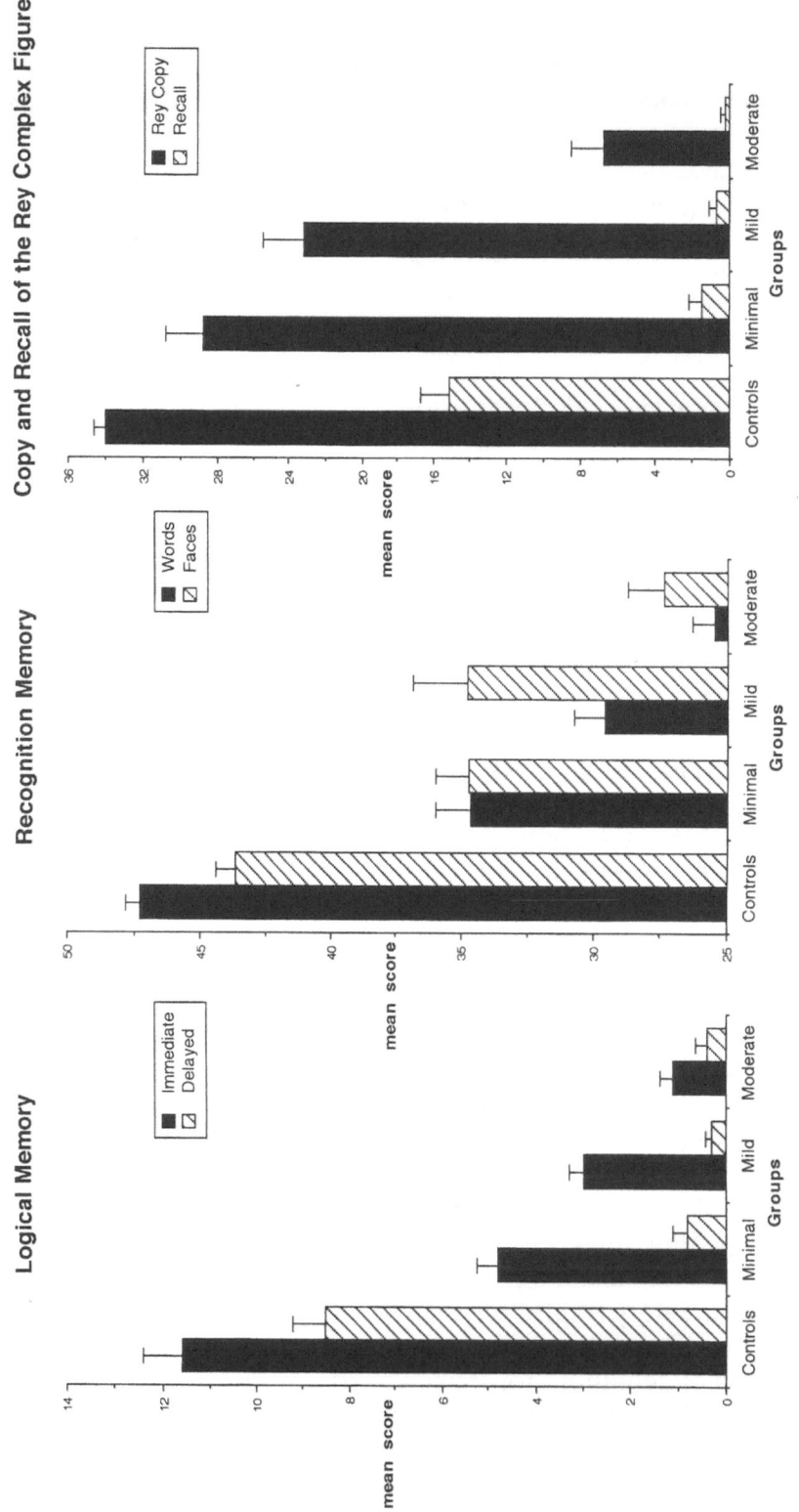

Fig. 1. Performance on control subjects and DAT patients (divided into three subgroups according to disease severity: minimal, mild and moderate) showing the groups' mean scores (±SE) on i) logical memory (story recall) subtest of the Wechsler Memory Scale-Revised (left), ii) Warrington's Recognition Memory Test — words and faces (centre) and iii) the Rey Complex Figure Test — copy and recall components (right)

tionate impairment in semantic category-based, as opposed to letter-based fluency tests (for review see Monsch et al., 1994; Rosser and Hodges, 1994). The underlying cause of the semantic deficit, at a cognitive level, has been a matter of controversy. Some researchers have claimed that the deficits found on tests of semantic memory may primarily reflect impaired access to semantic memory (for review see Bayles et al., 1991; Nebes, 1989); but the majority of investigators support the interpretation of a breakdown in the structure of semantic memory (Chan et al., 1993; Chertkow and Bub, 1990; Hodges et al., 1992b; Martin et al., 1985). Using a battery of tests of semantic memory all of which test knowledge about the same consistent set of 48 items, via differing modalities of sensory input and/or output, we have established that most patients presenting with even minimal AD (MMSE >24) show impairment on tests of semantic memory (Hodges and Patterson, 1995). This is, however, not a universal phenomenon: some patients may be severely amnesic yet perform normally on the entire semantic battery. Certainly as the disease progresses into the moderate stages (MMSE <18) breakdown in semantic memory is a ubiquitous finding which is reflected in the increasing anomia, emptiness of language and failure on general knowledge tests.

In contrast to the deficits in these major components of longer-term memory — episodic and semantic memory — patients with AD typically perform normally on tests of short-term or working memory, as exemplified by their normal digit or block-tapping span. Even on dual-performance tests, designed to tap the more demanding aspects of working memory, the so-called central executive, in which subjects are required to divide their attention between two simultaneously presented streams of information, performance in the very early stages of AD is typically unimpaired (Greene et al., 1995).

One final aspect of memory which until recently has been studied relatively little, perhaps due to the lack of quantifiable tests, is remote personal (or autobiographical) memory. Because patients often become preoccupied with, or indeed appear to "live in", the past, it is commonly believed that such memory is spared in AD. Recent research has shown, however, that most patients early in the course of the disease do, in fact, show impaired performance on tests of autobiographical memory, although the degree of impairment is certainly less than that seen on anterograde memory tests. This loss is temporally-graded with relative sparing of more distant memories; accounting, in part, for the clinical observation above. Moreover, there is no clear correlation between the degree of anterograde and retrograde memory deficit (Greene and Hodges, 1996; Kopelman, 1989; Sagar et al., 1988).

Pathological and anatomical correlates

From a theoretical standpoint, it is interesting to correlate the pattern of memory deficits with the anatomical locus of the pathological changes in the early stages of AD. It has been proposed by Braak and Braak (1991), on the basis of extensive neuropathological studies, that the characteristic neu-

rofibrillary tangles of AD first appear in the transentorhinal region (stages
I–II) and only later progress to involve limbic structures proper — entorhinal
cortex, subiculum and hippocampal zone CA1 — in stages III–IV. In the
final stages of the disease (V–VI), there are widespread changes in all cortical
association areas. The transentorhinal region is a complex transitional
zone located between the entorhinal region proper and the adjoining
temporal isocortex. Lesions in this region are critically placed to disrupt
connections to and from the hippocampal formation and would thus be expected to produce severe impairment in episodic memory, of the type found
in early AD.

Studies of primates with experimental ablations, and of humans with
surgically-induced or naturally occurring lesions, have established the primary
role of the hippocampus (and related medial temporal structures) and components of the diencephalon in the formation of new episodic memory traces
(for review see Squire, 1992). By comparison, we know much less about the
neural substrate of semantic memory. Current evidence, however, implicates
the temporal neocortex as the most important region. Patients with the syndrome of semantic dementia, in which there is progressive, yet selective, loss
of semantic memory with relative preservation of other linguistic and nonverbal cognitive abilities, have structural and/or functional changes involving
the infero-lateral temporal lobe especially on the left (Hodges et al., 1992a).
Similarly, patients with semantic memory deficits following Herpes Simplex
virus encephalitis typically show destruction of the temporal neocortex
(Sartori et al., 1993). The neuroanatomical basis of working memory is sur-
prisingly complex; regions of the dominant peri-sylvian cortex are critical for
the short-term maintenance of phonological material, whereas regions of the
frontal lobe are associated with central executive function (Vallar and
Papagno, 1995).

In early AD, the site of initial pathological involvement, the transentorhinal zone, is entirely in keeping with the profound deficit in new
learning ability found in patients. As soon as the disease progresses to
involve the temporal neocortex, however, impairment of semantic memory
should occur. Since the peri-sylvian cortex is relatively spared, the finding
of preserved auditory-verbal short-term memory is to be expected. Likewise deficits in dual-performance tasks would not be predicted in early
AD.

Non-amnestic deficits in AD

We have concentrated on aspects of memory in AD since this is the predominant cognitive deficit in early cases. There are, of course, other more widespread deficits which become more prominant as the disease progresses.
Impairment in visuo-spatial and perceptual abilities are common in the
middle stages of the disease, reflecting involvement of posterior higher-order
visual association and parietal regions (Kaskie and Storandt, 1995; Mendez et

al., 1990). The language disorder of AD is dominated by the semantic breakdown discussed above; the phonological and syntactical components of language remain relatively intact, at least until the late stages of the disease (Hart, 1988). Apraxia is found in patients with AD (Rapcsak et al., 1989) and may occasionally be severe enough to interfere with writing and other manual tasks.

A broad summary of the cognitive deficits in the successive stages of AD are given in Table 2.

In marked contrast to the profile of DFT (see below), basic aspects of personality, comportment, social interaction and behaviour are strikingly preserved in the early stages of AD and most patients retain at least partial insight into their predicament. Many of the features of DFT such as restlessness, perseverative behaviour and echolalia may occur in the late stages of the disease but are virtually never seen at presentation, but is notable that even in advanced cases of AD the Kluver-Bucy syndrome is very rare.

Atypical presentations of AD

Having stressed the amnesic presentation of AD, it is important to point out that there have been a number of case reports of patients with pathologically verified AD presenting with atypical features including progressive aphasia (Green et al., 1990 and in press; Kempler et al., 1990; Pogacar and Williams, 1984), visual apperceptual agnosia and Balint's syndrome (Berthier et al., 1991; Hof et al., 1990), or even progressive unilateral parietal syndrome (Crystal et al., 1982). There are, however, to the best of our knowledge, no convincing detailed case studies of patients with AD presenting with the picture of DFT, although a few such cases are included in the group studies reported by Gustafson et al. (1987).

Table 2. Stages of cognitive decline in AD

Stage I: Pure amnesic syndrome
  Severe impairment of anterograde episodic memory
  Variable and temporally-graded impairment of remote memory
  Sparing of immediate (working) memory

Stage II: Predominately posterior cortical syndrome
  Semantic memory impairment:
    Anomia, impaired category fluency, word comprehension etc.
  Visuo-perceptual and spatial disorders
  Apraxia
  Deficits in attention and problem solving

Stage III: Global dementia
  Impairment in all aspects of cognition
  Disintegration of personality

Dementia of frontal type

The history of DFT

Arnold Pick (1892), after describing patients with progressive aphasia as a result of progressive temporal lobe atrophy, was the first to report the syndrome of frontal dementia (Pick, 1906) The pathological features were reported a few years later by Alzheimer (1910–1911) who described Pick cells and Pick bodies in association with focal brain atrophy. Subsequently, however, it became apparent that only a minority of cases of frontal lobe degeneration were, in fact, accompanied by Pick cells and Pick bodies (Brun, 1987; Neary et al., 1986). As a consequence, a number of other terms were introduced including frontal lobe degeneration of non-Alzheimer's type (Brun, 1987) frontal lobe degeneration (Miller et al., 1991) and dementia of frontal type (Neary et al., 1987). Most recently, the Lund and Manchester groups (Brun et al., 1994) have introduced the term frontotemporal dementia and in the same paper have produced provisional diagnostic criteria, which await prospective validation. Since as yet there is no entirely consistent label for this condition, we have chosen to use the term dementia of frontal type (DFT).

Between the 1930's and 60's many single and small groups of patients with Picks disease (PD) were reported. The clinical symptomatology of these cases was described, often at some length, to characterise the presentation of PD and sometimes specifically to highlight differences between AD and PD (Goldstein and Katz, 1937; Robertson et al., 1958; Stengel, 1943; Thorpe, 1932). In 1943, Stengel stated that "many problems concerning AD and PD are still awaiting clarification" and that "the knowledge of the symptomatology of these conditions (AD & DFT) is still incomplete". More recent work has continued to compare the symptomatology of AD and DFT to assist clinicians in the differential diagnosis (Gustafson and Nilsson, 1982; Mendez et al., 1993). Although there has been considerable progress in our understanding of AD, as shown earlier in this paper, the statements of Stengel remain largely true regarding the neurobehavioural and psychiatric symptomatology of DFT.

Epidemiology of DFT

DFT is clearly much less common than AD, but estimates of the ratio of the two disease ranges from 1 in 5 to 1 in 20 (Hodges, 1994). These figures are however all biased by the source of the patients studied (usually hospital-based, and often from specialist units) and the mode of diagnosis. Of pathologically verified studies, one of the most comprehensive by Brun et al. (Brun, 1987) reported that 20 of their first 150 consecutive autopsied cases suffered from frontal or fronto-temporal degeneration. On clinical grounds alone, Neary et al. (1988) estimated that 19% of 130 cases seen in the neurological unit over 5 years met criteria for frontal lobe dementia. In the latter two studies, however, the mean age of the total patient population was unusually young which may well have led to an over representation of DFT patients. A definitive community-based clinico-pathological study of unselected demented patients is required to answer the question of the true prevalence of DFT.

Much less controversy surrounds the age of onset. There is no doubt that DFT affects younger patients than does AD. The peak age of onset is 45 to 65. Cases above 75 appear relatively rare (Miller et al., 1991). In our series of 15 patients, the age range was 37 to 74 with a mean of 62 years. Men and women appear to be equally affected.

Neurobehavioural features of DFT

In striking contrast to AD, the majority of patients with DFT are brought along to the clinic blissfully unaware of the major changes in personality and behaviour observed by their relatives. Patients may appear apathetic and withdrawn, or alternatively become socially disinhibited with facetiousness and inappropriate jocularity. Their ability to plan and organise complex activities (work, social engagements etc.) is almost invariably impaired, reflecting deficits in sustained attention, goal setting and attainment, mental set-shifting and flexibility. Mental rigidity and an inability to appreciate the more subtle aspects of language (irony, punning etc.) are common. There is often indifference to domestic and occupational responsibilities, a lack of empathy for family and friends and gradual withdrawal from all social interactions. A deterioration in self-care with a reluctance to bath, groom and change clothes is frequently reported. Many patients show a change in eating habits with an escalating desire for sweet food coupled with reduced satiety; the increasing gluttony may lead to enormous weight gain. The other components of the Klüver-Bucy syndrome (hypersexuality and oral exploratory behaviour) are much less commonly observed (Cummings and Duchen, 1981).

Language dysfunction is an early, but subtle, finding in many patients with DFT and consists of factually empty speech which is reduced in quantity. Articulation, phonology and syntax are typically preserved. Mild anomia may be present but repetition is normal. In terms of classical aphasic syndromes the picture corresponds to a transcortical motor or dynamic aphasia. Many patients develop spontaneous echolalia (a tendency to immediately repeat the examiner's last phrase) and other reiterative speech acts such as the repetition of phrases, words, syllables or sounds. In advanced cases, comprehension may become impaired. Finally, muteness supervenes.

Having described the characteristic presentation of DFT, it is important to emphasise a number of features which distinguish it from AD. Memory is typically intact in DFT and although patients may admit, when pressed, to "memory" difficulties, when this is explored further they usually have problems with concentration and immediate (working) memory, rather than the severe amnesia found in AD (see above). Visuospatial skills are also very well preserved in DFT.

Towards diagnostic criteria for DFT

Alzheimer's disease has well recognised diagnostic criteria used by clinicians and researchers e.g. DSM IV criteria (APA, 1994), or the NINCDS ADRDA criteria (McKhann et al., 1984), which have been validated against post-mortem results and shown to have approximately 80–90% accuracy (e.g., Morris et al., 1988). This is not yet the case with DFT. The most detailed work to date, is that of the Lund Manchester workers, who, in 1994, (Brun et al., 1994) published extensive diagnostic criteria for frontotemporal dementia, (see Table 3). It is not yet clear, however, how these should be used; whether all criteria are equally weighted and need to be present, in which case only advanced cases will be diagnosed: or alternatively whether some symptoms and signs may have greater significance so that only a certain number or cluster need be present to make a diagnosis of DFT.

Based on the literature, both old and recent (Gustafson, 1987; Gustafson and Nilsson, 1982; Miller et al., 1991; Neary et al., 1988; Robertson et al., 1958;

Table 3. Lund Manchester criteria — Core diagnostic features

Behavioural disorder	*Affective symptoms*
Insidious onset	Depression/Anxiety
Early loss of personal awareness	Delusion early & evanescent
Early loss of social awareness	Suicidal & fixed ideation
Disinhibition	Hypochondriasis
Mental rigidity	Bizarre somatic complaints
Hyperorality	Emotional unconcern
Stereotyped behaviour	Amimia
Utilisation behaviour	
Distractibility/impulsivity	*Physical signs*
Loss of insight	Early primitive reflexes
	Early incontinence
Speech disorder	Late akinesia/rigidity & tremor
Reduction in speech	Low & labile B.P.
Stereotypy	
Echolalia & perseveration	*Investigations*
Late mutism	Normal EEG
	Failure on frontal neuropsychological tests
	Abnormal imaging, structural &/or functional

Spatial orientation & Praxis preserved

Supportive diagnostic features
Onset before 65
Positive family history/Bulbar palsy, motor neurone disease

Diagnostic exclusion features	
Abrupt onset with ictal events	Myoclonus
Head trauma	Cortical bulbar and spinal deficits
Early severe amnesia	Choreoathetosis
Early spatial disorientation/apraxia	Cerebellar ataxia
Logoclonus speech	Early/severe pathological EEG

Stengel, 1943), experience of cases from the Memory and Cognitive Disorders Clinic (see above) and knowledge of symptomatology found in patients with non-degenerative frontal lobe disease, we developed our own local clinical criteria for the diagnosis of DFT, which we were using prior to the publication of the consensus criteria, (see Table 4). These were applied to the case notes of 12 patients in a retrospective study of DFT who had been referred to the Memory and Cognitive Disorders Clinic and who had been fully investigated and were being followed up at that clinic (Gregory and Hodges, in press). All patients had, at the time of diagnosis, at least 5 of the neurobehavioural features from the checklist. Based on these criteria we have developed an informant interview and are now using this interview and the clinical criteria prospectively. All 15 patients in the prospective study had at least 6 of the neurobehavioural symptoms and signs, the distribution of which is shown in Fig. 2.

The neuropsychology of DFT

In contrast to AD, memory is typically unaffected early in the course of the disease. In a recent (unpublished) study of 6 cases, who fulfilled the criteria outlined above, we found a striking lack of impairment on a comprehensive battery of episodic and semantic memory tests. Likewise, tests of visuospatial function may show no significant abnormality. Tasks aimed at specific evalu-

Table 4. Locally developed criteria for the diagnosis of dementia of frontal type

---

i) Presentation with an insidious and progressive disorder of personality and behaviour of at least six months duration characterised by at least 5 of the following features:
   loss of insight
   disinhibition
   restlessness
   distractibility
   emotional lability
   reduced empathy and unconcern for others
   lack of foresight and planning
   impulsivity
   social withdrawal
   apathy or lack of spontaneity
   poor self care
   reduced verbal output
   verbal stereotypes or echolalia
   perseveration (verbal or motor)
   features of the Klüver-Bucy syndrome (gluttony, pica, sexual hyperactivity)
ii) historical evidence of preserved memory for day-to-day events
iii) neuropsychological evidence of disproportionate frontal dysfunction
iv) absence of history of significant head injury, stroke, score >4 on the Hachinski scale, long-term alcohol abuse, diagnosis of parkinsonism or other movement disorder
v) psychiatric phenomena may be present

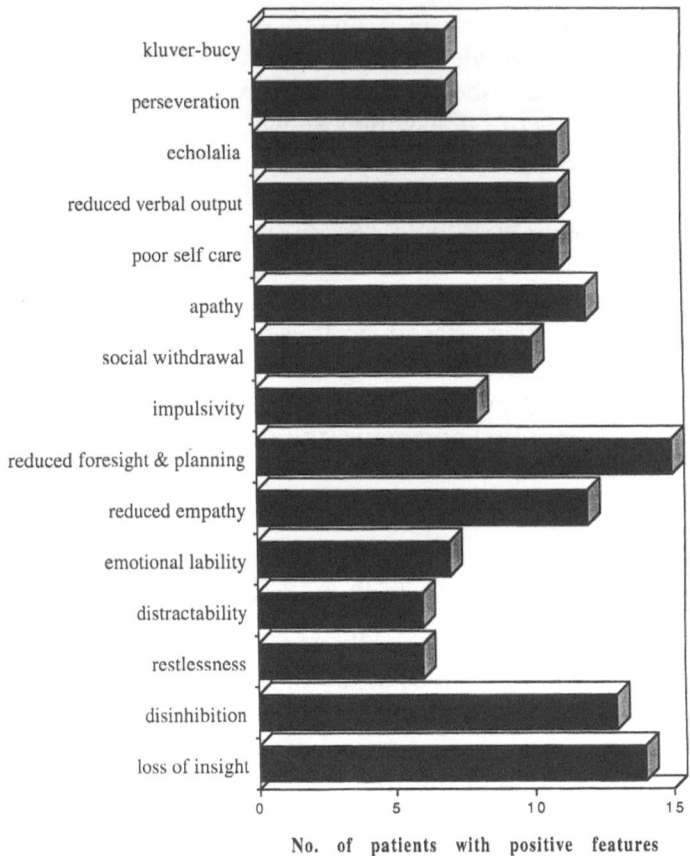

Fig. 2. Prevalence of neurobehavioural symptoms in a group of 15 prospectively assessed patients with DFT based on the checklist of symptoms and signs devised by Gregory and Hodges (1993)

ation of the frontal lobes (such as the Wisconsin Card Sorting Test, Trail Making Test, Stroop Test, Shallice's Cognitive Estimates Test and verbal fluency) will often show marked impairment (see Knopman et al., 1989; Miller et al., 1991; Neary et al., 1988), but it should be stressed that in some cases with marked neurobehavioural changes, sufficient to interfere with social relations and lead to premature retirement from work, there may be very little abnormality even after rigorous neuropsychological evaluation. We have seen a number of such patients who have a "full-house" of symptoms with eventually clear-cut frontal atrophy on MRI and a typical neuropsychological profile.

With disease progression, episodic memory deteriorates and visuospatial and perceptual functions are characteristically normal even late in the disease.

As mentioned above, the MMSE is insensitive in the very early amnesic phase of AD, but falls as patients enter even the mild stages of the disease. It is, however, an even less reliable indicator of DFT; as shown in Fig. 3, the majority of cases in our series of prospectively studied patients scored above the classic cut-off of 24, while approximately a third (6/15) obtained a maximum of 30/30.

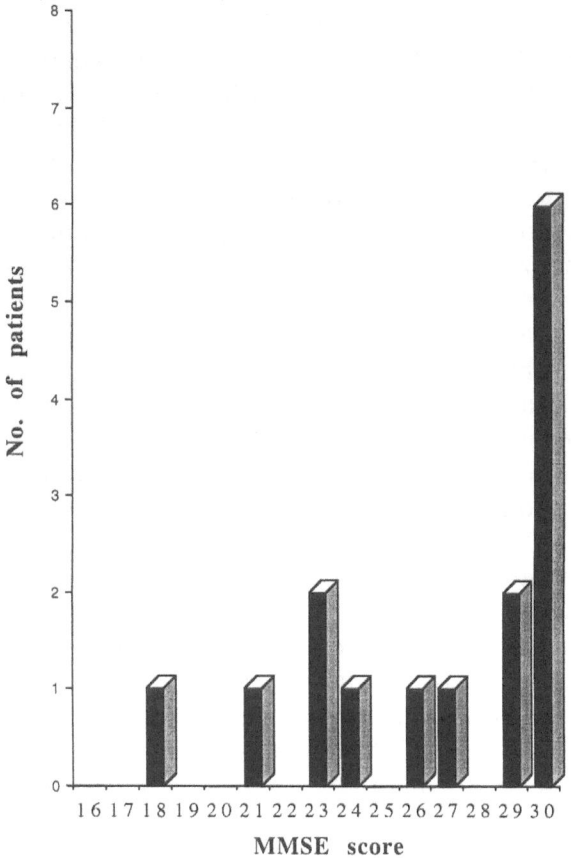

Fig. 3. Distribution of MMSE scores in a group of 15 prospectively asessed DFT patients

Psychiatric symptomatology in DFT

A wide range of psychiatric symptoms have been decribed in DFT. For instance, in an early report Goldstein and Katz (1937) described a pathologically proven PD patient who suffered frank visual hallucinations and delusions and was agitated and distressed about her deceased brother whom she believed to be going hungry. At the other extreme there are reports of patients in whom no emotional response was described (Robertson et al., 1958).

More recent work has continued to provide detailed reports of neurobehavioural features, but information regarding specific psychiatric symptoms remains scanty. Neary et al. (1988), reported on 7 patients, one was "hypochondriacally obsessed with pain in the perineum", a second had "paranoid ideas", while a third had a diagnosis of "agitated depression". Gustafson (1987), in a prospective study of dementia patients, stated that of 20 patients with DFT, six had psychotic episodes, but they provided little in the way of further information. In that same paper it was stated that one third had a mood change towards euphoria, and that a picture like depression (apathy, reduced speech and movement) or brief depressive reactions could be seen. Miller et al. (1991), reported 8 patients, three of whom had marked psychiatric symptomatology. One was depressed with psychotic features consisting of religious delusions, a second developed a delusional disorder as her frontal dementia progressed and a third became depressed following the death of her son, but subsequently developed marked behavioural and personality changes. Similarly, in a retrospective study of 21 patients with post-mortem verified PD, Mendez et al. (1993) comment that two patients had depressive symptoms which were felt to be severe enough to warrant ECT. None of these studies, however, state whether any standardised psychiatric assessment was used, or report on the changes in psychiatric symptomatology over time.

Our interest in the psychiatric symptoms of DFT lead us to first perform a retrospective investigation of 12 patients with a clinical diagnosis of DFT, as described above (Gregory and Hodges, in press). The case notes of these patients, all of whom had been seen by a consultant psychiatrist, were scrutinised. Seven (58%) initially presented to a psychiatrist, the other five were referred to a neurologist. One third, i.e., four patients received an initial psychiatric diagnosis: (i) schizophreniform psychosis, (ii) psychogenic memory impairment and depression, (iii) recurrence of a depressive illness with obsessional-compulsive features, and (iv) alcohol dependency with hypomanic features. Two of these three patients had a past history of depressive illness with one of the patients having a strong family history of psychiatric illness with three family members committing suicide (2 grandparents and an uncle).

A prospective study of the psychiatric symptomatology in DFT

The purpose of our present work, a prospective study of 15 DFT patients who are being followed by the clinic, is to look more closely at psychiatric symptomatology over time using the Comprehensive Psychiatric Rating Scale (CPRS) (Asberg et al., 1978), a semi-structured standardised clinical interview. This scale is designed to measure change in psychiatric symptomatology over time or with treatment. It consists of 40 self-reported items and 25 observer-rated items, (see Appendix 1). From both the self-reported and observer-rated items, clusters of symptoms and signs can be seen which allow diagnosis of psychiatric syndromes, e.g., depression, hypomania etc. The major results are summarised in Fig. 4.

Depressive symptoms: Three patients (20%) reported themselves as having a lowered mood, and 2 (13%) of these acknowledged pessimistic feelings (self-reproach, ideas of failure), fleeting suicidal thoughts and a number of other symptoms which would fulfil DSM IV criteria for major depression. Two of these patients appeared sad at times during the interview. The third patient appeared incongruously rather elated with mild pressure of speech and flight of ideas. Interestingly, five patients (33.3%) reported an inability to feel or experience emotion in the usual way, including two of the patients who felt low.

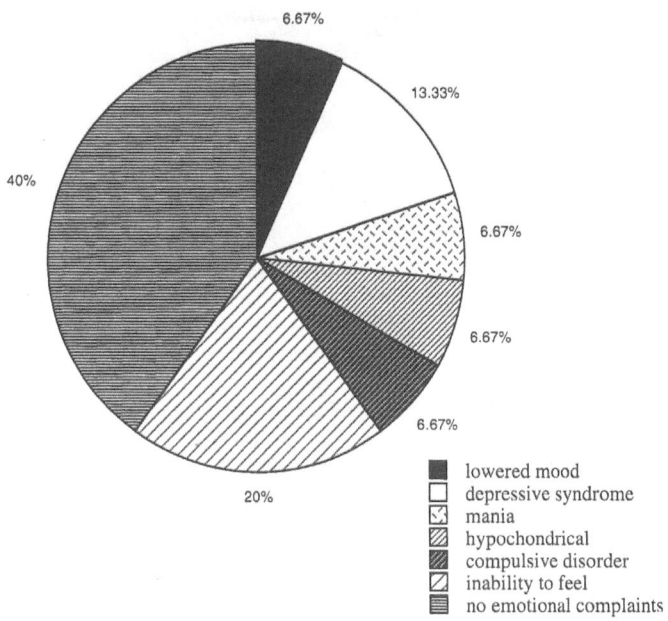

Fig. 4. Prevalence of subjective emotional complaints in 15 patients with DFT prospectively assessed using the CPRS (see text)

Elevated mood: Only one patient (6.7%) reported an elevated mood, describing feelings of well-being most of the time, this patient also reported ideas of grandeur stating that his memory was better than normal and that his "recall was great". He also reported some concentration difficulties. Objectively, he was markedly labile in mood, at times hostile and showed inappropriate emotional responses. However most striking, and negating a diagnosis of manic disorder, was a lengthy history of change in personality with social and occupational decline antedating his manic symptoms and his grossly abnormal speech with echolalia and perseveration.

Other neurotic symptomatology: One patient (6.7%) reported the development of compulsive counting. This patient had previously always checked the plugs several times at night and had, since the onset of the personality change reported by her husband, begun to count pictures in any room that she entered. This same patient also reported symptoms of "dizziness" that she continually sought explanation and investigation for. One other patient had also become hypochondriacal; she repeatedly brought the interview back to her concerns that her brain no longer appeared to work correctly and fears that she had a brain tumour.

Delusions and hallucinations: No patient to date in our prospective group has developed psychotic symptoms. However, as noted earlier one patient in our retrospective study developed a florid psychosis with delusions of reference, delusions of passivity and auditory hallucinations.

Physical and intellectual symptomatology (Fig. 5): Many patients had mild physical complaints, eight (53%) complaining of lassitude or physical fatigue,

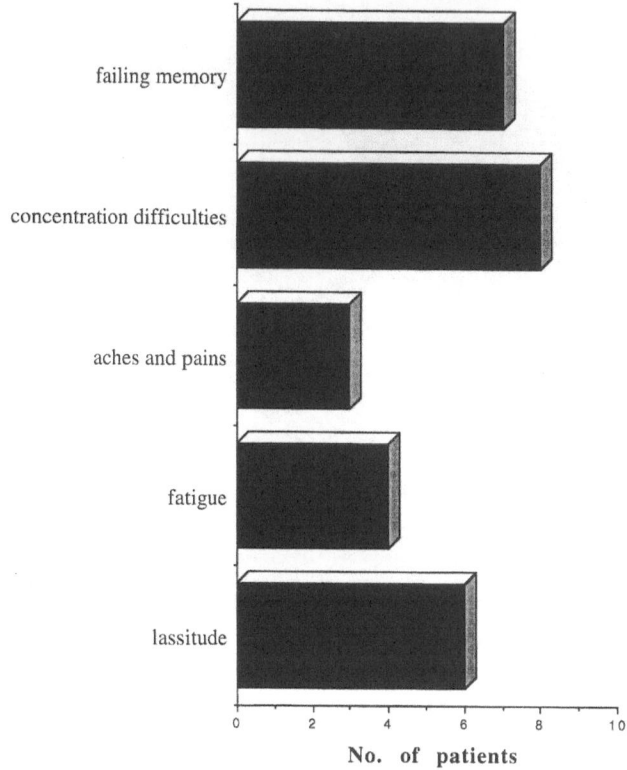

Fig. 5. Intellectual and physical complaints in 15 patients with DFT prospectively asssessed using the CPRS (see text)

three (20%) reporting generalised aches and pains, nine patients (60%) reporting either or both concentration and memory difficulties.

Psychiatric symptomatology in AD vs. DFT

How does the psychopathology of DFT compare with that of AD? There are now many studies which have looked at psychiatric symptomatology in AD. For instance, Berrios and Brook (1985) examined 100 patients with AD, multi-infarct dementia or mixed dementia referred to an old age psychiatry clinic. A half of patients with AD were deluded. Diagnostic criteria for the diagnosis of the dementing process were not identified, nor any standardised psychiatric interview applied. More recently, Burns et al. (1990a) examined 178 patients with AD as defined by the NINCDS-ADRDA criteria for probable and possible AD. Patients included had all been in contact with the old age psychiatry service. Delusions were rated if they had ever been present or were present at the time of interview and were classified as simple delusions (theft and suspicion), or other delusions (complex, multiple or bizarre) using the Geriatric Mental State schedule based on the Present State Examination. Sixteen percent had experienced delusions at some point in their illness and

20% had experienced ideas of persecution. Cognitive function was not related to presence or absence of psychosis, although there was a significant correlation between the degree of cerebral atrophy as judged by the Ventricular Brain ratio and presence of bizarre or complex delusions. In an analysis of the same group of patients, looking for disorders of perception (Burns et al., 1990b), 13% experienced visual hallucinations, and 10% auditory hallucinations with 30% suffering from misidentification syndromes. There was evidence to show that hallucinations were associated with a more rapid cognitive decline. It is of course of interest now whether some of the these patients with hallucinations and rapid decline may have had cortical Lewy body disease. Two-thirds of patients were found to have a least one depressive symptom, and 43% were felt to be depressed by a trained observer. Meanwhile elevated mood was uncommon (3.5%).

An earlier review of psychiatric symptoms in AD by Wragg and Jeste (1989) found widely disparate frequencies of psychiatric symptoms, no doubt in part related to the how the patient groups were ascertained, but also how rigorously symptoms were pursued. For example, the prevalence of depressed mood ranged from 0 to 87%, depressive syndrome from 0 to 86% and delusions from 10 to 73%.

Our DFT patients were ascertained from a specialist outpatient clinic. Referrals to this clinic are generally made to the behavioural neurologist and patients with more florid psychiatric symptomatology may be referred to alternative specialist psychiatric services. Nevertheless, it is interesting that in this group of patients affective symptoms are common, while psychotic phenomena appear to be rare. Despite reports in the literature that no changes in emotion are experienced by the patient, this is not our experience. In addition, other intellectual and physical symptoms are commonly reported. Objective assessment may be at odds with the reported mental state, and this plus the essential aspects of the informant history provide important diagnostic clues. Clearly further research into the prevalence of psychiatric symptoms in patients with AD and DFT which attempts to circumvent these referral biases is required.

Appendix 1

Comprehensive Psychopathological Rating Scale (Asberg et al., 1978)

Reported	Observed
Sadness	Apparent sadness
Elation	Elated mood
Hostile feelings	Hostility
Inability to feel	Labile emotional response
Pessimistic thoughts	Autonomic disturbances
Suicidal thoughts	Sleepiness
Hypochondriasis	Distractibility
Worrying over trifles	Withdrawal
Compulsive thoughts	Perplexity

Phobias
Rituals
Indecision
Lassitude
Fatiguability
Concentration difficulties
Failing memory
Reduced appetite
Reduced sleep
Increased sleep
Reduced sexual interest
Increased sexual movements
Autonomic disturbances
Aches and pains
Muscular tension
Loss of sensation or movement
Derealisation
Depersonalisation
Feeling controlled
Disrupted thoughts
Ideas of persecution
Ideas of grandeur
Delusional mood
Ecstatic experiences
Morbid jealousy
Other delusions
Commenting voices
Other auditory hallucinations
Visual hallucinations
Other hallucinations

Blank spells
Disorientation
Pressure of speech
Reduced speech
Specific speech deficits
Flight of ideas
Incoherent speech
Perseveration
Overactivity
Slowness of movement
Agitation
Involuntary movements
Muscular tension
Mannerisms and posture
Hallucinatory behaviour

Global rating of illness
Assumbed reliability of rating

References

Alzheimer A (1910–1911) Über eigenartige Krankheitsfälle des späteren Alters. Z Ges Neurol Psychiat 4: 356–385

APA (1994) Diagnostic and statistical manual of mental disorders, 4th edn. APA, Washington DC

Asberg M, Montgomery SC, Perris C, Schalling D, Sedvall G (1978) A comprehensive psychopathological rating scale. Acta Psychiatr Scand [Suppl] 271: 1–70

Bayles KA, Tomoeda CK, Kasniak AW, Trosset MW (1991) Alzheimer's disease effects on semantic memory: loss of structure or impaired processing. J Cogn Neurosci 3: 166–182

Berrios GE, Brook P (1985) Delusions and psychopathology of the elderly with dementia. Acta Psychiatr Scand 72: 296–301

Berthier ML, Leiguarda R, Starkstein SE, Sevlever G, Taratuto AL (1991) Alzheimer's disease in a patient with posterior cortical atrophy. J Neurol Neurosurg Psychiatry 54: 1110–1111

Braak H, Braak E (1991) Neuropathological staging of Alzheimer-related changes. Acta Neuropathol 82: 239–259

Brandt J, Rich JB (1994) Memory disorders in the dementias. In: Baddeley AD, Wilson BA, Watts F (eds) Handbook of memory disorders. Wiley, Chichester, pp 243–271

Brun A (1987) Frontal lobe degeneration of non-Alzheimer's type. I. Neuropathology. Arch Gerontol Geriatr 6: 209–233

Brun A, Englund B, Gustafson L, Passant U, Mann DMA Neary D, Snowden JS (1994) Consensus statement. Clinical and neuropathological criteria for frontotemporal dementia. Lund and Manchester groups. J Neurol Neurosurg Psychiatry 57: 416–418

Burns A, Jacoby R, Levy R (1990a) Psychiatric phenomena in Alzheimer's disease. I. Disorders of thought content. Br J Psychiatry 157: 72–76

Burns A, Jacoby R, Levy R (1990b) Psychiatric phenomena in Alzheimer's disease. II. Disorders of perception. Br J Psychiatry 157: 76–91

Chan AS, Butters N, Paulson JS, Salmon DP, Swenson M, Maloney L (1993) An assessment of the semantic network in patients with Alzheimer's disease. J Cogn Neurosci 5: 254–261

Chertkow H, Bub D (1990) Semantic memory loss in dementia of Alzheimer's type. Brain 113: 397–417

Cooper B (1991) The epidemiology of dementia. In: Jacoby R, Oppenheimer C (eds) Psychiatry in the elderly. Oxford University Press, Oxford, pp 574–585

Crystal HA, Horoupian DS, Katzman R, Jotkowitz S (1982) Biopsy-proved Alzheimer disease presenting as a right parietal lobe syndrome. Ann Neurol 12: 186–188

Cummings JL, Duchen LW (1981) Kluver-Bucy syndrome in Pick's disease: clinical and pathological correlations. Neurology 31: 1415–1422

Goldstein K, Katz SE (1937) The psychopathology of Pick's disease. Arch Neurol Psychiatry 38: 473–490

Grady CL, Haxby JV, Horwitz B, Sundaram M, Berg G, Schapiro M, Friedland RP, Rapoport SI (1988) Longitudinal study of the early neuropsychological and cerebral metabolic changes in dementia of the Alzheimer type. J Clin Exp Neuropsychol 10: 576–596

Green J, Morris JC, Sandson J, McKeel DW, Miller JW (1990) Progressive aphasia: a precursor of global dementia? Neurology 40: 423–429

Greene JDW, Hodges JR (1996) Identification of famous faces and famous names in early Alzheimer's disease: relationship to anterograde episodic and general semantic memory. Brain 119: 111–128

Greene JDW, Baddeley AD, Hodges JR (1995) Autobiographical memory and executive function in early dementia of Alzheimer type. Neuropsychologia 33: 1647–1670

Greene JDW, Hodges JR, Baddeley AD (1996) Recall and recognition of verbal and nonverbal material in early Alzheimer's disease: applications of the Doors and People Test. Neuropsychologia (in press)

Greene JDW, Miles K, Hodges JR (1996) The use of neuropsychology and SPECT imaging in diagnosis and staging dementia of Alzheimer type. J Neurol 243: 175–190

Greene JDW, Patterson K, Xuereb J, Hodges JR (1996) Alzheimer's disease presenting with nonfluent progressive aphasia. Arch Neurol (in press)

Gregory CA, Hodges JR (1993) Dementia of frontal type and the focal lobar atrophies. Int Rev Psychiatry 5: 397–406

Gregory CA, Hodges JR (1996) Dementia of frontal type: use of consensus criteria and prevalence of psychiatric features. Neuropsychiatry Neuropsychol Behav Neurol (in press)

Gustafson L (1987) Frontal lobe degeneration of non-Alzheimer type. II. Clinical picture and differential diagnosis. Arch Gerontol Geriatr 6: 209–233

Gustafson L, Nilsson L (1982) Differential diagnosis of presenile dementia on clinical grounds. Acta Psychiatr Scand 65: 194–209

Hart S (1988) Language and dementia: a review. Psychol Med 18: 99–112

Heindel WC, Salmon DP, Butters N (1993) Cognitive approaches to the memory disorders of demented patients. In: Sutker PB, Adams HE (eds) Comprehensive handbook of psychopathology. Plenum Press, New York, pp 735–761

Hodges JR (1994) Pick's disease. In: Burns A, Levy R (eds) Dementia. Chapman and Hall, London, pp 739–752

Hodges JR, Patterson K (1995) Is semantic memory consistently impaired early in the course of Alzheimer's disease? Neuroanatomical and diagnostic implications. Neuropsychologia 33: 441–459

Hodges JR, Ratterson K, Oxbury S, Funnell E (1992a) Semantic dementia; progressive fluent aphasia with temporal lobe atrophy. Brain 115: 1783–1806

Hodges JR, Salmon DP, Butters N (1992b) Semantic memory impairment in Alzheimer's disease: failure of access or degraded knowledge? Neuropsychologia 30: 310–314

Hof PR, Bouras C, Constantinidis J, Morrison JH (1990) Selective disconnection of specific visual association pathways in cases of Alzheimer's disease presenting with Balint's syndrome. J Neuropathol Exp Neurol 49: 168–184

Jorm AF, Korten E, Henderson AS (1987) The prevalence of dementia; a quantitative integration of the literature. Acta Psychiatr Scand 76: 465–479

Kaskie B, Storandt M (1995) Visuospatial deficit in dementia of Alzheimer type. Arch Neurol 52: 422–425

Kempler D, Metter EJ, Riege WH, Jackson CA, Benson DF, Hanson WR (1990) Slowly progressive aphasia: three cases with language, memory, CT and PET data. J Neurol Neurosurg Psychiatry 53: 987–993

Knopman DS, Christensen KJ, Schut LJ, Harbaugh RE, Reeder RN, Ngo T, Frey W (1989) The spectrum of imaging and neuropsychological findings in Pick's disease. Neurology 39: 362–368

Knopman DS, Mastri AR, Frey WH, Sung JH, Rustan T (1990) Dementia lacking distinctive histological features: a common non-Alzheimer degenerative disease. Neurology 40: 251–256

Kopelman MD (1985) Rates of forgetting in Alzheimer-type dementia and Korsakoff's syndrome. Neuropsychologia 23: 623–638

Kopelman MD (1989) Remote and autobiographical memory, temporal context memory and frontal atrophy in Korsakoff and Alzheimer patients. Neuropsychologia 27: 437–460

Martin A, Brouwers P, Cox C, Fedio P (1985) On the nature of the verbal memory deficit in Alzheimer's disease. Brain Lang 25: 323–341

McKhann G, Drachman D, Folstein M, Katzman R, Price D, Stradlan EM (1984) Clinical diagnosis of Alzheimer's disease. Neurology 34: 939–944

Mendez MF, Mendez MA, Martin R, Smyth KA, Whitehouse PJ (1990) Complex visual disturbances in Alzheimer's disease. Neurology 40: 439–443

Mendez MF, Selwood A, Mastri AR, Frey WH (1993) Pick's disease versus Alzheimer's disease: a comparison of clinical characteristics. Neurology 43: 289–292

Miller BL, Cummings JL, Villanueva-Meyer J, Boone K, Mehringer CM, Lesser IM, Mena I (1991) Frontal lobe degeneration: clinical, neuropsychological, and SPECT characteristics. Neurology 41: 1374–1382

Monsch AU, Bondi MW, Butters N, Pauslen JS, Salmon DP, Brugger P, Swenson MR (1994) A comparison of category and letter fluency in Alzheimer's disease and Huntington's disease. Neuropsychologia 8: 25–30

Morris J, McKeel DWJ, Fulling K, Torack RM, Berg L (1988) Validation of clinical diagnostic criteria for Alzheimer's disease. Ann Neurol 24: 17–22

Neary D, Snowden JS, Bowen DM, Sims NR, Mann DMA, Benton JS, Northen, B, Yates PO, Davison AN (1986) Neuropsychological syndromes in presenile dementia due to cerebral atrophy. J Neurol Neurosurg Psychiatry 49: 163–174

Neary D, Snowden JS, Mann DMA (1993) The clinical pathological correlates of lobar atrophy. Dementia 4: 154–159

Neary D, Snowden JS, Northen B, Goulding P (1988) Dementia of frontal lobe type. J Neurol Neurosurg Psychiatry 51: 353–361

Neary D, Snowden JS, Shields RA, Burjan AWI, Northen B, MacDermott N, Prescott MC, Testa HJ (1987) Single photon emission tomography using 99mTc-HM-PAO in the investigation of dementia. J Neurol Neurosurg Psychiatry 50: 1101–1109

Nebes RB (1989) Semantic memory in Alzheimer's disease. Psychol Bull 106: 377–394

Patterson K, Graham N, Hodges J (1994) Reading in Alzheimer's type dementia: a preserved ability? Neuropsychologia 8: 395–407

Pick A (1892) Über die Beziehungen der senilen Hirnatrophie zur Aphasie. Prag Med Wochenschr 17: 165–167

Pick A (1906) Über einen weiteren Symptomenkomplex im Rahmen der Dementia senilis, bedingt durch umschriebene stärkere Hirnatrophie (gemische Apraxie). Mschr Psychiat Neurol 19: 97–108

Pogacar S, Williams RS (1984) Alzheimer's disease presenting as slowly progressive aphasia. Rhode Island Med J 67: 181–185

Rapcsak SZ, Croswell SC, Rubens A (1989) Apraxia in Alzheimer's disease. Neurology 39: 664–668

Robertson EE, Le Roux A, Brown JH (1958) The clinical differentiation of Pick's disease. J Ment Sci 104: 1000–1024

Rosser A, Hodges JR (1994) Initial letter and semantic category fluency in Alzheimer's disease, Huntington's disease and progressive supranuclear palsy. J Neurol Neurosurg Psychiatry 57: 1389–1394

Sagar HA, Cohen NJ, Sullivan EV, Corkin S, Growdon JH (1988) Remote memory function in Alzheimer's disease and Parkinson's disease. Brain 111: 185–206

Sartori G, Job R, Miozzo M, Zago S, Marchiori G (1993) Category-specific form-knowledge deficit in a patient with Herpes Simples virus encephalitis. J Clin Exp Neuropsychol 15: 280–299

Squire LR (1992) Memory and the hippocampus: a synthesis from findings with rats, monkeys, and humans. Psychol Rev 99: 195–231

Stengel E (1943) A study on the symptomatology and differential diagnosis of Alzheimer's disease and Pick's disease. J Ment Sci 539: 1–20

Thorpe FT (1932) Pick's disease (circumscribed senile atrophy) and Alzheimer's disease. J Ment Sci 78: 302–314

Tulving E (1987) Multiple memory systems and consciousness. Hum Neurobiol 6: 67–80

Vallar G, Papagno C (1995) Neuropsycholigical impairments of shortterm memory. In: Baddeley AD, Wilson BA, Watts FN (eds) Handbook of memory disorders. Wiley, Chichester, pp 135–165

Warrington EK, Shallice T (1984) Category specific semantic impairments. Brain 107: 829–854

Welsh K, Butters N, Hughes J, Mohs R, Heyman A (1991) Detection of abnormal memory decline in mild cases of Alzheimer's disease using CERAD neuropsychological measures. Arch Neurol 48: 278–281

Welsh KA, Butters N, Hughes JP, Mohs RC (1992) Detection and staging of dementia in Alzheimer's disease: use of the neuropsychological measures developed for the Consortium to Establish a Registry for Alzheimer's disease. Arch Neurol 49: 448–452

Wragg RE, Jeste DV (1989) Overview of depression and psychosis in Alzheimer's disease. Am J Psychiatry 146: 577–587

Authors' address: Dr. J. R. Hodges, Addenbrooke's Hospital, Box 165, Hills Road, Cambridge CB2 2QQ, United Kingdom.

J Neural Transm (1996) [Suppl] 47: 125–132

Frontal lobe dementia and motor neuron disease

P. R. Talbot

Cerebral Function Unit, Department of Neurology, The Royal Infirmary,
Manchester, United Kingdom

Summary. Frontal lobe dementia (FLD) (syn. frontotemporal dementia and dementia of frontal type) is a generic term that describes a clinical syndrome in which patients manifest a profound breakdown in personality and social conduct, together with adynamic spontaneous speech, culminating in mutism. This pattern of cognitive impairment implicates bilateral frontal lobe dysfunction, an assumption supported by functional neuroimaging findings of anterior cerebral abnormality.

Patients with FLD can go on to develop motor neuron disease (FLD-MND), although the clinical features of MND may accompany or occasionally precede the onset of dementia. The emergence of MND is responsible for death within 3 years of onset. Frontotemporal lobar pathology in FLD-MND is characterized by loss of large cortical neurons, spongiform change and mild astrocytic gliosis. Ubiquitinated (but not tau-positive) inclusions are present within the frontal cortex. There is severe nigral cell loss (without Lewy bodies), and marked hypoglossal and spinal motor neuron degeneration, together with ubiquitinated (but not tau-positive) inclusions within the spinal neurons. Some authors suggest that FLD-MND is a separate disease entity, whereas others suggest it represents an interface between FLD and "classic" (non-dementing) motor neuron disease (CMND). An association with CMND is supported by findings in these patients of failure in tasks sensitive to "frontal lobe" dysfunction, and patterns of functional neuroimaging abnormality which are identical in distribution, but less severe than those encountered in FLD-MND. However, the nosological status of FLD-MND remains enigmatic in the absence of defined pathological and molecular markers.

Introduction

Over recent years, an association between frontal lobe dementia and motor neuron disease (FLD-MND) has been increasingly recognized (Mitsuyama et al., 1979, 1984, 1993; Hudson, 1981; Morita et al., 1987; Neary et al., 1990). However, the nosological status of this disorder remains a matter of controversy. Whereas some authors suggest that FLD-MND is a separate disease entity (Morita et al., 1987; Mitsuyama et al., 1993), others suggest it represents an interface between frontal lobe dementia (FLD) and "classic" (non-dementing) motor neuron disease (CMND) (Hudson, 1981; Neary et al., 1990). In order to address these nosological issues, the following review summarizes the clinical, functional neuroimaging and pathological findings in patients with FLD-MND, and compares findings to those of patients with FLD alone and those with CMND.

Frontal lobe dementia-motor neuron disease

Clinical features

Frontal lobe dementia-motor neuron disease (FLD-MND) is a rare disorder which is usually sporadic in nature, but can be familial (Neary et al., 1990; Mitsuyama et al., 1993). Men appear to be affected slightly more often than women. The mean age of onset is 55 years, and duration of illness is usually less than 3 years.

The disorder usually presents as a profound breakdown in personality and social conduct (Neary et al., 1990). Initial behavioural change comprises a spectrum with disinhibition, overactivity and inappropriate affect contrasting with an apathetic inert state. With disease progression, patients manifesting disinhibition and restlessness become increasingly apathetic and inert, but not *vice versa*. In additional to motor preserverations of an elementary type, stereotypic behaviour and repetitive rituals of hoarding, dressing, wandering and toileting are seen. Patients over-eat, exhibit hyperoral tendencies and develop food fads. Spontaneous speech is adynamic in type, culminating in mutism but frank dysphasic errors of a phonological or semantic type are usually absent. Visuospatial and executive skills are maintained throughout the illness and memory performance is variable. This pattern of neuropsychological breakdown implicates bilateral frontal lobe dysfunction, an assumption supported by functional neuroimaging findings of anterior cerebral abnormality (Fig. 1) (Neary et al., 1990; Mitsuyama et al., 1993; Talbot et al., 1995).

Clinical signs of motor neuron involvement usually follow, but may accompany (or occasionally precede) the onset of dementia (Mitsuyama et al., 1993). MND usually manifests with muscular weakness, wasting and fasciculation in the upper and lower limbs, together with progressive bulbar palsy. Signs of upper motor neuron involvement are typically less prominent (Neary et al., 1990; Mitsuyama et al., 1993). Akinesia and rigidity may emerge in a minority of FLD-MND patients (Morita et al., 1987).

Pathological findings

There is a predominantly frontal and anterior temporal distribution of cerebral atrophy (Fig. 2) (Mann et al., 1993; Mann and South, 1993; Mitsuyama et al., 1993; Brun et al., 1994). The underlying histological changes are characterized by loss of large cortical neurons, spongiform change and mild astrocytic

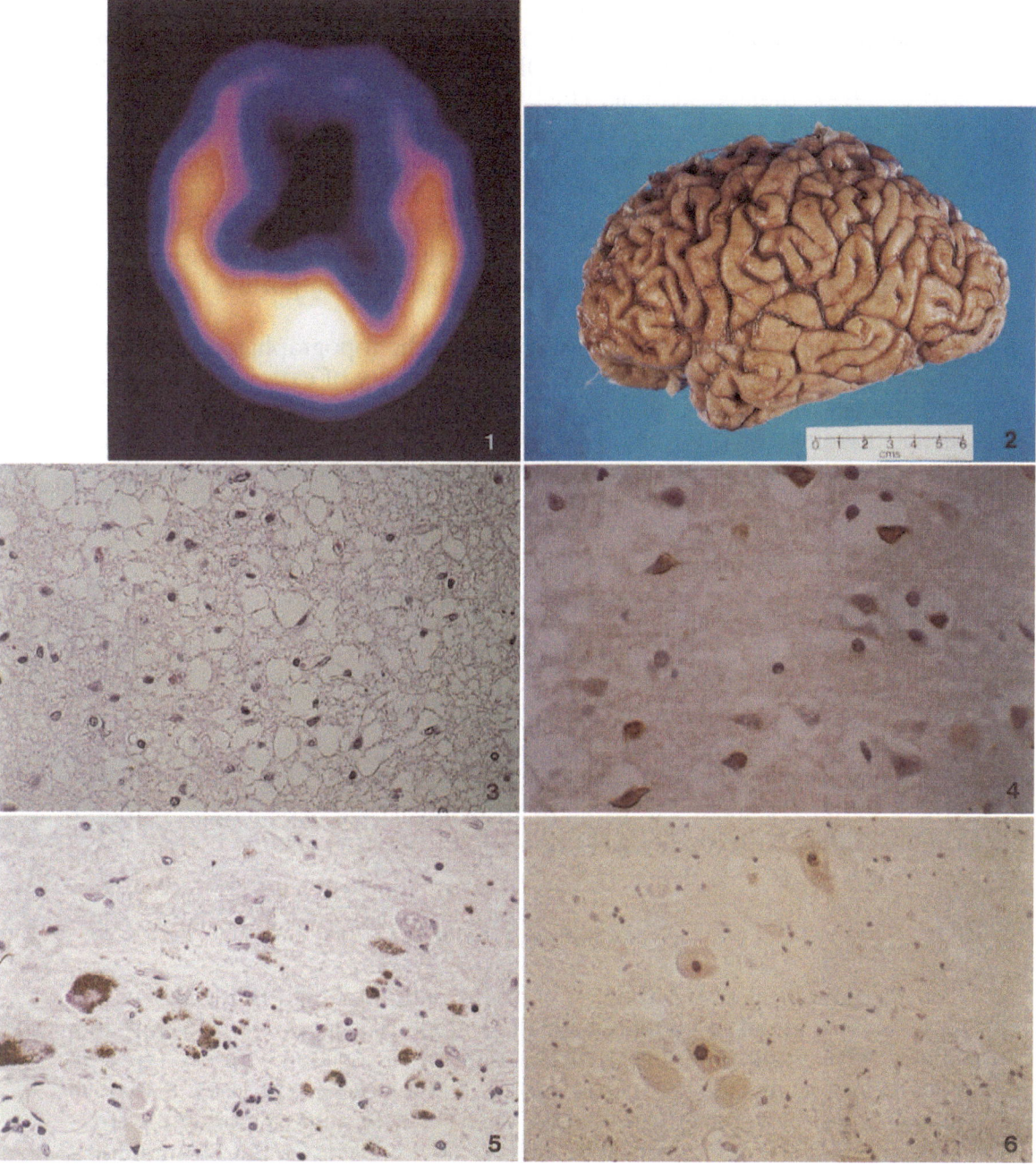

Fig. 1. Bilateral anterior cerebral abnormality in a patient with frontal lobe dementia-motor neuron disease (^{99m}Tc-HMPAO SPECT scan-transaxial section)

Fig. 2. Anterior cerebral atrophy (Lateral view of the brain of a patient with frontal lobe dementia-motor neuron disease)

Fig. 3. Spongiform change in layer II of the frontal cortex (frontal lobe dementia-motor neuron disease) (Haematoxylin-eosin × 200)

Fig. 4. Ubiquitinated intra-neuronal inclusions in layer II of the frontal cortex (frontal lobe dementia-motor neuron disease) (Anti-ubiquitin × 200)

Fig. 5. Loss and degeneration of nerve cells in substantia nigra (frontal lobe dementia-motor neuron disease) (Haematoxylin-eosin × 200)

Fig. 6. Ubiquitinated inclusions in the anterior horn cells of the spinal cord (frontal lobe dementia-motor neuron disease) (Anti-ubiquitin × 200)

gliosis (Fig. 3) (Mann et al., 1993; Mann and South, 1993). Ubiquitinated (but not tau-positive) inclusions are present within the frontal cortex (Fig. 4) and dentate gyrus of the hippocampus (Okamoto et al., 1992; Mann et al., 1993; Lowe, 1994). Inflated neurons (Pick cells) and inclusions which are both ubiquitin- *and* tau-positive (Pick bodies) are typically absent, although this is not invariably the case (Tissot et al., 1985). The Betz cells of the precentral gyrus are largely preserved in number and there is relatively little corticospinal tract involvement. However, there is severe nigral cell loss (without Lewy bodies) (Fig. 5), and marked hypoglossal and spinal motor neuron degeneration, together with ubiquitinated (but not tau-positive) inclusions within the spinal neurons (Fig. 6).

The clinical features of FLD-MND reflect the topographical distribution of cerebral pathology. However, the relative paucity of extrapyramidal signs in FLD-MND contrasts with the severe degree of nigral involvement. It seems likely, therefore, that the rapid progression of FLD-MND and early death pre-empts the emergence of such signs (Neary et al., 1990).

Frontal lobe dementia-motor neuron disease in relation to frontal lobe dementia alone

Clinical features

The pattern of neuropsychological breakdown encountered in FLD-MND is the same as that found in FLD alone (Gustafson, 1987; Neary et al., 1988; Gustafson, 1993; Brun et al., 1994). This observation is supported by ^{99m}Tc-HMPAO SPECT findings which show an identical pattern of anterior cerebral abnormality in both conditions (Talbot et al., 1995).

Pathological findings

The topographical distribution of cerebral pathology in FLD-MND is the same as that found in patients with FLD alone, but less severe (Mann and South, 1993; Mann et al., 1993). FLD is typically associated with two types of histological change (Brun et al., 1994). The commonest pathology is that of neuronal loss and spongiform change, together with mild to moderate astrocytic gliosis in the outer cortical layers (Fig. 7), and is designated frontal lobe degeneration (Brun et al., 1994). The latter term serves to distinguish histological changes from those characterized by intense astrocytic gliosis with or without tau- *and* ubiquitin-positive inclusion bodies (Pick bodies) (Fig. 8 and 9) and swollen neurons (Pick cells) (Fig. 10) (Brun et al., 1994).

Thus, the histological changes found in FLD-MND show similarities with those of frontal lobe degeneration. However, the presence of ubiquitinated (but not tau-positive) inclusions within frontal cortical neurons in FLD-MND appears to set this disorder apart, not only from frontal lobe degeneration, but also from Pick"s disease in which neuronal inclusions are both tau- *and*

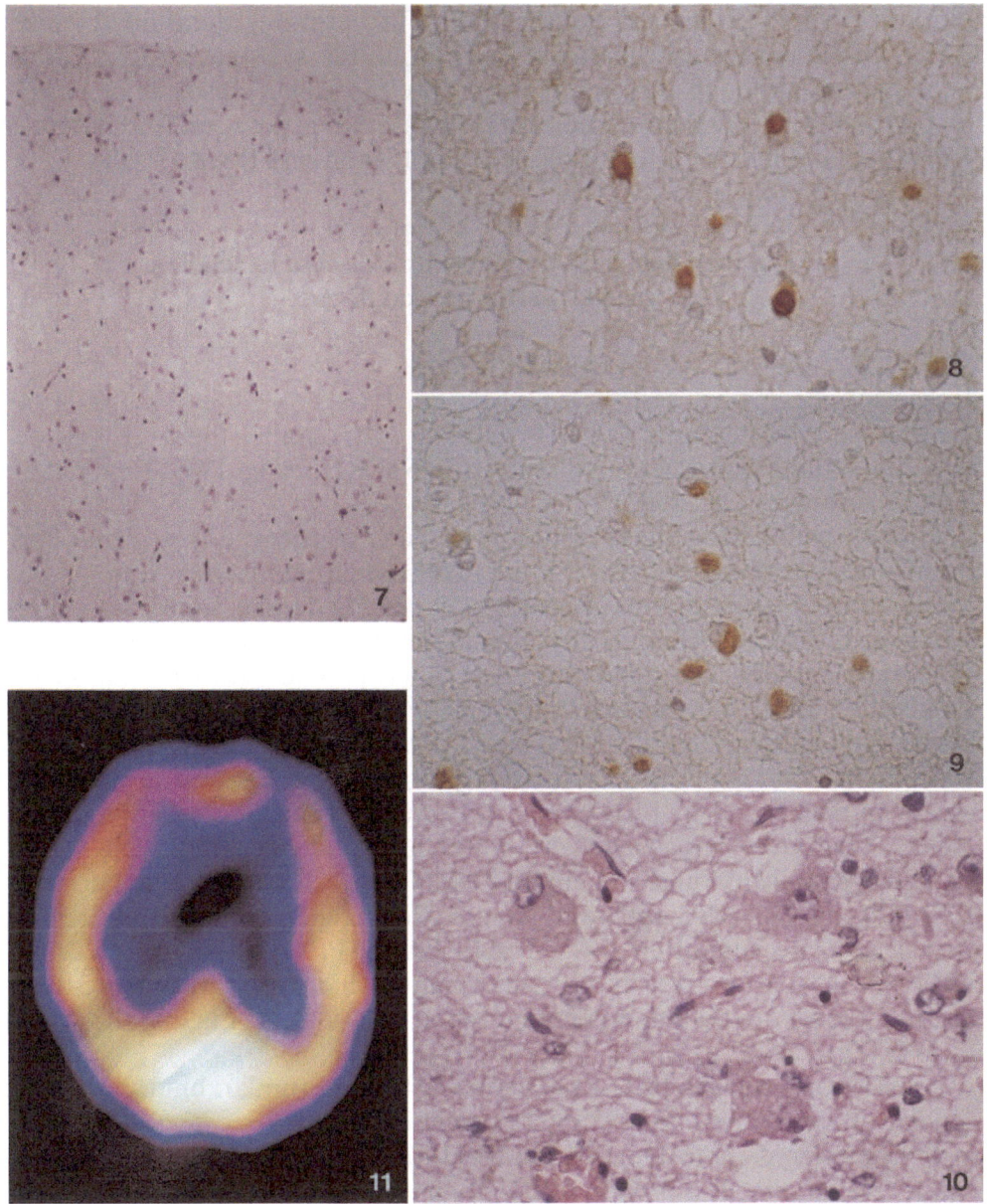

Fig. 7. Spongiform change in layer II of the frontal cortex (frontal lobe dementia) (Haematoxylin-eosin × 200)

Fig. 8. Pick bodies in the frontal cortex showing tau immunoreactivity (frontal lobe dementia) (Anti-tau × 400)

Fig. 9. Pick bodies in the frontal cortex showing ubiquitin immunoreactivity (frontal lobe dementia) (Anti-ubiquitin × 400)

Fig. 10. Pick cells in the frontal cortex (frontal lobe dementia) (Haematoxylin-eosin × 400)

Fig. 11. Bilateral anterior cerebral abnormality in a patient with "classic" non-dementing) motor neuron disease (^{99m}Tc-HMPAO SPECT scan-transaxial section)

ubiquitin-positive (Mann and South, 1993). Furthermore, nigral involvement in FLD-MND is severe, whereas in FLD alone the substantia nigra is relatively spared, although this is not invariably the case (Tissot et al., 1985). Hypoglosssal and spinal motor neuron degeneration is not usually a feature of FLD alone, but has been found on occasion (Mann and South, 1993).

Frontal lobe dementia-motor neuron disease in relation to "classic" motor neuron disease

Clinical features

The demographic features of FLD-MND closely parallel those of "classic" (non-dementing) motor neuron disease (CMND) (Hudson, 1981; Neary et al., 1990; Mitsuyama et al., 1993).

Patients with CMND have traditionally been considered free from cognitive impairment (Hudson, 1981). Evidence is emerging, however, to suggest that cognitive impairment may occur, albeit of mild degree, implicating more widespread cerebral abnormality extending beyond motor cortices and corticospinal tracts. The most consistent neuropsychological finding in patients with CMND is failure in tasks sensitive to "frontal lobe" dysfunction (David and Gillham, 1986; Ludolph et al., 1992; Kew et al., 1993; Talbot et al., 1995). Hence, the nature of cognitive impairment encountered in CMND is similar to that found in FLD-MND, differing only in degree. Whereas in CMND cognitive impairment is mild and evident only on formal neuropsychological evaluation, in FLD-MND psychological breakdown is profound and clinically apparent, manifesting as dementia. These clinical observations are supported by ^{99m}Tc-HMPAO SPECT findings in CMND which reveal a pattern of cerebral abnormality which is identical in distribution, but less severe than that encountered in FLD-MND (Fig. 11) (Talbot et al., 1995).

Neurological signs in FLD-MND and CMND are similar, but they are not identical. Whereas muscle wasting, fasciculation and bulbar involvement are usually prominent clinical features in FLD-MND, signs of upper motor neuron involvement are less pronounced than in CMND (Mitsuyama et al., 1993).

Pathological findings

The topographical distribution of cerebral pathology in CMND has similarities with that found in patients with FLD-MID. In CMND, anterior cerebral involvement is relatively mild and encountered in only a minority of patients (Hudson, 1981), whereas in FLD-MND, frontotemporal lobar pathology is profound. Substantia nigra degeneration (without Lewy bodies) is a feature of CMND (Burrow and Blumbergs, 1992), but to a lesser degree compared to that found in FLD-MND (Neary et al., 1990). Hypoglossal and spinal motor neuron degeneration is a feature of both conditions, whereas motor cortex and corticospinal tract involvement in FLD-MND is relatively mild in comparison to that found in CMND. Ubiquitinated (but not tau-positive) inclusions are present in the spinal neurons of both conditions (Mann et al., 1993; Okamoto et al., 1992), which are similar to those found in the frontal cortical neurons of patients with FLD-MND (Okamoto et al., 1992; Mann et al., 1993).

Conclusion

FLD-MND shares similarities with both FLD and CMND with regard to clinical features, demographic characteristics, functional neuroimaging findings and pathology. All three disorders share a common pattern of cognitive impairment implicating bilateral frontal lobe dysfunction. This is reflected in the findings of functional neuroimaging which reveal an identical pattern of anterior cerebral abnormality in all three conditions. Histological findings of ubiquitinated (but not tau-positive) inclusions in the frontal cortex of patients with FLD-MND provide support for a link with CMND, but appear to separate FLD-MND from FLD. However, it is possible that the histological features associated in these disorders represent stages in, rather than departures from, a common disease process. Overall, clinical, demographic, functional neuroimaging and pathological findings provide support for the concept that FLD, FLD-MND, and CMND represent overlapping clinical manifestations of a multi-system disorder, the nature of which is dictated by the topographical distribution of cerebral pathology. However, further work is required before it is possible to "lump" or "split" these disorders on a more rational basis. In the meantime, the nosological status of FLD-MND remains enigmatic in the absence of defined pathological and molecular markers.

Acknowledgement

I wish to thank Dr. D. Mann for providing the pathology illustrations.

References

Burrow JN, Blumbergs PC (1992) Substantia nigra degeneration in motor neuron disease: a quantitative study. Aust NZ J Med 22: 469–472

Brun A, England B, Gustafson L, Passant U, Mann DMA, Neary D, Snowden JS (1994) Clinical and neuropathological criteria for frontotemporal dementia. J Neurol Neurosurg Psychiatry 57: 416–418

David AS, Gillham RA (1986) Neuropsychological study of motor neuron disease. Psychosomatics 27: 441–445

Gustafson L (1987) Frontal lobe degeneration of non-Alzheimer type. II. Clinical picture and differential diagnosis. Arch Gerontol Geriatr 6: 193–208

Gustafson L (1993) Clinical picture of frontal lobe degeneration of non-Alzheimer type. Dementia 4: 143–148

Hudson AJ (1981) Amyotrophic lateral sclerosis and its association with dementia, parkinsonism and other neurological disorders: a review. Brain 104: 217–247

Kew JJM, Leigh PN, Playford ED, Passingham RE, Goldstein LH, Frackowiak RSJ, Brooks DJ (1993) Cortical function in amyotrophic lateral sclerosis: a positron emission study. Brain 116: 655–680

Lowe J (1994) New pathological findings in amyotrophic lateral sclerosis. J Neurol 124: 38–51

Ludolph AC, Langen KJ, Regard M (1992) Frontal lobe function in amyotrophic lateral sclerosis: a neuropsychologic and positron emission tomography study. Acta Neurol Scand 85: 81–89

Mann DMA, South PW (1993) The topographical distribution of brain atrophy in frontal lobe dementia. Acta Neuropathol 85: 334–340

Mann DMA, South PW, Snowden JS, Neary D (1993) Dementia of frontal lobe type: neuropathology and immunohistochemistry. J Neurol Neurosurg Psychiatry 56: 605–614

Miller BL, Cummings JL, Villanueva-Meyer J, Boone K, Mehringer CM, Lesser IM, Mena I (1991) Frontal lobe degeneration: clinical, neuropsychological, and SPECT characteristics. Neurology 41: 1374–1382

Mitsuyama Y, Takamiya S (1979) Presenile dementia with motor neuron disease in Japan. A new entity? Arch Neurol 36: 592–593

Mitsuyama Y (1984) Presenile dementia with motor neuron disease in Japan: clinico-pathological review of 26 cases. J Neurol Neurosurg Psychiatry 47: 953–959

Mitsuyama Y (1993) Presenile dementia with motor neuron disease. Dementia 4: 137–142

Morita K, Kaiya H, Ikeda T, Namba M (1987) Presenile dementia combined with amyotrophy: a review of 34 Japanese cases. Arch Gerontol Geriatr 6: 263–246

Neary D, Snowden JS, Shields RA, Burjan AWI, Northen B, MacDermott N, Prescott MC, Testa HJ (1987) Single photon emission tomography using ^{99m}Tc-HM-PAO in the investigation of dementia. J Neurol Neurosurg Psychiatry 50: 1101–1109

Neary D, Snowden JS, Northen B, Goulding P (1989) Dementia of frontal lobe type. J Neurol Neurosurg Psychiatry 51: 353–361

Neary D, Snowden JS, Mann DMA, Northen B, Goulding PJ, Macdermott N (1990) Frontal lobe dementia and motor neuron disease. J Neurol Neurosurg Psychiatry 53: 23–32

Okamoto K, Murakami N, Yoshida H, Hashizume M, Nakazato Y, Matsubara E, Hirai S (1992) Ubiquitin-positive intraneuronal inclusions in the extramotor cortices of presenile dementia patients with motor neuron disease. J Neurol 239: 426–430

Starkstein SE, Migliorelli R, Teson A, Sabe L, Vascuez S, Turjanski M, Robinson RG, Leiguarda R (1994) Specificity of changes in cerebral blood flow in patients with frontal lobe dementia. J Neurol Neurosurg Psychiatry 57: 790–796

Talbot PR, Goulding PJ, Lloyd JJ, Snowden JS, Neary D, Testa HJ (1995) Inter-relation between "classic" motor neuron disease and frontotemporal dementia: neuropsychological and single photon emission computed tomography study. J Neurol Neurosurg Psychiatry 58: 541–547

Tissot R, Constantinidis J, Richard J (1985) Pick"s disease. Handb Clin Neurol 2: 233–245

Authors' address: Dr. P. R. Talbot, Cerebral Function Unit, Department of Neurology, Manchester Royal Infirmary, Manchester M13 9WL, United Kingdom.

J Neural Transm (1996) [Suppl] 47: 133–141

Clinical and pathological characteristics of primary progressive aphasia and frontal dementia

A. Kertesz[1] and **D. Munoz**[2]

[1]Department of Clinical Neurological Sciences, St. Joseph's Health Centre, University of Western Ontario, and [2]Department of Pathology, Division of Neuropathology, University of Western Ontario, London, Ontario, Canada

Summary. The recently described conditions of primary progressive aphasia and frontal lobe dementia overlap clinically and pathologically to a considerable extent with each other and with clinical and pathological descriptions of Pick's disease. Our clinical and neuropathological experience is summarized, leading us to the conclusion that the degree of overlap justifies the concept of "Pick complex" to include, in addition to the above, corticobasal ganglionic degeneration and some instances motor neuron disease with dementia.

Introduction

Arnold Pick's (1892) report of a patient with progressive aphasia became the basis of the concept of Pick's disease (PD). He concluded, "a more or less circumscribed type of aphasia could result from a single circumscribed atrophic process" and established the concept of focal atrophy causing a specific behavioral syndrome. Some subsequent descriptions of PD emphasized aphasia (Caron, 1934; Lüers, 1947), while others considered the progressive loss of fluency leading to mutism, a nonaphasic phenomenon (Tissot et al., 1985) and this found its way to the DSM-III-R (1987) definition of PD. Other cases of progressive aphasia without widespread dementia were also described to have PD (Rosenfeld, 1909; Wechsler, 1977; Holland et al., 1985). A series of six patients with progressive language disorder without additional intellectual or behavioral disturbances was reported and named "primary progressive aphasia" (PPA) (Mesulam, 1982, 1987). A cortical biopsy in one case of PPA showed nonspecific findings, consisting of gliosis, neuronal loss and spongiform degeneration mainly in layer II of the frontotemporal cortex. These features were found in other cases of PPA as well. Subsequently, more specific abnormalities were described, such as neuronal achromasia in ballooned cells containing phosphorylated neurofilament epitopes (Lippa et al., 1991; Kertesz et al., 1994). Similar pathology, including neuronal achromasia was described in PD, corticonigral or corticobasal degeneration (CBD)

(Rebeiz et al., 1968; Riley et al., 1990; Thompson and Marsden, 1992), and frontal lobe dementia (FLD) (Brun, 1987).

Two European centres have recently described FLD as an important and relatively frequent entity, distinct from Alzheimer's disease (AD). Although the groups from Lund and Manchester (1994) acknowledged that it clinically resembled PD, they considered the pathology different. The Manchester group studied biopsy material (Neary et al., 1986), and the Lund group (Brun, 1987; Gustafson, 1987) a large series of autopsied patients from a psychiatric institution. Reports of neuronal loss, gliosis, superficial spongiosis, and the occasional ballooned cells (Pick cells) resembled many of the pathological descriptions of PPA, but also variants of PD (Constantinidis, 1974). Both groups observed a clinical picture dominated by personality change, apathy, lack of insight, and various forms of disinhibition. A progressive anomia and adynamic aphasia ending in mutism was often described in the cases published as examples. Memory and spatial functions were comparatively spared. Positive family history for dementia was reported in 50% of the cases compared with 30% of the AD reference group. They promoted the idea of FLD being a distinct entity, suggesting a profound failure of frontal lobe tests without severe amnesia, aphasia or perceptual spatial disorder was diagnostic of the profile (Lund/Manchester group, 1994). Subsequently, case reports began to appear elsewhere in the literature. Neuroimaging studies with CT, MRI, and SPECT scans were considered confirmatory and in some series played an important role in the selection of patients (Neary et al., 1987; Jagust et al., 1989; Miller et al., 1991; Starkstein et al., 1994). It has also been recognized that some cases of dementia described with motor neuron disease (MND) resemble FLD more than AD. Several series of cases of combined FLD and MND (Neary et al., 1990), and PPA and MND appeared (Caselli et al., 1993). The clinical and pathological overlap between frontotemporal dementia and CBD and PD has been also increasingly recognized (Kosaka et al., 1991; Lang et al., 1994; Rinne et al., 1994).

Clinical features of PPA

We initially reported a 10% incidence of prominent aphasic presentation in a dementia clinic (Kertesz et al., 1986). Since our published series of 10 patients with probable PPA (Karbe et al., 1993) and 3 cases of pathologically examined cases (Kertesz et al., 1994), we have examined 34 patients with this entity. This group of patients was seen in a cognitive neurology clinic from a population of 360 patients with a comprehensive clinical, neuropsychological and imaging assessment. We made a distinction of possible and probable cases of PPA because aphasia is common in AD and differentiation from PPA can be problematic. Case descriptions of PPA have been variable in the literature. Mesulam's suggested guidelines of progressive aphasia for two years without other cognitive domains being involved are only relative, and the interpretation of symptoms such as early forgetfulness that often reflects early anomia are problematic. The variable extent to which other cognitive domains are examined is difficult to standardize. Nevertheless, we used those guidelines to identify probable cases of PPA. We also used a neuroimaging confirmation and longitudinal follow-up to establish the diagnosis in these individuals. We considered those cases who had a logopenic, anomic toward nonfluent aphasic presentation for several years before other cognitive domains were involved as "probable PPA." Cases who had a fluent paraphasic aphasia with significant comprehension difficulty (Wernicke's aphasia), or transcortical sensory aphasia (also described as "semantic aphasia") or only anomia were considered as possible PPA. Patients whose history suggested memory loss simultaneously with aphasia at the onset are only placed in the possible PPA category if their aphasia is prominent, progressive, and their behavior and nonverbal performance are relatively intact, otherwise they are considered probable AD with aphasia.

In the course of the follow-up of these patients one of the pathologically examined cases was observed to have motor neuron disease (Kertesz et al., 1994) and two others had prominent dysphagia, without any other manifestations of motor neuron disease. Limb and verbal apraxia was prominent in 8 cases, and verbal apraxia with stuttering behavior was striking at early stages in 3 others. Some degree of verbal apraxia or articulatory dysfunction tends to occur in the majority of the nonfluent cases with increasing severity as the disease progresses.

Neuroimaging often showed striking asymmetrical, usually left temporal, central parietal and ventricular atrophy (Fig. 1). At times, mostly temporal or central atrophy is seen selectively affecting the language areas (Fig. 2).

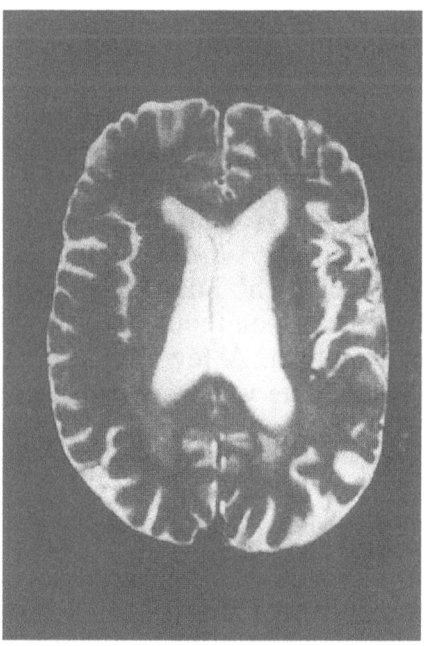

Fig. 1. Ventricular and sulcal asymmetry in a typical case of primary progressive aphasia with anomic, logopenic presentation

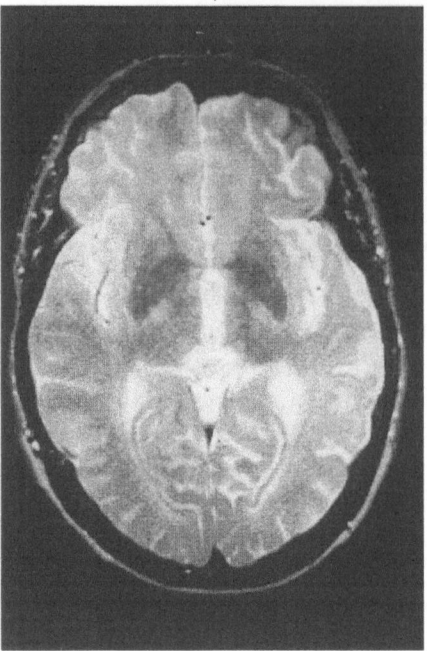

Fig. 2. Predominantly temporal atrophy in a case of primary progressive aphasia. Asymmetry of inferior frontal and occipital sulci is also noticeable

Patients with possible PPA have a lesser degree of asymmetrical atrophy. Neuropsychological testing in the early cases showed only articulatory language difficulties (reading and writing were also affected) with preservation of memory, although construction was involved at early times.

At later stages, a number of the PPA patients develop with behavioral changes indicative of FLD. Apathy, and irritability were common, but these findings are not very specific and can be seen, of course, in other dementias. One of the pathologically examined patients received psychiatric treatment for a combination of depression and uncharacteristic aggression toward his wife, while another one developed classical "utilization behavior", or "hypermetamorphosis" picking up stones and other objects in the street. Eventually, many PPA patients who initially were quite intact, except their language, became unable to carry on their daily activities because of increasingly severe apraxia, and mutism. A few others developed extrapyramidal symptoms, including two patients with asymmetrical rigidity, suggesting an overlap with CBD.

Clinical features of FLD

We also had experience with 12 cases of frontal lobe dementia presenting characteristically with alterations of behavior and personality. Some of these early changes were very disturbing to the families, but not usually to the patient, since they uniformly lacked insight. Erratic driving, impulsive spending of money, disinhibited, socially inappropriate behavior, aggression, perseveration, overeating were dramatic symptoms bringing the patients to the psychiatrist, or to our cognitive and behavioral neurology clinic. Other patients had apathy, aspontaneity, and social withdrawal and were treated for depression unsuccessfully. Logopenia and anomia were common and one patient became mute shortly after the development of irritability and aggression, and really represent a transitory form of FLD and PPA. One of the FLD cases also developed classical motor neuron disease and his decline was more rapid. Another case with pathological confirmation also had terminal rigidity. Both these groups were younger than AD controls, in particular the FLD patients.

In an effort to quantitate the behavioral symptoms and to operationalize diagnostic criteria, we constructed a Frontal Behavioral Inventory (FBl) (Kertesz et al., 1995) selecting items from our experience and the Lund/Manchester consensus (1994). Caregivers were asked about 24 behaviors, 12 negative items of some deficiency of behavior and 12 positive items of some excess of behavior (disinhibition phenomenon). This frontal behavioral inventory distinguished FLD patients with a high degree of specificity from Alzheimer patients (100%) at a similar duration of illness, and from patients with depressive dementia. Only 2/12 patients with manic depressive illness had borderline high scores overlapping with two of the FLD patients. Patients obtaining scores above 29 on the FBI all had FLD and all FLD patients had scores above 27. We consider these scores on the brief FBI (average administration — 15 minutes) diagnostic and part of our operational criteria of FLD. Other criteria require the exclusion of depression and vascular disease, par-

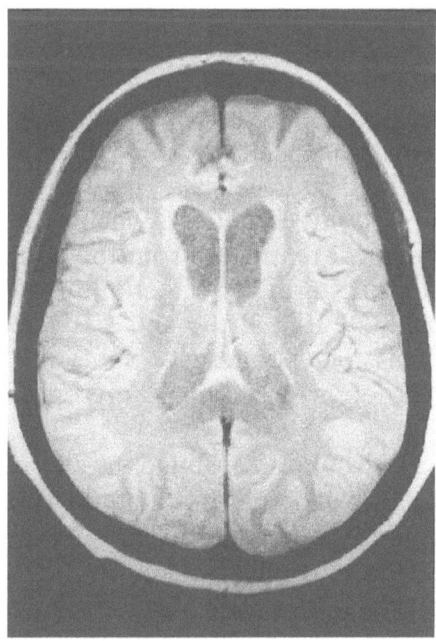

Fig. 3. Atrophy of frontal horns and frontopolar cortex in a patient with apathy — disinhibition type of frontal dementia. Memory and language are preserved

ticularly subcortical, frontal, arteriosclerotic encephalopathy (Binswanger's disease). This is usually accomplished by CT or MRI. An example of frontal atrophy confirming frontal lobe dementia is shown in Fig. 3.

Pathological features of PPA and FLD

The pathological changes in PPA and FLD were quite similar and also resembled the description of the cortical changes in CBD (Rebeiz et al., 1968; Riley et al., 1990). The cortical atrophy may not be as marked as in PD. In PPA, it may be restricted to the dominant frontotemporal region. In FLD it may be bilateral or nondominant frontal lobe only. The cortical atrophy in CBD tends to be frontoparietal, often asymmetrical (Thompson and Marsden, 1992).

Microscopically, in addition to neuronal loss, gliosis, and superficial cortical spongiosis, there are scattered ballooned, achromatic neurons, best identified by the use of antibodies to phosphorylated neurofilaments (Lippa et al., 1991; Kertesz et al., 1994). Several, but not all cases, demonstrate neuronal cytoplasmic argyrophilic inclusions of somewhat irregular shape, contrasting with the perfect roundness of the inclusions of classical PD. Furthermore, most cases of PPA and FLD do not show Pick bodies in dentate granular cells or hippocampal pyramidal neurons. A common feature of our PPA cases was the expression of tau immunoreactivity in glial cells. In the neocortex, this takes the form of "glial plaques" associated with astrocytes, whereas in the white matter the expression of tau occurs predominantly in oligodendrocytes. Unlike the oligodendroglial inclusions of multiple system atrophy those in PPA are not detectable on H & E sections. Finally, argyrophilic grains, described by Braak and Braak (1989) are present in the hippocampus in all cases.

Other entities, described under various terminologies, such as Hereditary dysphasic dementia (Morris et al., 1984) and "Dementia lacking distinctive histological features" (Knopman et al., 1990), Disinhibition, dementia, parkinsonism, and amyotrophy complex (Lynch et al., 1994) seem to have similar pathology and clinical features. From these clinical and pathological similarities, we suggested the term, "Pick complex" to recognize its relationship to PD and to include FLD, PPA, and CBD in a spectrum with PD (Kertesz et al., 1994). This allows to reserve the term "Pick's disease" for the pathologically proven variety with globular argyrophilic inclusion and severe lobar atrophy.

The concept of focal atrophies causing a variety of progressive cognitive and behavioral syndromes, which has originated with Arnold Pick (1892), is becoming increasingly important again. Frontotemporal atrophy or FLD and PPA are examples of focal atrophies which are likely associated with Pick complex or PD. Since classical PD is a relatively infrequent pathological finding, the often retrospective clinical description of PD has been variable, influenced by chance observations of patients having atrophy in one or other cortical locations. Focal frontal atrophy bilaterally would likely produce a clinical phenotype of frontal lobe dementia. Progressive aphasic disturbance would be prominent with dominant hemisphere frontotemporal atrophy. Right frontotemporal atrophy is less frequently described than the left sided one, but this may be related to a case finding bias due to the dramatic aphasic symptomatology. Recent studies show the same pathology can be found with progressive dominant hemisphere temporoparietal atrophy producing the picture of "semantic aphasia" (Snowden et al., 1992; Hodges et al., 1992). Descriptions of posterior cortical atrophy (Benson et al., 1988) and right focal parietal atrophy have less specific pathology and they have not been described with Pick complex or Pick's disease yet. Alzheimer's disease (Pogacar and Williams, 1984; Tariska, 1970) and Creutzfeldt-Jakob disease (Mandell et al., 1989) has been described as having focal presentation, such as PPA. However, Pogacar and Williams' case had concomittant early memory change and this does not fit the strict criteria of PPA. Some of the cases of Creutzfeldt-Jakob disease with PPA may have had Pick variant pathology, similar to one of our cases of FLD published previously, as a case of familial spongiform encephalopathy (Rice et al., 1980). However, prion proteins were not found, and a recent review of the pathology with modern histochemistry in this case also revealed Pick complex. Other cases reported as AD with PPA had only senile plaques and no neurofibrillary tangles, and the neuronal loss, gliosis and superficial spongiosis were suggestive of Pick complex (Benson and Zaias, 1991).

In summary, it appears FLD, PPA, frontotemporal atrophies, circumscribed parietal atrophy, CBD, hereditary dysphasic dementia, "dementia without specific pathology", and dementia with motor neuron disease may have certain similarities clinically and pathologically with PD and all form a spectrum that may be justifiably called "Pick's complex" (Kertesz et al., 1994). The expanded concept of PD has already gained acceptance in Europe by some (Constantinidis et al., 1974), although others are less willing to recognize the cohesion of the spectrum. New biochemical and genetic evidence of the relationship may allow less reliance on the pathological variations to provide a link. The incidence of FLD is considered 15–25% of dementia in various series (with classical PD included). Similarly, in our estimation, PPA represents approximately 10% of patients seen in dementia clinics. Even considering that in some centres the same patient may be described as FLD and in others as PPA, the combined incidence of the two presentations (recently called frontotemporal atrophy) is likely to exceed 20–25% of all degenerative dementias. Therefore, Pick complex, including classical and atypical varieties of PD, may be one of the largest nosological entities after AD to cause dementia, particularly in the presenile age group. This may have important implication in the future research of the biology and treatment of dementias.

References

Alzheimer A (1907) Über eine eigenartige Erkrankung der Hirntinde. Allg Z Psychiatrie 64: 146–148

American Psychiatric Association (1987) Diagnostic and statistical manual of mental disorders (DSM-III-R). American Psychiatric Association, Washington DC

Benson DF, Davis RJ, Snyder J (1988) Posterior cortical atrophy. Arch Neurol 45: 789–793

Benson DF, Zaias BW (1991) Progressive aphasia: a case with postmortem correlation. Neuropsychiatr Neuropsychol Behav Neurol 4: 115–223

Braak H, Braak E (1989) Cortical and subcortical argyrophilic grains characterize a disease associated with adult onset dementia. Neuropathol Appl Neurobiol 15: 13–26

Brun A (1987) Frontal lobe degeneration of non-Alzheimer type. I. Neuropathology. Arch Gerontol Geriatr 6: 193–208

Caron M (1934) Etude clinique de la maladie Pick. Vigot, Paris

Caselli RJ, Windebank AJ, Petersen RC, Komori T, Parisi JE, Okazaki E, Iverson R, Dinapoli RP, Graff-Radford NR, Stein SD (1993) Rapidly progressive aphasic dementia and motor neuron disease. Ann Neurol 33: 200–207

Constantinidis J, Richard J, Tissot R (1974) Pick's disease. Histological and clinical correlations. Eur Neurol 11: 208–217

Gustafson L (1987) Frontal lobe degeneration of non-Alzheimer type. II. Clinical picture and differential diagnosis. Arch Gerontol Geriatr 6: 209–223

Hodges JR, Patterson K, Oxbury S, Funnell E (1992) Semantic dementia. Progressive fluent aphasia with temporal lobe atrophy. Brain 115: 1783–1806

Holland AL, McBurney DH, Moossy J, Reinmuth OM (1985) The dissolution of language in Pick's disease with neurofibrillary tangles: a case study. Brain Lang 24: 36–58

Jagust WJ, Reed BR, Seab JP, Kramer JH, Budinger TF (1989) Clinical-physiologic correlates of Alzheimer's disease and frontal lobe dementia. Am J Physiol Imag 4: 89–96

Karbe H, Kertesz A, Polk M (1993) Profiles of language impairment in primary progressive aphasia. Arch Neurol 50: 193–201

Kertesz A, Appell J, Fisman M (1986) The dissolution of language in Alzheimer's disease. Can J Neurol Sci 13: 415–418

Kertesz A, Davidson W, Fox H (1995) Clinical and behavioral criteria in the diagnosis of frontal lobe dementia. Neurology 45 [Suppl 4]: A273

Kertesz A, Hudson L, Mackenzie IRA, Munoz DG (1994) The pathology and nosology of primary progressive aphasia. Neurology 44: 2065–2072

Knopman DS, Mastri AR, Frey II WH, Sung JH, Rustan T (1990) Dementia lacking distinctive histologic features: a common non-Alzheimer degenerative dementia. Neurology 40: 251–256

Kosaka K, Ikeda K, Kobayashi K, Mehraein P (1991) Striatopallidonigral degeneration in Pick's disease. J Neurol 238: 151–160

Lang AE, Bergeron C, Pollanen MS, et al (1994) Parietal Pick's disease mimicking corticobasal ganglionic degeneration. Neurology 44: 1436–1440

Lippa CF, Cohen R, Smith TW, Drachman DA (1991) Primary progressive aphasia with focal neuronal achromasia. Neurology 41: 882–886

Lüers T (1947) Ueber den Verfall der Sprache bei der Pickschen Krankheit (umschniebene Atrophie der Grosshirnrinde). Z Ges Neurol Psychiatrie 179: 94–131

Lynch T, Sano M, Marder KS, et al (1994) Clinical characteristics of a family with chromosome 17 linked disinhibition-dementia-parkinsonism-amyotrophy complex. Neurology 44: 1878–1884

Mandell AM, Alexander MP, Carpenter S (1989) Creutzfeldt-Jakob disease presenting as isolated aphasia. Neurology 39: 55–58

Mesulam MM (1982) Slowly progressive aphasia without dementia. Ann Neurol 11: 592–598

Mesulam MM (1987) Primary progressive aphasia — differentiation from Alzheimer's disease. Ann Neurol 22: 533–534

Miller BL, Cummings JL, Villanueva-Meyer J, Boone K, Mehringer CM, Lesser IM, Mena I (1991) Frontal lobe degeneration: clinical, neuropsychological, and SPECT characteristics. Neurology 14: 1374–1382

Morris JC, Cole M, Banker BQ, Wright D (1984) Hereditary dysphasic dementia and the Pick-Alzheimer spectrum. Ann Neurol 16: 455–466

Neary D, Snowden JS, Bowen DM, Sims NR, Mann DMA, Benton JS, Northen B, Yates PO, Davison AN (1986) Neuropsychological syndromes in presenile dementia due to cerebral atrophy. J Neurol Neurosurg Psychiatry 49: 163–174

Neary D, Snowden JS, Mann DMA, Northen B, Goulding PJ, MacDermott N (1990) Frontal lobe dementia and motor neurone disease. J Neurol Neurosurg Psychiatry 53: 23–32

Neary D, Snowden JS, Shields RA, Burjan AWI, Northen B, MacDermott N, Prescott MC, Testsa HJ (1987) Single photon emission tomography using 99m Tc-AM-PM in the investigation of dementia. J Neurol Neurosurg Psychiatry 50: 1101–1109

Pick A (1892) Über die Beziehungen der senilen Hirnatrophie zur Aphasie. Prag Med Wochenschr 17: 165–167

Pogacar S, Williams RG (1984) Alzheimer's disease presenting as slowly progressive aphasia. RI Med J 67: 181–185

Rebeiz JJ, Kolodny EH, Richardson EP Jr (1968) Corticodentatonigral degeneration with neuronal achromasia. Arch Neurol 18: 20–33

Rice GPA, Paty DW, Ball MJ, Tatham R, Kertesz A (1980) Spongiform encephalopathy of long duration: a family study. Can J Neurol Sci 7: 171–175

Riley DE, Lang AE, Lewis A, Resch L, Ashby P, Horneykiewicz O, Black SI (1990) Cortical-basal ganglionic degeneration. Neurology 40: 1203–1212

Rinne JO, Lee MS, Thompson PD, et al (1994) Corticobasal degeneration. A clinical study of 36 cases. Brain 117: 1183–1196

Rosenfeld M (1909) Die partielle Grosshirnatrophie. J Psychol Neurol 14: 115–130

Snowden JS, Goulding PJ, Neary D (1989) Semantic dementia: a form of circumscribed cerebral atrophy. Behav Neurol 2: 167–182

Starkstein SE, Migliorelli R, Teson A, Sabe L, Vazquez S, Turjanski M, Robinson RG, Leiguarda R (1994) Specificity of changes in cerebral blood flow in patients with frontal lobe dementia. J Neurol Neurosurg Psychiatry 57: 790–796

Tariska I (1970) Circumscribed cerebral atrophy in Alzheimer's disease: a pathological study. In: Wolstenhome GEW, O'Connor M (eds) Alzheimer disease and related conditions. Churchill, London, pp 51–69

The Lund and Manchester Groups (1994) Clinical and neuropathological criteria for frontotemporal dementia. J Neurol Neurosurg Psychiatry 57: 416–418

Thompson PD, Marsden CD (1992) Corticobasal degeneration. In: Bailliere's clinical neurology, vol 1. Bailliere-Tindall, London, pp 677–687

Tissot R, Constantinidis J, Richard J (1985) Pick's disease. In: Fredcriks JAM (ed) Handbook of clinical neurology, vol 2 (46). Neurobehavioural disorders. Elsevier, Amsterdam, pp 233–246

Wechsler AF (1977) Presenile dementia presenting as aphasia. J Neurol Neurosurg Psychiatry 40: 303–305

Authors' address: Dr. A. Kertesz, Department of Clinical Neurological Sciences, St. Joseph's Health Centre, University of Western Ontario, London, Ontario N6A 4V2, Canada.

J Neural Transm (1996) [Suppl] 47: 143–153

MR-imaging of non-Alzheimer's dementia

F. Aichner, M. Wagner, Ch. Kremser, and **S. Felber**

Department of Neurology and Magnetic Resonance, University Hospital,
Innsbruck, Austria

Summary. Up to now, computerized tomography (CT) and MR-imaging
have been used for the morphological assessment of dementia patients, while
MRI has become the structure imaging modality of choice. With the advent of
fast and ultrafast sequences provided by higher gradient field strenghts, functional MR studies like diffusion, perfusion and activation studies become
available

The greatest advantage of MR is its versatility including MR-imaging, 3D
postprocessing, MR-volumetry, MR-spectroscopy, MR-angiography, MR-
perfusion and diffusion imaging as well as functional MRI activation studies.
The application of the multimodal MR-technology in dementia disorders has
already began and has to be validated in clinical practice. The multimodality
of MR represents a diagnostic challenge for the future with the hope, that the
diagnostic efficacy, which has to be proven, is also followed by an improvement of patients care and prognosis.

Introduction

In the evaluation of the dementia patient a careful history, review of family
disorders, consideration of any drugs, assessment of mental status, neurological and physical examination are the critical first steps. Different laboratory
tests should be included, and CT or MRI of the brain should be requested, if
a diagnosis is not established by the history and laboratory tests. Recently, the
American health care guidelines have given the following statement and
recommendation: "MRI is the best way to evaluate the brain when acute
hemorrhage is not an issue. If MRI is available and not contraindicated, CT
should be omitted in all other circumstances". This is even true for the workup
of the dementia patient. Electroencephalography, lumbar puncture, HIV-
antibody test, single photon emission computed tomography (SPECT),
positron emission tomography (PET), and other specialized tests should be
requested, when the clinical finding suggest that they will provide useful
information.

Hardly an issue of a self respecting neurological journal appears without
an article on changes that may be shown by detailed analysis of expensive

investigations like CT, MRI, SPECT or PET in demented patients. Few of these have shown any useful reliable correlation between structural or even functional imaging and specific causes of dementia. Indeed, in most published studies, the accepted diagnosis is that made on clinical and psychometric grounds (Mosely, 1995). Neurological, psychiatric and neuropsychological findings represent the basis of any diagnostics of dementia and with them an 80% detection reliability may be obtained. With application of the CT, MRI, SPECT and PET, as well as of different laboratory parameters the etiology of dementia can be attributed to a definite pathology in approximately 95% of the cases (Aichner et al., 1993). In the following, some forms of non-Alzheimer's dementia are described in respect to their MR-imaging features.

Vascular dementia

Vascular dementia (VD) is a clinical syndrome of intellectual decline produced by ischemic, hypoxic or hemorrhagic brain lesions. The diagnosis requires, apart from the presence of dementia, cerebral vascular disease manifested by neurological signs with neuroimaging evidence of stroke or ischemic brain injury and a temporal relation between the dementia and the vascular disease. MR-imaging may detect the following major morphological types of VD (Jellinger and Bancher, 1994):

1. classical multiinfarct encephalopathy with multiple large infarcts in the cortex and white matter / basal ganglia in territories of large cerebral arteries, frequently involving both hemispheres;
2. strategic infarct dementia with small or medium-sized infarcts in regions as the thalamus, the basal forebrain, angulate gyrus;
3. microangiopathic dementia caused by subcortical arteriosclerotic encephalopathy or by multiple small infarcts in basal ganglia and hemispheral white matter with preservation of cerebral cortex; or caused by multiple microinfarcts (lacunes) or caused by granular cortical atrophy due to multiple small infarctions within the border zones between ACA and MCA in one or both hemispheres;
4. hemorrhagic dementia caused by multiple intracranial hematomas in idiopathic cerebral amyloid angiopathy or in superficial siderosis (SS) of the CNS.

In recent years, attention has been focused on white matter changes. MR is more sensitive in detecting white matter changes than CT, but the changes are more difficult to interpret. White matter changes have been analysed often only as present or absent and the location, extent and type of these changes have not always been studied in detail. As white matter changes are rather nonspecific and do not indicate the underlying pathology, the term leukoaraiosis for the patchy or diffuse white matter areas of altered signal intensity seen both on CT and on MRI is widely used (Erkinjuntti and Hachinski, 1993).

Several different types of periventricular hyperintensities are seen on T_2 weighted MR-images in elderly patients: triangle-shaped "caps" around the frontal horns; thin, smooth, periventricular rims and patchy periventricular hyperintenties. Leukoaraiosis in normal subjects ranges from 22% to 96%, but more extensive changes have been seen in less than 10% of normal aged subjects. The white matter changes have usually been correlated with age. Leukoaraiosis in normal individuals has been related to arterial hypertension, cardiovascular disorders, cerebral vascular disorders, Hachinski's ischemic score, and with diabetes. From a clinical and neuroradiological point of view, it seems likely that the tiny hyperintensities around the frontal and occipital horns, narrow periventricular linings as well as a few small dot-like hyperintensities in subcortical white matter do not have clinical significance (Erkinjuntti and Hachinski, 1993).

In patients with probable Alzheimer's disease (AD) periventricular white matter changes have been reported in 40% to 100%, being of moderate or severe degree in 33% to 50%. Deep and subcortical white matter hyperintensities have been seen in 50% to 93% of cases, but more extensive changes in about 30%. The white matter changes on MRI in patients with AD, although prevalent, are of mild degree, without significant correlation between the degree of dementia and white matter changes seen on MRI (Aichner et al., 1994).

Patients with VD usually show broad white matter changes on MRI extending to the deep white matter, especially in cases with more subcortically

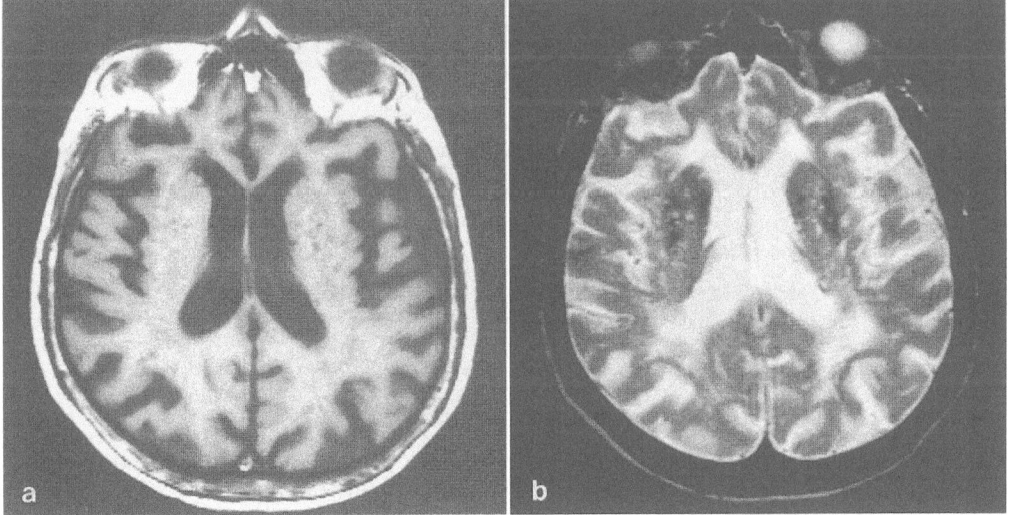

Fig. 1. a Axial, T_1 weighted MR image showing diffuse brain volume reduction with enlargement of the subarachnoid spaces bilaterally and dilatation of the lateral ventricles. Within the basal ganglia small dark areas are visible. **b** The corresponding axial T_2 weighted MR image shows in addition periventricular and white matter signal hyperinsensities. The MR-features are in accordance with the neuroimaging term of leuko-araiosis and with the clinical diagnosis of subcortical arteriosclerotic encephalopathy presenting as vascular dementia

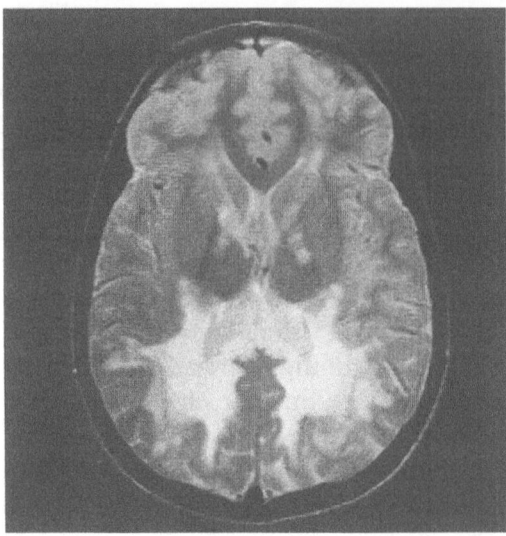

Fig. 2. The T_2 weighted axial MR image demonstrates diffuse signal hyperintensity within the posterior region of the white matter in a case of a juvenile form of adrenoleucodystrophy. These findings indicate symmetric white matter demyelination in the peritrigonal regions. The 17 year old patient presented with seizures, hearing loss, corticospinal tract involvement and cognitive decline

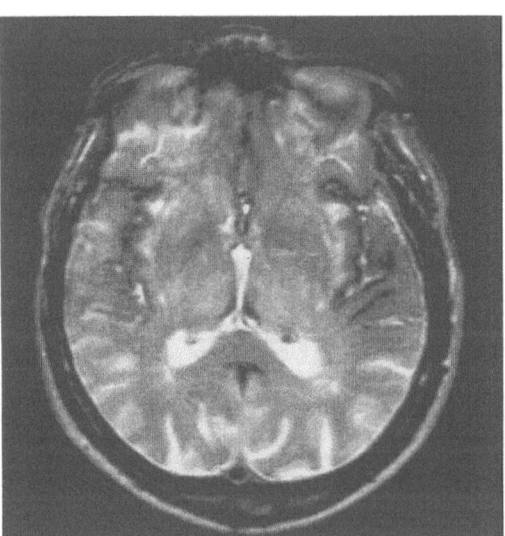

Fig. 3. T_2 weighted axial MR image of the brain in a 58 year old patient suffering from superficial siderosis of the CNS is shown. Abnormal T_2 shortening causes a hypointense rim at the surface of the brain within the Sylvian fissure bilaterally

accentuated symptoms. In most studies patients with VD show more extensive white matter changes than those with AD's (Fig. 1a,b).

Patchy or diffuse white matter changes are also observed in many other disorders including, for example, leukodystrophies (Fig. 2), mitochondrial encephalomyopathies, hyperintense encephalopathy, hydrocephalus, brain irradiation, intrathecal methotrexate treatment, cerebral amyloid angiopathy, multiple sclerosis, the AIDS-complex, Creutzfeldt-Jakob disease, progressive multifocal leukencephalopathy, systemic lupus erythematosus, polymyalgia rheumatica and temporal arteriitis, Behçet disease, and a number of other conditions.

As an example of hemorrhagic dementia, superficial siderosis (SS) of the CNS is described. Typical signs of SS are progressive cerebellar ataxia, spasticity, hearing loss and in the later stage of the disease dementia. Deposition of free iron and hemosiderin in pial and subpial structures leads to intoxication of the CNS and represents the pathophysiological mechanisms of SS. Hypointensity of the marginal zones of CNS on T_2 weighted MRI, indicates an iron-induced susceptibility effect and seems pathognomonic for SS (Fig. 3). In almost all previous described cases SS was verified by biopsy or autopsy. Today, MRI enables diagnosis at an early stage of the disease. Therapeutic management requires the elimination of any potential source of bleeding (Willeit et al., 1992).

Non-Alzheimer degenerative dementia

Dementia with Parkinson's disease (PD)

30 to 40% of patients with PD have an overt dementia and up to 70% have some degree of cognitive impairment. Demonstration by high field MRI of putative changes in brain iron distribution in Parkinsonism has been very enthusiastically promoted some years ago, but has since spectaculary failed to change clinical practice. Iron is a trace element involved in brain function. Iron is essential for cellular respiration, neurotransmitter synthesis, brain development, and maturation. It is easily detected on MR scans because magnetic susceptibility causes preferential T2 shortening. In normal adults, iron is localized in specific brain regions. Highest concentrations are found in globus pallidus, red nuclei and substantia nigra where iron concentration exceeds that found in the liver. Signal attenuation on MRI is detected in those areas that contain the highest concentration of iron (Olanow, 1992).

Although tissue iron and ferritin concentrations are elevated in PD in most cases, they do not cause detectable significant T_2 shortening. In patients with PD there is a decreased width of the substantia nigra as estimated by the distance between the substantia nigra and the red nuclei. These changes are suggested to result from atrophy of the pars compacta of the substantia nigra and deposition of iron or other pigments. However, similar changes have been also observed in normal aging. Small areas of increased white matter signal intensity within the internal capsule, cerebral hemisphere white matter have been identified in PD patients more often than in controls. These changes are probably vascular in nature, but it is unknown, whether they are related to the dementia found in some patients with PD.

Proton MR-spectroscopy of the brain in patients with PD revealed an increase of lactate, especially in cases with dementia. These findings support the hypothesis that PD is a systemic disorder characterized by an impairment of oxydative energy metabolism. If the presence of elevated lactate is confirmed in further studies, then therapeutic clinical trials of drugs that lower lactate levels could be undertaken as is now beeing done for Huntington patients with MR-spectroscopy used to monitor changes in cerebral lactate in vivo (Bowen et al., 1995).

Huntington's disease

It has been hoped that modern imaging might prove more helpful than invasive techniques in diagnosis of early Huntington's disease, but clinical features and family history and DNA-analysis seem to be better guides. It has been suggested, however, that the degree of atrophy of the caudate nucleus may be a guide to prognosis (Fig. 4a,b) (Wardlaw and Sellar, 1991).

Other disorders

Some disorders, such as *Hallervorden-Spatz-disease*, have highly suggestive MRI-findings, namely, the "eye of the tiger sign" within the globus pallidus and substantia nigra (Fig. 5a, b) (Savoiardo et al., 1993).

The findings in *Wilsons disease*, however, are variable, inconstant and do not necessarily correlate with clinical status or response to treatment. They may serve to strengthen a clinical diagnosis, but clearly do not replace metabolic investigations. The atrophic changes seen in "multiple system atrophy" are similarly non-specific and bolster clinical impressions rather than throwing

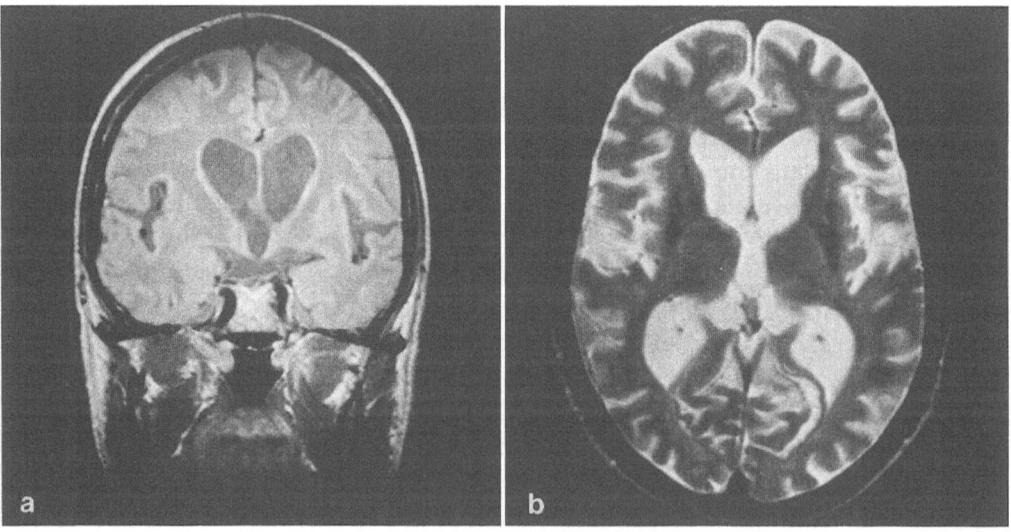

Fig. 4. a,b The coronal PD and axial T$_2$ weighted MR images are taken from a teenage boy with a declining IQ and progressive chorea and dysarthria. The caudate nuclei and putamina are noted to be atrophic

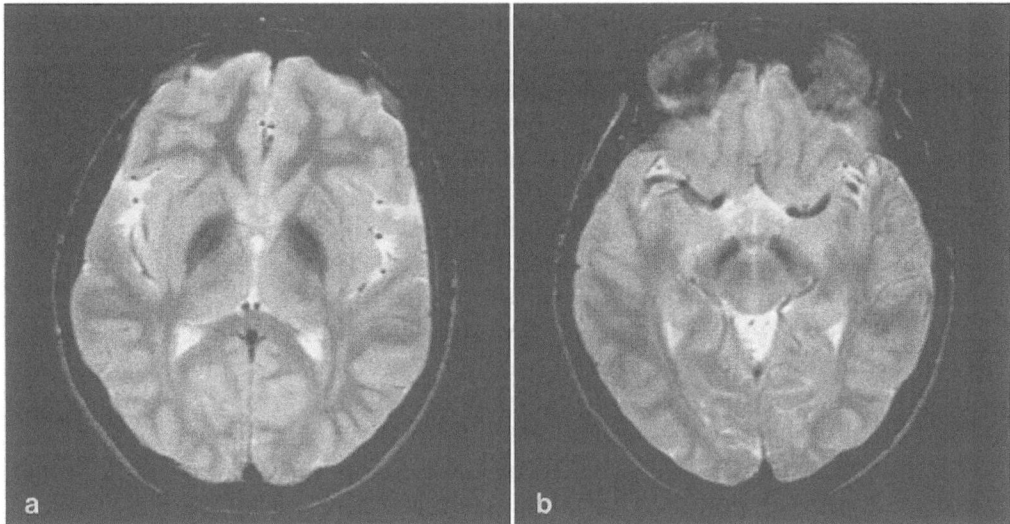

Fig. 5. a,b The T_2 weighted axial MR slices demonstrate signal loss within the globus pallidus and substantia nigra symmetrically. These MRI findings are highly suggestive for Hallervorden-Spatz disease ("Eye of the tiger" sign)

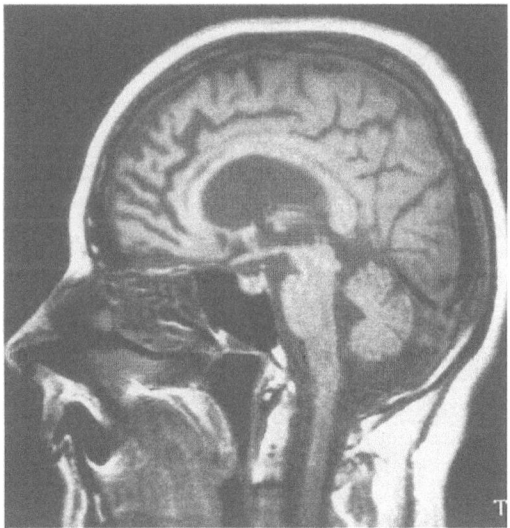

Fig. 6. The sagittal T_1 weighted image of a 62 year old man with a frontal lobe syndrome indicates frontal lobe atrophy

up an unsuspected diagnosis (Willeit et al., 1992). Regrettable, static imaging methods concerned with structure rather than function, have contributed little to clinical investigation of involuntary movements.

Pick's disease is morphologically featured by frontal and temporal lobe atrophy. Similar lesions without Pick bodies are seen in frontal lobe dementia. Both disorders show similar volume loss and may be difficult to separate from Alzheimer's disease (Fig. 6).

Aids-dementia complex

Clinical staging of HIV-infection distinguishes patients with asymptomatic infection or persistent generalized lymphadenopathy from those, who have certain diseases associated with immunosupression and low CD 4 count (<200 cells/mm³) which define the acquired immunodeficiency syndrome (AIDS). The nervous system is commonly infected by HIV early in the course of systemic infection. Neurological dysfunction can result from direct nervous system involvement and/or from concomitant immunosupression.

In AIDS-patients with classic HIV encephalopathy, cerebral atrophy is the most common MR-imaging abnormality. White matter changes, which are typically patchy or confluent periventricular areas of hyperintensity, are less common (Fig. 7). Taken together, these diffuse abnormalities occur in over 50% of such patients. The severity of the abnormalities and frequency of occurrence roughly parallel clinical neurological deteriorioration. The antiviral agent zidovudine has been reported to cause partial resolution of the white matter abnormalities on MR-imaging and to improve cognitive function. Interestingly, the most common and distinctive histological feature of HIV encephalopathy at autopsy is white matter pallor, which appears to result

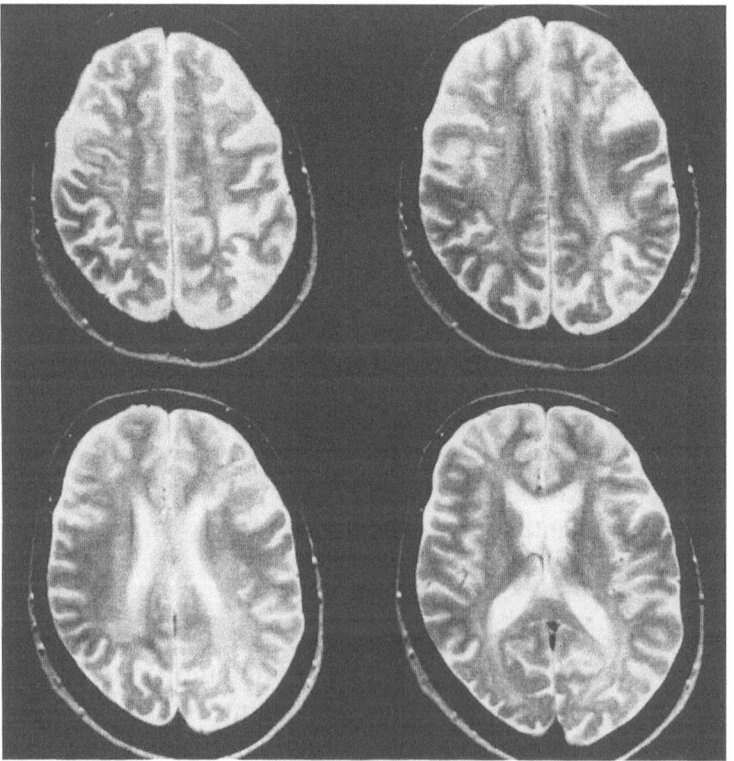

Fig. 7. Four axial T_2 weighted MR images of a 27 year old HIV infected encephalopathic man show atrophic changes and marked diffuse as well as patchy signal intensity abnormalities in the white matter

from perivascular demyelination primarily in the periventricular and central white matter accompanied by astrocytic reaction. In asymptomatic patients, abnormalities (cerebral atrophy and/or white matter signal hyperintensities without mass effect) are minor and are present in only 13% of subjects compared to 46% of the symptomatic subjects (Fig. 7). The number and size of the white matter lesions are greater in the symptomatic group. It appears that routine screening of the very early stage asymptomatic group will yield few positive imaging findings (Chong et al., 1993).

Measurement of T1 and T2 relaxation times for cerebral white matter in neurologically asymptomatic and symptomatic subjects may similarly provide quantitative evidence to support the qualitative imaging findings regarding white matter lesions. Functional MR-imaging studies may allow early detection of HIV encephalopathy.

Proton MR-spectroscopy reportedly has greater sensitivity than imaging in distinguishing neurological symptomatic from asymptomatic subjects and, combined with imaging results, is highly specific for the late stages of HIV encephalopathy. 1H MR-spectroscopy studies of the brain have demonstrated reduced NAA levels on semiquantitative analysis. Changes are most marked in the frontal lobe white matter. Increased total choline ratios have also been demonstrated as well as increases in peaks in the 2.1.–2.2. ppm range representing levels of excitatory aminoacids. 31 phosphor MR-spectroscopy studies of the brain have shown reductions in high energy phosphate metabolites. MR-spectroscopy abnormalities have been shown to correlate with both the cognitive and motor manifestations of this disease. MR-spectroscopy has been shown to bee more sensitive than MRI and may prove to be the most sensitive indicator of the disease (Jarvik et al., 1993).

The primary role of spinecho MR-imaging in HIV-infection is to exclude the possibility that neurological symptoms are due to treatable opportunistic infections, tumors or cerebral vascular diseases. There may be lesions associated with mass-effect: parasitic (toxoplasma gondii), fungal (cryptococcus neoformans) and bacterial (mycobacterium tuberculosis) infections as well as CNS neoplasms (primary lymphoma). Furthermore, there may be lesions not associated with mass-effect (excluding HIV encephalopathy): viral infections, such as progressive multifocal leucencephalopathy, and those due to herpes viruses (cytomegaly virus, herpes simplex and varicella zoster). Last not least, vascular occlusive lesions may also occur (neurosyphilis/treponema pallidum and granulomatous angiitis).

Other brain diseases

Hydrocephalus

Three possible mechanisms account for the development of hydrocephalus: With the exception of hydrocephalus caused by choroid plexus tumors, hydrocephalus is caused by obstructed CSF flow, decreased CSF absorption or a combination of both.

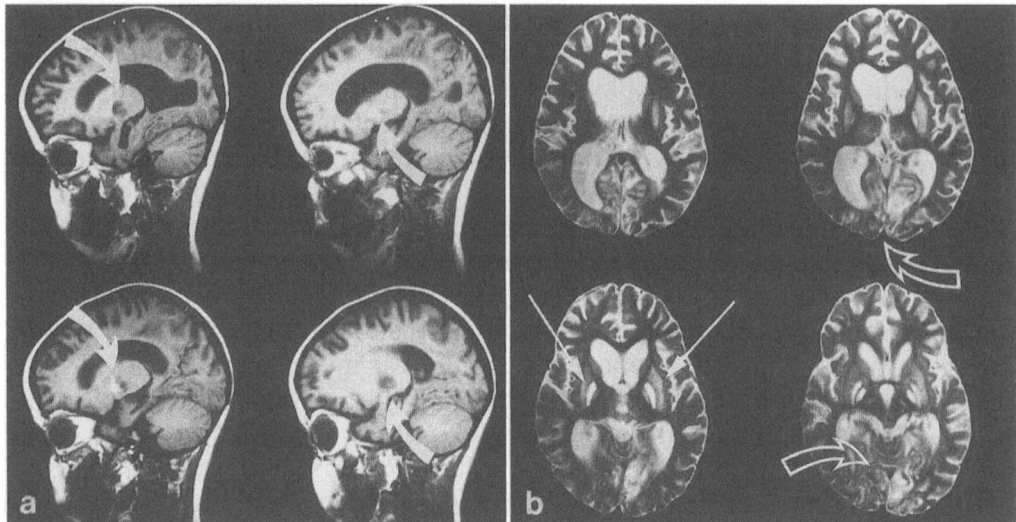

Fig. 8. Six year old child. MRI nine weeks after drowning accident. **a** Sagittal T_1 weighted MR image revealed bilateral cystic-hemorrhagic lesions of the nuclei lentiformis and moderate enlargement of ventricle size. **b** Axial T_2 weighted MR slices show cystic lesions of the nuclei lentiformis (arrows). In addition, bilateral infarctions in the calcarina region are present

Normal pressure hydrocephalus (NPH) is differentiated from generalized atrophy by ventricular dilatation out of proportion to sulcal enlargement on CT on MR scans. Some investigators report CSF flow through the cerebral aqueduct hyperdynamic, producing an accentuated CSF flow void. Others suggested that symptoms of NPH (memory loss, gait disturbances, urinary incontinence) relate not to ventricular dilatation but rather to impingement of the corpus callosum by the falx cerebri (George, 1991).

Hypoxic encephalopathy

Images of hypoxic encephalopathy vary with length and severity of the insult, patient age, individual cerebral circulatory pattern and the inherent vulnerability of certain anatomic regions and cell types to hypoxic ischemic injury. Hypoxic encephalopathy in adults typically results in borderzone infarctions and bilateral selective neuronal necrosis within the globus pallidus, putamen caudate nuclei, thalamus, parahippocampal gyrus, hippocampus, cerebellum, and brain stem nuclei (Fig. 8a,b) (Birbamer et al., 1991).

References

Aichner FT (1993) Clinical value of magnetic resonance imaging in the diagnosis of demential diseases. Psychiat Danub 5: 177–187

Aichner FT, Felber SR, Birbamer GG (1994) Computed tomography and magnetic resonance imaging in the diagnosis of Alzheimer's disease. In: Jellinger KA, Ladurner G, Windisch M (eds) New trends in the diagnosis and therapy of Alzheimer's disease. Springer, Wien New York, pp 41–51

Birbamer G, Aichner F, Felber S, Kampfl A, Berek K, Schmutzhard E, Gerstenbrand F (1991) MRI of cerebral hypoxia. Neuroradiology 33 [Suppl]: 53–55

Bowen BC, Block RE, Sanchez-Ramos J, Pattany PM, Lampman DA, Murdoch JB, Quencer RM (1995) Proton MR spectroscopy of the brain in 14 patients with Parkinson's disease. Am J Neuroradiol 16: 61–68

Chong WK, Sweeney B, Wilkinson ID, Paley M, Hall-Craggs MA, Kendall BE, Shepard JK, et al (1993) Proton spectroscopy of the brain in HIV infection: correlation with clinical, immunologic, and MR imaging findings. Radiology 188: 119–124

Erkinjuntti T, Hachinski VC (1993) Rethinking vascular dementia. Cerebrovasc Disord 3: 3–23

George AE (1991) Chronic communicating hydrocephalus and periventricular white matter disease: a debate with regard to cause and effect. Am J Neuroradiol 12: 42–44

Jarvik JG, Lenkinski RE, Grossman RI, Gomori JM, Schnall MD, Frank I (1993) Proton MR spectroscopy of HIV-infected patients: characterization of abnormalities with imaging and clinical correlation. Radiology 186: 739–744

Jellinger K, Bancher C (1994) Classification of dementia based on functional morphology. In: Jellinger KA, Ladurner G, Windisch M (eds) New trends in the diagnosis and therapy of Alzheimer's disease. Springer, Wien New York, pp 9–39

Mosely I (1995) Imaging the adult brain. J Neurol Neurosurg Psychiatry 58: 7–21

Olanow CW (1992) Magnetic resonance imaging in parkinsonism. Neurol Clin 10: 405–420

Patel MR, Siewert B, Warach S, Edelman RR (1995) Diffusion and perfusion imaging techniques. In: MR Angiography of the central nervous system. MRI Clin North Am 3: 425–438

Savoiardo M, Halliday WC, Nardocci N, Strada L, D'Incerti, Angelini L, et al (1993) Hallervorden-Spatz disease. MR and pathological findings. Am J Neuroradiol 14: 155–162

Wardlaw JM, Sellar RJ (1991) Early caudate nucleus atrophy in Huntington's disease: does it correlate with presenting symptoms? Neuroradiology 33: 238–240

Willeit J, Aichner F, Felber S, Berek K, Deisenhammer F, Kiechl SG, Gerstenbrand F (1992) Superficial siderosis of the central nervous system: report of three cases and review of the literature. J Neurol Sci 111: 20–25

Willeit J, Kiechl G, Birbamer G, Schmidauer C, Felber S, Aichner F (1992) Morbus Wilson mit primärer ZNS-Manifestation — aktueller Stand in Diagnostik und Therapie. Fortschr Neurol Psychiat 60: 237–245

Authors' address: Prof. Dr. F. Aichner, Department of Neurology and Magnetic Resonance, University Hospital, Anichstrasse 35, A-6020 Innsbruck, Austria.

J Neural Transm (1996) [Suppl] 47: 155–167
© Springer-Verlag 1996

Functional imaging techniques in the diagnosis of non-Alzheimer dementias

D. J. Brooks

MRC Cyclotron Unit, Hammersmith Hospital, London, United Kingdom

Summary. Functional imaging (positron emission tomography — PET, single photon emission tomography — SPECT, magnetic resonance spectroscopy — MRS) enables regional cerebral function to be assessed in vivo in dementias. There are three basic approaches to examining the patterns of cerebral function associated with specific disorders: First, abnormalities in resting levels of regional cerebral metabolism and blood flow can be examined. Second, patients can be asked to perform cognitive tasks with a view to demonstrating aberrations in their pattern of cerebral activation. Third, resting dysfunction of brain pharmacology can be revealed. The bulk of the research on non-Alzheimer dementias has been performed with PET and SPECT and this review will concentrate on these two modalities.

Introduction

PET measurements are performed by administering a tracer tagged with a short-lived positron-emitting isotope. These isotopes are usually generated by a cyclotron and those most frequently employed are ^{15}O ($t_{1/2}$ 2.03 mins), ^{11}C ($t_{1/2}$ 20.4 mins), and ^{18}F ($t_{1/2}$ 110 mins). The subject is scanned and axial tomographic maps of regional cerebral tracer uptake are obtained. By comparing the kinetics of tracer accumulation in different brain regions with that in arterial plasma, regional cerebral tracer uptake can be quantitatively related to metabolism, blood flow, integrity of nerve terminal function, or receptor binding. SPECT tracers are longer lived and are usually labelled with either ^{123}I or ^{99m}Tc. As a scatter correction cannot be performed SPECT measurements are less sensitive and currently semi-quantitative. Commonly used PET and SPECT tracers and their biological applications are detailed in Table 1.

In order to assess the contribution of functional imaging towards the diagnosis of the non-Alzheimer dementias, it is convenient to divide these disorders into cortical and subcortical degenerations — see Table 2.

Other causes of non-Alzheimer dementia, such as multi-infarct and prion disease, will be reviewed in detail in other chapters. The purpose of this

Table 1. PET and SPECT tracers in common use for studying dementia

Biological application	Tracer
Blood flow	$H_2^{15}O$, ^{99m}Tc-HMPAO, ^{133}Xe
Oxygen metabolism	$^{15}O_2$
Glucose metabolism	^{18}F-2-fluoro-2-deoxyglucose (FDG)
Dopamine storage	^{18}F-6-fluorodopa (F-dopa)
Dopamine reuptake sites	^{11}C-CFT, ^{123}I-CIT
Dopamine D_2 sites	^{11}C-raclopride (RAC)
	^{123}I-iodobenzamide (IBZM)

Table 2. Non-Alzheimer dementias studied with PET

Degenerative:	(a) cortical:	Cortical Lewy body disease
		Pick's disease
		Spongioform/ALS
		Creuzfeldt-Jakob syndrome
		Lobar degenerations
		Corticobasal degeneration
	(b) subcortical:	Progressive supranuclear palsy
		Subcortical gliosis
		Huntington's disease

chapter is primarily to compare the findings in cortical and subcortical dementias.

Lewy body disease

Parkinson's disease (PD) is characterised by degeneration of the pigmented and other brain stem nuclei, the ventrolateral substantia nigra compacta projections to putamen in particular being targeted (German et al., 1989; Spokes et al., 1979; Fearnley and Lees, 1991). Degenerating neurones contain Lewy bodies and in a recent pathological series all PD patients examined with an antibody stain to ubiquitin were found to have occasional cortical, as well as brainstem, Lewy bodies (Hughes et al., 1992). When cortical involvement becomes extensive the condition is termed Diffuse Lewy body disease (DLBD), rather than PD, but currently it remains unclear whether DLBD and PD are part of a spectrum or separate disorders (Kosaka, 1990). Frequently DLBD co-exists with Alzheimer pathology. Most cases of pure DLBD present as levodopa responsive parkinsonism and then go on to develop dementia but this condition can manifest as an isolated dementia indistinguishable from Alzheimer's disease (Byrne et al., 1989). Severity of dementia has been found to correlate with cortical Lewy body density in some, but not all, series (Byrne et al., 1989).

Looking at the problem from the opposite viewpoint, dementia is thought to develop in 10–20% of patients with PD. Clinicopathological correlations have generally implicated co-existent AD or DLBD but on occasion have found no associated cortical pathology. It has been suggested that DLBD may differ clinically from AD in that patients show fluctuating severity of dementia, are more prone to hallucinations, have early gait difficulties, and show profound neuroleptic sensitivity (McKeith et al., 1992). It has also been suggested that DLBD cases are more prone to show atypical parkinsonian features (lack of L-dopa response, voluntary gaze difficulties) than their non-demented PD counterparts (Sage et al., 1990).

Resting metabolic studies

PET measurements of regional cerebral oxygen and glucose metabolism with $^{15}O_2$ and ^{18}FDG primarily reflect the metabolism of nerve terminal synaptic vesicles. Consequently, levels of metabolism in brain structures reflect the metabolic activity of afferent projections to those regions and of intrinsic inter-neurons rather than that of efferent projections. Using PET, increased resting oxygen and glucose metabolism can be demonstrated in the lentiform nucleus contralateral to the affected limbs in non-demented hemiparkinsonian patients (Miletich et al., 1988; Wolfson et al., 1985). By the time the parkinsonism has become bilateral, metabolism of the lentiform nucleus has generally normalised.

PET studies on hemiparkinsonian patients, early into their disease, have shown small but significant decreases in resting prefrontal blood flow and metabolism contralateral to their affected limbs (Wolfson et al., 1985; Perlmutter and Raichle, 1985). Covariance analysis more sensitively demonstrates this abnormal inverse relationship between resting lentiform and frontal function (Eidelberg et al., 1994). Bilaterally affected non-demented PD patients may show a more diffuse cortical hypometabolism, levels of glucose utilisation correlating with their psychometric performance (Kuhl et al., 1984b; Peppard et al., 1988). ^{18}FDG scans of frankly demented PD patients show an Alzheimer pattern of impaired brain glucose utilisation, posterior parietal and temporal association areas being most severely affected (Kuhl et al., 1984a, 1985; Wolfson et al., 1985; Otsuka et al., 1991). SPECT studies have shown normal cortical blood flow in non-demented PD and either frontal or fronto-temporo-parietal decreases in demented cases (Sawada et al., 1992). Only one demented PD patient, to date, has had pathological findings correlated with functional imaging. He showed an Alzheimer ^{18}FDG pattern of uptake but, while brainstem Lewy body disease was present, neither Alzheimer changes or Lewy bodies were evident in the cortex (Schapiro et al., 1990). As a consequence, it currently remains unclear whether the pattern of glucose hypometabolism in demented PD patients reflects coincidental Alzheimer's disease, cortical Lewy body disease, loss of cholinergic projections, or some other degenerative process. As lesions of the nucleus basalis of Meynert in primates result in only transient diffuse cortical hypometabolism (Kiyosawa et al., 1989), loss of cholinergic projections seems unlikely to be responsible for the Alzheimer pattern of reduced ^{18}FDG uptake found in demented PD patients.

We have recently started to perform resting [18]FDG PET scans on PD cases who fulfill the clinical criteria for the presence of cortical Lewy bodies. The first three patients studied all had rest tremor, rigidity, and bradykinesia that was levodopa responsive. They experienced intermittent disorientation and confusion and one would confabulate at times. Despite this, none were frankly demented. Two of the patients had visual hallucinations and limb apraxia. PET findings were compared with those obtained for 15 age-matched controls using statistical parametric mapping (SPM) to demonstrate the localisation of focal reductions in resting glucose metabolism. Figure 1 shows the SPM findings for one of the cases. Decreases in glucose metabolism were found in prefrontal, inferior and mesial temporal, and inferior parietal cortex bilaterally. The other two cases also showed reduced metabolism in frontal and temporal association areas. These preliminary findings are, therefore, similar to those seen in Alzheimer's disease though the early frontal involvement despite the absence of frank dementia may distinguish true DLBD from PD-AD cases. Further studies are required to confirm this initial impression.

Activation studies

In normal subjects stereotyped movements of a joystick in a forward direction with the right hand result in contralateral rCBF increases in the lentiform nucleus and sensorimotor cortex (SMC), and bilateral increases in caudal anterior cingulate, supplementary motor area (SMA), and lateral premotor

[18]FDG decreases in DLBD

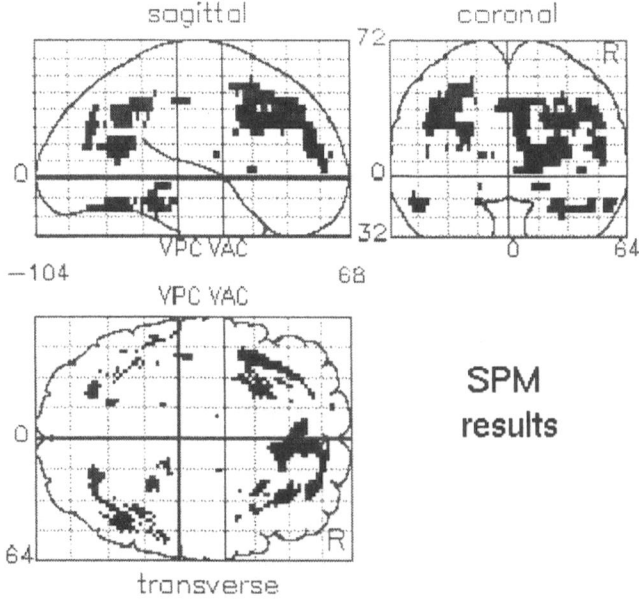

SPM
results

Fig. 1

cortex (PMC) (Playford et al., 1992). Joystick movements in freely selected directions result in additional bilateral activation of rostral anterior cingulate, SMA, PMC, parietal association areas, and dorsolateral prefrontal cortex (DLPFC). When PD patients, scanned after cessation of treatment for 12 hours, perform the same joystick tasks normal activation of SMC, PMC, and lateral parietal association areas occurs, but there is selectively impaired activation of the contralateral lentiform nucleus, and of the anterior cingulate, SMA, and DLPFC, that is those cortical areas that receive their main input from the basal ganglia.

It is thought that the SMA and DLPFC play a crucial role in generating volitional motor programmes while parietal association and lateral premotor cortex are responsible for generating motor responses to external cues (Thaler and Passingham, 1989; Goldberg, 1985; Mushiake et al., 1990; Goldman-Rakic, 1987). An inability to activate SMA and DLPFC in PD could explain the difficulty these patients experience in initiating motor actions. Jenkins et al. (1992) have demonstrated that when apomorphine, a combined D_1 and D_2 agonist, is given subcutaneously to PD patients resolution of their akinesia is associated with a significant increase in SMA blood flow, providing further evidence for the role of this structure in the generation of motor programmes. Similar findings have been reported using ^{133}Xe SPECT (Rascol et al., 1992). It can be seen, therefore, that patients with Diffuse Lewy body disease effectively suffer from a double hit phenomenon. The loss of dopaminergic fibres deafferents frontal areas while there is also direct involvement of parieto-temporal and frontal association areas.

Progressive supranuclear palsy

This condition is generally taken to refer to Steele-Richardson-Olszewski syndrome, and is characterised pathologically by neurofibrillary tangle formation and neuronal loss in the basal ganglia and brainstem nuclei (Steele et al., 1964). The full clinical syndrome of PSP comprises an akinetic-rigid syndrome which is poorly levodopa responsive in association with axial dystonia, a supranuclear down-gaze palsy, bulbar dysfunction, and dementia of frontal type. In the early stages of the disease, however, the patient may simply present as an akinetic-rigid syndrome making a clear distinction from other parkinsonian disorders difficult (Maher and Lees, 1986; Jackson et al., 1983).

Metabolic studies

Several series have reported on resting regional cerebral glucose and oxygen metabolism in patients with probable PSP, some of whom have later had the diagnosis confirmed at autopsy (D'Antona et al., 1985; Blin et al., 1990a; Foster et al., 1988; Leenders et al., 1988; Goffinet et al., 1989). Cortical metabolism is globally depressed in this condition, prefrontal and premotor areas being particularly targeted. Frontal levels of metabolism have been shown to correlate with performance on psychometric tests of frontal function (Blin et al., 1990a). Hypofrontality is not specific for PSP and can also be seen in striatonigral degeneration (De Volder et al., 1989), progressive subcortical gliosis (Foster et al., 1992), and Pick's disease (Kamo et al., 1987). Striatal metabolism is also depressed in PSP and cerebellar and thalamic metabolism may also be affected. ^{18}FDG PET, therefore, provides a valuable way of distinguishing PSP from PD as striatal metabolism is preserved in the latter disorder.

Pharmacological studies

Striatal ^{18}F-dopa uptake in PSP is significantly reduced, putamen and caudate being similarly affected (Leenders et al., 1988; Bhatt et al., 1991; Brooks et al., 1990). These PET findings suggest that the nigra is uniformly involved in PSP and this is in agreement with pathological reports (Jellinger et al., 1980; Kish et al., 1985). In contrast, PD patients with a similar degree of locomotor disability show significant sparing of caudate ^{18}F-dopa uptake. Striatal dopamine D_2 receptor binding in PSP has been studied with PET and SPECT in a number of centres. Mean binding is invariably reduced although a significant minority of these cases still retain normal indices (Baron et al., 1986; Wienhard et al., 1990; Brooks et al., 1992). In view of this, it is likely that in PSP degeneration of pallidal and brainstem projections is responsible for the poor L-dopa responsiveness of this akinetic-rigid syndrome rather than a primary loss of dopamine receptors. Most recently, opioid binding has been studied in PSP with ^{11}C-diprenorphine PET. These cases show a severe equivalent loss of caudate and putamen binding in contrast to PD where striatal binding is preserved (Burn et al., 1995).

Corticobasal degeneration

This syndrome, also known as corticodentatonigral degeneration and neuronal achromasia, presents as an akinetic-rigid syndrome with associated dyspraxia or alien limb behaviour (Riley et al., 1990). Cortical sensory loss, dysphasia, myoclonus, supranuclear gaze problems, and bulbar dysfunction may also be evident. Intellect is spared until late. Eventually all four limbs become involved and the condition is invariably poorly L-dopa responsive. The pathology consists of collections of swollen, achromatic, tau-positive cells, without argyrophilic inclusion bodies, concentrated in the posterior frontal, inferior parietal, and superior temporal lobes, and the substantia nigra (Gibb et al., 1989).

There have been three reports of PET studies on patients with the clinical syndrome of CBD. Sawle et al. (1991) studied six patients with $^{15}O_2$ PET. As might be predicted from the distribution of the pathology, cortical oxygen metabolism (rCMRO$_2$) was most significantly reduced in posterior frontal, inferior parietal, and superior temporal regions. Again these rCMRO$_2$ reductions were strikingly asymmetrical, being most severe contralateral to the more affected limbs. The authors felt that these PET findings distinguished CBD from Alzheimer's and Pick's disease, where posterior parietal and inferior frontal hypometabolism predominate respectively, and from PSP, where frontal and striatal metabolism are more symmetrically reduced. This metabolic pattern of dysfunction, however, has been reported in the lobar atrophies associated with progressive dyspraxia and dysphasia (Tyrrell et al., 1990). In Sawle et al's. (1991) patients ^{18}F-dopa PET showed strikingly asymmetrical striatal ^{18}F-dopa uptake and caudate and putamen tracer uptake were equally severely depressed in CBD in contrast to PD. Mesial frontal ^{18}F-dopa uptake was also significantly depressed.

Eidelberg et al. (1991) have studied five CBD patients with PET. They found that inferior parietal, hippocampal, and thalamic glucose metabolism, and striatal ^{18}F-dopa uptake, were significantly depressed contralateral to the more affected limbs compared to ipsilateral values. This contrasted with PD patients who had symmetrical levels of regional cerebral glucose metabolism. Blin et al. (1990b) have reported similar asymmetric reductions in inferior parietal and thalamic FDG uptake in CBD. A single SPECT study has reported asymmetrical reduction of striatal D_2 dopamine receptor binding in this condition.

Huntington's disease

Huntington's disease (HD) presents with involuntary movements or an akinetic-rigid syndrome in association with dementia and behavioural changes (Martin and Gusella, 1986). The pathology of HD involves loss of spiny neurones from the striatum and dentate nuclei. Those patients with predominant chorea show selective loss of striato-lateral pallidal projections, while those with akinetic-rigid syndromes show additional severe loss of striato-medial pallidal fibres (Albin et al., 1990). The condition is dominantly inherited and associated with increased CAG triplet repeats (>38) in the IT15 gene on the short arm of chromosome 4. The disorder dentatorubropallidoluysian atrophy (DRPLA), associated with excess CAG triplet repeats in a gene on chromosome 12, and neuroacanthocytosis (NA) are also associated with chorea and dementia.

Metabolic studies

Affected HD patients have severely reduced caudate and lentiform nucleus glucose and oxygen metabolism and this is present in early disease when CT and MRI are generally normal (Kuhl et al., 1982; Hayden et al., 1986; Leenders et al., 1986). Levels of striatal glucose metabolism correlate with the locomotor function of these patients (Young et al., 1986). In early disease cortical metabolism is preserved in HD but subsequently declines as dementia becomes prominent, the frontal cortex being targeted (Kuhl et al., 1984b;

Kuwert et al., 1990). While caudate hypometabolism is a characteristic of HD, its presence is not specific for this condition. Caudate glucose utilisation is also reduced in DRPLA and NA (Dubinsky et al., 1989; Hosokawa et al., 1987).

The sensitivity of PET for the detection of sub-clinical caudate hypometabolism in adult subjects carrying the HD gene is still controversial. Grafton et al. (1990) reported [18]FDG PET findings for 54 at-risk subjects for HD and found low caudate metabolism in twelve cases, nine of whom were identified as high-risk from either DNA linkage studies or subsequent development of the disease. Young et al. (1987), however, found no abnormalities of caudate metabolism in 29 at-risk subjects, while Hayden et al. (1987) reported reduced caudate glucose utilisation in three out of eight high-risk subjects. Present evidence suggests that [18]FDG PET detects striatal dysfunction in around one third of asymptomatic adult HD gene carriers. More interestingly, Grafton et al. (1992) showed that striatal glucose metabolism falls at a rate of ≈3% per annum in HD gene carriers. [18]FDG PET, therefore, provides an objective means of monitoring disease progression and, in the future, or measuring the effects of putative neuroprotective agents and tissue transplants.

The dopaminergic system

A number of PET an SPECT series have reported reduced striatal D_2 receptor binding in symptomatic HD cases (Wong et al., 1985; Hagglund et al., 1987; Leenders et al., 1986; Wienhard et al., 1990; Brücke et al., 1991). The finding of reduced striatal D_2 site binding potential, like that of reduced caudate metabolism, is not specific for HD. Brooks et al. (1991) have reported a mean 70% reduction of striatal ^{11}C-raclopride binding in three neuroacanthocytosis patients. Reduced striatal D_1 and D_2 binding can also be demonstrated in around 50% of asymptomatic adult HD gene carriers (Weeks et al., 1995). This finding suggests that HD progression can also be objectively monitored by following striatal dopamine receptor binding as well as glucose metabolism.

Table 3. PET findings in dementia

	Alzheimer	Lewy body	Pick's	PSP	CBD	HD
Cortical metabolism	low PT	low PTF	low F	low F	low IP, ST	normal
Striatal metabolism	normal	normal	low	low	low	low
F-dopa uptake	normal	low	normal	low	low	normal
Striatal D_2 sites	normal	normal	normal	low	low	low

P parietal, *T* temporal, *F* frontal, *IP* inferior parietal, *ST* superior temporal

Conclusions

Table 3 details functional imaging findings in various cortical and subcortical dementias.

References

Albin RL, Reiner A, Anderson KD, Penney JB, Young AB (1990) Striatal and nigral neuron subpopulations in rigid Huntington's disease: implications for the functional anatomy of chorea and rigidity-akinesia. Ann Neurol 27: 357–365

Baron JC, Maziere B, Loc'h C, Cambon H, Sgouropoulos P, Bonnet M, Agid Y (1986) Loss of striatal (76Br)bromospiperone binding sites demonstrated by positron tomography in progressive supranuclear palsy. J Cereb Blood Flow Metab 6: 131–136

Bhatt MH, Snow BJ, Martin WRW, Peppard R, Calne DB (1991) Positron emission tomography in progressive supranuclear palsy. Arch Neurol 48: 389–391

Blin J, Baron JC, Dubois P, Pillon B, Cambon H, Cambier J, Agid Y (1990a) Positron emission tomography study in progressive supranuclear palsy. Arch Neurol 47: 747–752

Blin J, Vidhailhet M, Bonnet AM, Dubois P, Pillon P, Syrota A, Agid Y (1990b) PET study in corticobasal degeneration. Mov Disord 5 [Suppl 1]: 19

Brooks DJ, Ibañez V, Sawle GV, Quinn N, Lees AJ, Mathias CJ, Bannister R, Marsden CD, Frackowiak RSJ (1990) Differing patterns of striatal ^{18}F-dopa uptake in Parkinson's disease, multiple system atrophy and progressive supranuclear palsy. Ann Neurol 28: 547–555

Brooks DJ, Ibanez V, Playford ED, Sawle GV, Leigh PN, Kocen RS, Harding AE, Marsden CD (1991) Presynaptic and postsynaptic striatal dopaminergic function in neuroacanthocytosis: a positron emission tomographic study. Ann Neurol 30: 166–171

Brooks DJ, Ibanez V, Sawle GV, Playford ED, Quinn N, Mathias CJ, Lees AJ, Marsden CD, Bannister R, Frackowiak RSJ (1992) Striatal D_2 receptor status in Parkinson's disease, striatonigral degeneration, and progressive supranuclear palsy, measured with ^{11}C-raclopride and PET. Ann Neurol 31: 184–192

Brücke T, Podreka I, Angelberger P, Wenger S, Topitz A, Kufferle B, Muller C, Deecke L (1991) Dopamine D2 receptor imaging with SPECT: studies in different neuropsychiatric disorders. J Cereb Blood Flow Metab 11: 220–228

Burn DJ, Rinne JO, Quinn NP, Lees AJ, Marsden CD, Brooks DJ (1995) Striatal opioid receptor binding in Parkinson's disease, striatonigral degeneration, and Steele-Richardson-Olszewski syndrome: an ^{11}C-diprenorphine PET study. Brain 118: 951–958

Byrne E, Lennox G, Lowe J, Godwin-Austin RB (1989) Diffuse Lewy body disease: clinical features in 15 cases. J Neurol Neurosurg Psychiatry 52: 709–717

D'Antona R, Baron JC, Samson Y, Serdaru M, Viader F, Agid Y, Cambier J (1985) Subcortical dementia: frontal cortex hypometabolism detected by positron tomography in patients with progressive supranuclear palsy. Brain 108: 785–800

De Volder AG, Francard J, Laterre C, Dooms G, Bol A, Michel C, Goffinet AM (1989) Decreased glucose utilisation in the striatum and frontal lobe in probable striatonigral degeneration. Ann Neurol 26: 239–247

Dubinsky RM, Hallett M, Levey R, Di Chiro G (1989) Regional brain glucose metabolism in neuroacanthocytosis. Neurology 39: 1253–1255

Eidelberg D, Dhawan V, Moeller JR, Sidtis JJ, Ginos JZ, Strother SC, Cederbaum J, Greene P, Fahn S, Powers JM, Rottenberg DA (1991) The metabolic landscape of cortico-basal ganglionic degeneration: regional asymmetries studies with positron emission tomography. J Neurol Neurosurg Psychiatry 54: 856–862

Eidelberg D, Moeller JR, Dhawan V, Spetsieris P, Takikawa S, Ishikawa T, Chaly T, Robeson T, Margouleff D, Przedborski S, Fahn S (1994) The metabolic topography of parkinsonism. J Cereb Blood Flow Metab 14: 783–801

Fearnley JM, Lees AJ (1991) Ageing and Parkinson's disease: substantia nigra regional selectivity. Brain 114: 2283–2301

Foster NL, Gilman S, Berent S, Morin EM, Brown MB, Koeppe RA (1988) Cerebral hypometabolism in progressive supranuclear palsy studied with positron emission tomography. Ann Neurol 24: 399–406

Foster NL, Gilman S, Berent S, Sima AAF, D'Amato C, Koeppe RA, Hicks SP (1992) Progressive subcortical gliosis and progressive supranuclear palsy can have similar clinical and PET abnormalities. J Neurol Neurosurg Psychiatry 55: 707–713

German DC, Manaya K, Smith WK, Woodward DJ, Saper CB (1989) Midbrain dopaminergic cell loss in Parkinson's disease: computer visualization. Ann Neurol 26: 507–514

Gibb WRG, Luthert P, Marsden CD (1989) Corticobasal degeneration. Brain 112: 1171–1192

Goffinet AM, De Volder AG, Gillain C, Rectem D, Bol A, Michel C, Cogneau M, Labar D, Laterre C (1989) Positron tomography demonstrates frontal lobe hypometabolism in progressive supranuclear palsy. Ann Neurol 25: 131–139

Goldberg G (1985) Supplementary motor area structure and function: review and hypotheses. Behav Brain Sci 8: 567–616

Goldman-Rakic PS (1987) Circuitry of primate prefrontal cortex and regulation of behaviour by representational memory. In: Plum F (ed) The nervous system: higher functions of the brain. American Physiology Society, Bethesda, pp 373–417

Grafton ST, Mazziotta JC, Pahl JJ, St. George-Hyslop P, Haines JL, Gusella J, Hoffman JM, Baxter LR, Phelps ME (1990) A comparison of neurological, metabolic, structural, and genetic evaluations in persons at risk for Huntington's disease. Ann Neurol 28: 614–621

Grafton ST, Mazziotta JC, Pahl JJ, St. George-Hyslop P, Haines JL, Gusella, J, Hoffman JM, Baxter LR, Phelps ME (1992) Serial changes of cerebral glucose metabolism and caudate size in persons at risk for Huntington's disease. Arch Neurol 49: 1161–1167

Hagglund J, Aquilonius SM, Eckernas SA, Hartvig P, Lundquist H, Gullberg P, Langstrom B (1987) Dopamine receptor properties in Parkinson's disease and Huntington's chorea evaluated by positron emission tomography using 11C-N-methyl-spiperone. Acta Neurol Scand 75: 87–94

Hayden MR, Martin WRW, Stoessl AJ, Clark C, Hollenberg S, Adam MJ, Ammann W, Harrop R (1986) Positron emission tomography in the early diagnosis of Huntington's disease. Neurology 36: 888–894

Hayden MR, Hewitt J, Martin WRW, Clark C, Amman A (1987) Studies in persons at risk for Huntington's disease. N Engl J Med 317: 382–383

Hosokawa S, Ichiya Y, Kuwabara Y, Ayabe Z, Mitsuo K, Goto I, Kato M (1987) Positron emission tomography in cases of chorea with different underlying diseases. J Neurol Neurosurg Psychiatry 50: 1284–1287

Hughes AJ, Daniel SE, Kilford L, Lees AJ (1992) The accuracy of the clinical diagnosis of Parkinson's disease: a clinicopathological study of 100 cases. J Neurol Neurosurg Psychiatry 55: 181–184

Jackson JA, Jankovic J, Ford J (1983) Progressive supranuclear palsy: clinical features and response to treatment in 16 patients. Ann Neurol 13: 273–278

Jellinger K, Riederer P, Tomananga M (1980) Progressive supranuclear palsy: clinico-pathological and biochemical studies. J Neural Transm [Suppl 16]: 111–128

Jenkins IH, Fernandez W, Playford ED, Lees AJ, Frackowiak RSJ, Passingham RE, Brooks DJ (1992) Impaired activation of the supplementary motor area in

Parkinson's disease is reversed when akinesia is treated with apomorphine. Ann Neurol 32: 749–757

Kamo H, McGeer PL, Harrop R, McGeer EC, Calne DB, Martin WRW, Pate BD (1987) Positron emission tomography and histopathology in Pick's disease. Neurology 37: 439–445

Kish SJ, Chang LJ, Mirchandani LJ, Shannak K, Hornykiewicz O (1985) Progressive supranuclear palsy: relationship between extrapyramidal disturbances, dementia, and brain neurotransmitter markers. Ann Neurol 18: 530–536

Kiyosawa M, Baron JC, Hamel E, Pappata S, Duverger D, Riche D, Mazoyer B, Naquet R, MacKenzie ET (1989) Time course of effects of unilateral lesions of the Nucleus Basalis of Meynert on glucose utilisation by the cerebral cortex. Positron emission tomography in baboons. Brain 112: 435–455

Kosaka K (1990) Diffuse Lewy body disease in Japan. J Neurol 237: 197–204

Kuhl DE, Phelps ME, Markham CH, Metter EJ, Riege WH, Winter EJ (1982) Cerebral metabolism and atrophy in Huntington's disease determined by 18FDG and computed tomographic scans. Ann Neurol 12: 425–434

Kuhl DE, Metter EJ, Riege WH (1984a) Patterns of local cerebral glucose utilisation determined in Parkinson's disease by the 18F-fluorodeoxyglucose method. Ann Neurol 15: 419–424

Kuhl DE, Metter EJ, Riege WH, Markham CH (1984b) Patterns of cerebral glucose utilisation in Parkinson's disease and Huntington's disease. Ann Neurol 15 [Suppl]: S119–S125

Kuhl DE, Metter EJ, Benson DF, Ashford JW, Riege WH, Fujikawa DG, Markham CH, Mazziotta JC, Maltese A, Dorsey DA (1985) Similarities of cerebral glucose metabolism in Alzheimer's and Parkinsonian dementia. J Cereb Blood Flow Metab 5: S169–S170 (Abstract)

Kuwert T, Lange HW, Langen KJ, Herzog H, Aulich A, Feinendegen LE (1990) Cortical and subcortical glucose consumption measured by PET in patients with Huntington's disease. Brain 113: 1405–1423

Leenders KL, Frackowiak RSJ, Quinn N, Marsden CD (1986) Brain energy metabolism and dopaminergic function in Huntington's disease measured in vivo using positron emission tomography. Mov Disord 1: 69–77

Leenders KL, Frackowiak RS, Lees AJ (1988) Steele-Richardson-Olszewski syndrome. Brain energy metabolism, blood flow and flurorodopa uptake measured by positron emission tomography. Brain 111: 615–630

Maher ER, Lees AJ (1986) The clinical features and natural history of the Steele-Richardson-Olszewski syndrome (progressive supranuclear palsy). Neurology 36: 1005–1008

Martin JB, Gusella JF (1986) Huntington's disease: pathogenesis and management. N Engl J Med 315: 1267–1276

McKeith I, Fairbairn A, Perry R, Thompson P, Perry E (1992) Neuroleptic sensitivity in patients with senile dementia of Lewy body type. BMJ 305: 673–678

Miletich RS, Chan T, Gillespie M, Di Chiro G, Stein S (1988) Contralateral basal ganglia metabolism is abnormal in hemiparkinsonian patients. An FDG-PET study. Neurology 38: S260

Mushiake H, Inase M, Tanji J (1990) Selective coding of motor sequence in the supplementary motor area of the monkey cerebral cortex. Exp Brain Res 82: 208–210

Otsuka M, Ichiya Y, Hosokawa S, Kuwabara Y, Tahara T, Fukumura T, Kato M, Masuda K, Goto I (1991) Striatal blood flow, glucose metabolism, and ^{18}F-dopa uptake: difference in Parkinson's disease and atypical parkinsonism. J Neurol Neurosurg Psychiatry 54: 898–904

Peppard RF, Martin WRW, Guttman M, McGeer PL, Walsh EM, Carr GD, Phillips AG, Grochowski E, Okada J, Tsui JKC, Mak E, Ruth T, Adam MJ, Calne DB (1988) The relationship of cerebral glucose metabolism to cognitive dificits in Parkinson's disease. Neurology 38 [Suppl 1]: 364

Perlmutter JS, Raichle ME (1985) Regional blood flow in hemiparkinsonism. Neurology 35: 1127–1134

Playford ED, Jenkins IH, Passingham RE, Nutt J, Frackowiak RSJ, Brooks DJ (1992) Impaired mesial frontal and putamen activation in Parkinson's disease: a PET study. Ann Neurol 32: 151–161

Rascol O, Sabatini U, Chollet F, Celsis P, Montastruc J-L, Marc- Vergnes J-P, Rascol A (1992) Supplementary and primary sensory motor area activity in Parkinson's disease. Regional cerebral blood flow changes during finger movements and effects of apomorphine. Arch Neurol 49: 144–148

Riley DE, Lang AE, Lewis A, Resch L, Ashby P, Hornykiewicz O, Black S (1990) Cortical-basal ganglionic degeneration. Neurology 40: 1203–1212

Sage JI, Miller DC, Golbe LI, Walters A, Duvoisin RC (1990) Clinically atypical expression of pathologically typical Lewy-body parkinsonism. Clin Neuropharmacol 13: 36–47

Sawada H, Udaka F, Kameyama M, Seriu N, Nishinaka K, Shindou K, Kodama M, Nishitani N, Okumiya K (1992) SPECT findings in Parkinson's disease associated with dementia. J Neurol Neurosurg Psychiatry 55: 960–963

Sawle GV, Brooks DJ, Marsden CD, Frackowiak RSJ (1991) Corticobasal degeneration: a unique pattern of regional cortical oxygen metabolism and striatal fluorodopa uptake demonstrated by positron emission tomography. Brain 114: 541–556

Schapiro MB, Grady C, Ball MJ, DeCarli C, Rapoport SI (1990) Reductions in parietal/temporal cerebral glucose metabolism are not specific for Alzhemier's disease. Neurology 40 [Suppl] 1: 152

Spokes EGS, Bannister R, Oppenheimer DR (1979) Multiple system atrophy with autonomic failure. Clinical, histological, and neurochemical observations on four cases. J Neurol Sci 43: 59–62

Steele JC, Richardson JC, Olszewski J (1964) Progressive supranuclear palsy. A heterogeneous degeneration involving the brain stem, basal ganglia, and cerebellum, with vertical gaze and pseudobulbar palsy. Arch Neurol 10: 333–359

Thaler DE, Passingham RE (1989) The supplementary motor cortex and internally directed movement. In: Crossman AR, Sambrook M (eds) Neural mechanisms in disorders of movement. Libby, London, pp 175–181

Tyrrell PJ, Warrington EK, Frackowiak RSJ, Rossor MN (1990) Heterogeneity in progressive aphasia due to focal cortical atrophy; a clinical and PET scan study. Brain 113: 1321–1336

Weeks RA, Harding AE, Brooks DJ (1996) PET demonstrates a parallel loss of D_1 and D_2 dopamine receptors in asymptomatic mutation carriers of Huntington's disease. Ann Neurol (in press)

Wienhard K, Coenen HH, Pawlik G, Rudolf J, Laufer P, Jovkar S, Stocklin G, Heiss WD (1990) PET studies of dopamine receptor distribution using [18F]fluoroethylspiperone: findings in disorders related to the dopaminergic system. J Neural Transm 81: 195–213

Wolfson LI, Leenders KL, Brown LL, Jones T (1985) Alterations of regional cerebral blood flow and oxygen metabolism in Parkinson's disease. Neurology 35: 1399–1405

Wong DF, Links JM, Wagner HNJr, Folstein SE, Suneja S, Dannals RF, Ravert HT, Wilson AA, Tune LE, Pearlson G, Folstein MF, Bice A, Kuhar NJ (1985) Dopamine and serotonin receptors measured in-vivo in Huntington's disease with C-11 N-methylspiperone PET imaging. J Nucl Med 26: P107

Young AB, Penney JB, Starosta-Rubinstein S, Markel DS, Berent S, Giordani B, Ehrenkaufer R (1986) PET scan investigations of Huntington's disease: cerebral metabolic correlates of neurological features and functional decline. Ann Neurol 20: 296–303

Young AB, Penney JB, Starosta-Rubinstein S, Markel D, Berent S, Rothley J, Betley A, Hichwa R (1987) Normal caudate glucose metabolism in persons at-risk for Huntington's disease. Arch Neurol 44: 254–257

Author's address: Prof. D. J. Brooks, MRC Cyclotron Unit, Hammersmith Hospital, Du Cane Rd, London W12 0NN, United Kingdom.

J Neural Transm (1996) [Suppl] 47: 169–181

Quantitative EEG in frontal lobe dementia

C. Besthorn, H. Sattel, F. Hentschel, S. Daniel, R. Zerfaß, and H. Förstl

Central Institute of Mental Health, Mannheim, Federal Republic of Germany

Summary. A study on quantitative EEG in 14 patients with frontal lobe dementia (FLD), 14 patients with Alzheimer's disease (AD), and 14 healthy controls was conducted using a complete set of EEG parameters: band power, coherence and fractal dimension. Contrary to earlier studies, we observed higher theta power and sagittal interactions in higher frequency bands in the FLD than in the control group. Lateral interactions of coherence and two indices of fractal dimension were lower in FLD than in controls. There was greater electrophysiological resemblance between the control group and FLD than between any of these groups and AD. This was documented by the results of a discriminant analysis which led to a correct overall classification of 66% of the subjects with misclassifications occurring primarily between control and FLD group.

Introduction

A wealth of papers has documented the electro-physiological characteristics of Alzheimer's disease (AD) as the most prevalent form of dementia (Besthorn et al., 1994, 1995; Szelies et al., 1994; Coben et al., 1990), but little is known about electroencephalographic changes in frontal lobe dementia (FLD). Since in terms of clinical diagnoses FLD can not be distinguished from Pick's disease, reports on the effects of this diagnosis on EEG parameters may be included, though there are certain differences (Baldwin and Förstl, 1993).

Most of the rare original papers on EEG in FLD (Neary et al., 1988; Stigsby et al., 1981; Förstl et al., 1996) and several reviews (Fenton, 1986; Giannitrapani and Collins, 1988) mentioned normal EEG findings in FLD, whereas a decrease of alpha and beta power together with an increase of delta and theta power has been reported consistently in AD (Brenner et al., 1988; Penttilä et al., 1985; Soininen et al., 1991; Hooijer et al., 1990).

We have carried out an extensive analysis of quantitative EEG parameters from 17 EEG locations in FLD including band power, coherence and two indices of EEG fractal dimension. FLD patients are compared with normal controls and AD patients.

Methods

Sample

FLD Patients were identified from consecutive new referrals to the Central Institute of Mental Health. AD patients and controls were recruited from an ongoing longitudinal study (Förstl et al., 1993) and were matched for gender and age with the FLD patients. FLD patients (n = 14) were diagnosed according to standard clinical criteria, i.e. a score > 5 on the scale by Gustafson and Nilsson (1982) was required. AD Patients (n = 14) were diagnosed as probable AD following NINCDS-ADRDA criteria (McKhann et al., 1984). Controls (n = 14) were free of neurological or psychiatric disorders.

Standard psychometric tests (see below) and cranial computed tomography (CT) were carried out. Descriptive data of the sample are given as mean ± SD: FLD patients: n = 14, age = 58.9 ± 6.4, Mini Mental State Examination (MMSE) (Folstein et al., 1975) = 16.0 ± 10.7, Clinical Dementia Rating (CDR) (Hughes et al., 1982) = 1.7 ± 1.3. AD patients: n = 14, age = 60.3 ± 3.8, MMSE = 13.6 ± 6.1, CDR = 1.6 ± 0.8. Controls: n = 14, age = 59.7 ± 4.1, MMSE = 29.3 ± 0.7, CDR = 0.0 ± 0.0 . A a more detailed description of clinical and research criteria is given in Förstl et al. (1995).

EEG recording

Resting EEG was recorded with eyes closed and with eyes open. 17 EEG locations (all of the 10–20 system exept for Fp1 and Fp2) were amplified against common reference on a Nihon Kohden 4321 G using a time constant of 1.0 sec and a high frequency cut-off of 70 Hz. Common reference was the middle of a 20 kOhm voltage divider between the left and the right ear. This "shunted earlobes"-reference (Katznelson, 1981) is slightly superior to the traditional linked ears method (Nunez, 1991). Data (120 sec) were digitized online at 200 Hz on a PC-AT as laboratory computer.

Twenty sec EEG epochs were drawn by minimization of EOG power (Möcks et al., 1984) as an indicator of the subjects' relaxation. Vertical and horizontal EOG was recorded, in order to compute an EOG correction in a combined time and frequency domain approach (Möcks et al., 1989).

Bandpower

EEG Power was computed according to Matousek and Petersèn (1973) in six frequency bands: delta 1.5 — 3.5 Hz, theta 3.5 — 7.5 Hz, alpha1 7.5 — 9.5 Hz, alpha2 9.5 — 12.5 Hz, beta1 12.5 — 17.5 Hz and beta2 17.5 — 25.0 Hz. A frequency band (50.5 — 69 Hz) indicative of muscle activity was computed following Schellberg et al. (1993; see also O'Donnel et al., 1974) and integrated as covariate in the topographic ANOVAs (see below). This approach served as a control for muscle artifacts in higher frequency bands. Bandpower was log transfomed prior to analyses to approximate the normal distribution (Gasser et al., 1982).

Coherence

Coherence was computed in the above mentioned frequency bands according to Besthorn et al. (1994) by averaging the coherences between one electrode and all surrounding electrodes, e.g. for C4 the following coherences were averaged: C4-Fz, C4-F4, C4-F8, C4-T4, C4-T6, C4-P4, C4-Pz, C4-Cz. At the margin of the 10–20 system, the set of neighbouring electrodes is necessarily incomplete, e.g. coherences of F7 were only averaged over F7-F3, F7-C3 and F7-T3.

Coherences were averaged for two reasons. The influence of interelectrode distance on coherence (Bullock and McClune, 1989) was held constant by integrating the information from all electrodes being one "10–20 unit" apart from each other. Additionally, combinatorial explosion of channel pairs (in our data (17 * 16)/2 = 136 coherences for one frequency band) was avoided.

The resulting scores are interpreted as average synchrony with respect to neighbouring cortex areas. Averaged coherences were transformed towards normal distribution by arcsin(sqrt(x)) following Gasser et al. (1985).

Grassberger-Procaccia dimension

Fractal dimension or dimensional complexity is an application of chaos theory (Peitgen et al., 1992) towards empirically measured time series. A multidimensional reconstruction of the phase space of an EEG time series is conducted. Within the phase space the dimension of the subspace of the most frequently used orbits is determined, and this is called fractal dimension, attractor dimension or — following Pritchard et al. (1991) — dimensional complexity. The most common algorithm to compute the fractal dimension was given by Grassberger and Procaccia (1983). Using the multidimensional reconstruction the Grassberger-Procaccia dimension gives an index of dimensional complexity for each unidimensional EEG time series on input.

The interpretation of this parameter is system complexity: EEG with eyes open has a higher dimensional complexity than with eyes closed, mental tasks increase the complexity and during sleep it is reduced (Lutzenberger et al., 1992; Röschke and Aldenhoff, 1991; Pritchard and Duke, 1992). The fast algorithm being used is given in Besthorn (1992) and details of the application to EEG data and the estimation of parameters can be found in Besthorn et al. (1995).

Dvorak dimension

Since the estimation of Grassberger-Procaccia dimensions has been critisized (Jansen, 1992; Theiler, 1991), we used the Dvorak dimension as a another examination of the fractal dimension.

The Dvorak algorithm (Dvorak, 1990) is partly similar to the Grassberger-Procaccia algorithm. The multidi-mensional reconstruction from a unidimensional time series (Takens, 1981) with its inborn problems (Frank et al., 1990; Caputo et al., 1986) is replaced by a multidimensional time series as input. In our data 17 EEG channels were used as input. Further calculations are similar to the Grassberger-Procaccia algorithm, i.e. multidimensional distances between all points were determined and the dimension is estimated from the CD(r) curve.

The program for the Dvorak dimension was derived from the Grassberger-Procaccia program mentioned above. All 17 time series (length 4096 points) were standardized ($\mu = 0$, $\mu = 1$) and filtered (0.5 Hz to 30.0 Hz bandpass, see Besthorn et al., 1995): The radii r were set automatically. The log C(r) curve was computed and two times differentiated. The scaling region was automatically recognized where y'' was zero.

The Dvorak algorithm converges better (Dvorak, 1990), though fitting a kind of a "global brain attractor" to all EEG channels together appears to be artificial.

Topographical ANOVA

Using a set of 6 frequency bands and 17 channels one would expect 5 significant results from multiple univariate tests. In order to avoid multiple testing on one side and an excessively conservative Bonferroni correction on the other side, we applied repeated measurements analysis of variance (rANOVA). The diagnosis effect reflects FLD vs. AD patients vs. controls, whereas the multiple electrodes are regarded as repeated measurements being obtained within two trial factors ("lateral" = left versus right and "sagittal" = frontal vs. occipital). Since the trial factors can be interpreted in terms of topography, it is called "topographical ANOVA".

The trial factors are always significant, since they are modeling only natural modulations of the distribution of power in a given frequency band over the head. Trial factors themselves have no meaning for the evaluation of group differences and are not given in the ANOVA tables. Thus, the relevant terms are only the grouping factor (diagnosis) and its interactions with topography factors (sagittal and lateral). Additionally, the three way interaction (patient versus control * sagittal * lateral) was not specified.

Results

Band power

Conventional band power indices were tested by "topographical ANOVA" and the p-values are given in Table 1. In both conditions, eyes closed and eyes open, there was no significant effect for the delta band, but a significant main effect for the theta band. FLD patients had higher theta power than controls, and AD patients had a theta power above FLD patients. Means of the theta band from condition eyes open are displayed as an example in Fig. 1. For the alpha and beta bands in both conditions interactions were found between the factors diagnosis (control vs. FLD vs. AD) and sagittal (frontal vs. occipital). In order to display the interaction, all frontal, central, parietal and occipital electrodes were averaged together, respectively. As an example, these means of the alpha2 band in condition eyes closed are displayed in the lower half of Fig. 1. FLD patients start in frontal locations at the level of AD patients, and reach the level of controls in occipital locations.

Table 1. Topographical ANOVA for band power

		delta	theta	alpha1	alpha2	beta1	beta2
Eyes closed	Diag	.11	.002	.56	.34	.12	.04
	Diag*Sagit	.47	.19	.006	.001	.004	.05
	Diag*Lat	.83	.54	.14	.25	.14	.06
Eyes open	Diag	.06	.0005	.24	.53	.35	.09
	Diag*Sagit	.94	.71	.02	.0005	.007	.29
	Diag*Lat	.49	.73	.40	.54	.30	.32

P-values from repeated measures ANOVA for band power parameters in conditions EEG at rest with eyes closed and open. "Diag" is the main effect (Control vs. FLD vs. AD) (see methods for further description of "topographical ANOVA")

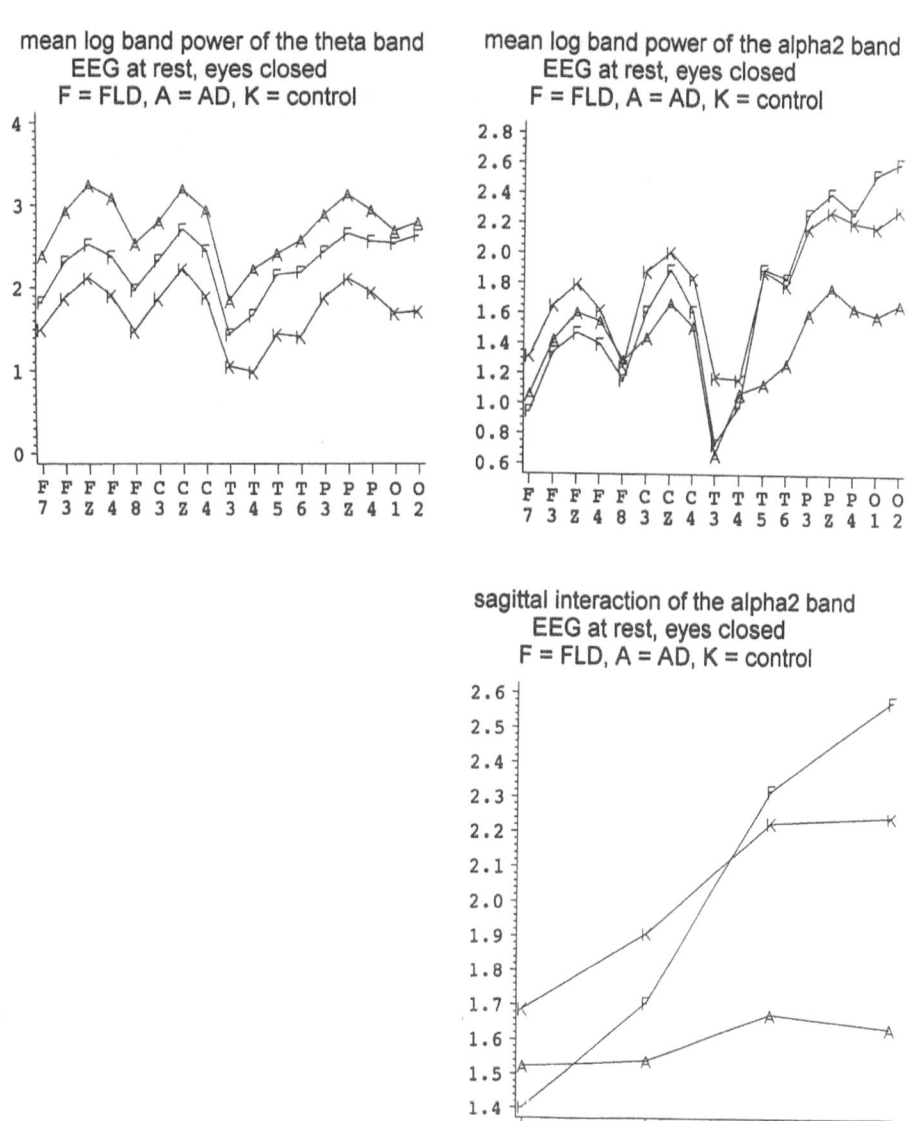

Fig. 1. Means for band power

Coherence

Coherences were submitted to topographical ANOVA and resulting p-values can be found in Table 2. There were no main effects, but a few significant interactions diagnosis * sagittal and several interactions diagnosis * lateral. The two selected frequency bands being displayed in Fig. 2 showed no pattern, that could be interpreted easily. This results from the fact, that coherence is restricted to values between 0.0 and 1.0 and that the means of the three groups were lying close together. The graphs became clearer, when

Table 2. Topographical ANOVA for coherence

		delta	theta	alpha1	alpha2	beta1	beta2
Eyes closed	Diag	.91	.86	.65	.94	.75	.39
	Diag*Sagit	.02	.004	.57	.59	.04	.04
	Diag*Lat	.39	.04	.01	.04	.0002	.02
Eyes open	Diag	.68	.30	.92	.73	.72	.36
	Diag*Sagit	.02	.22	.35	.37	.02	.09
	Diag*Lat	.58	.09	.008	.09	.002	.28

P-values from repeated measures ANOVA for coherences in conditions EEG at rest with eyes closed and open. "Diag" is the main effect (Control vs. FLD vs. AD)

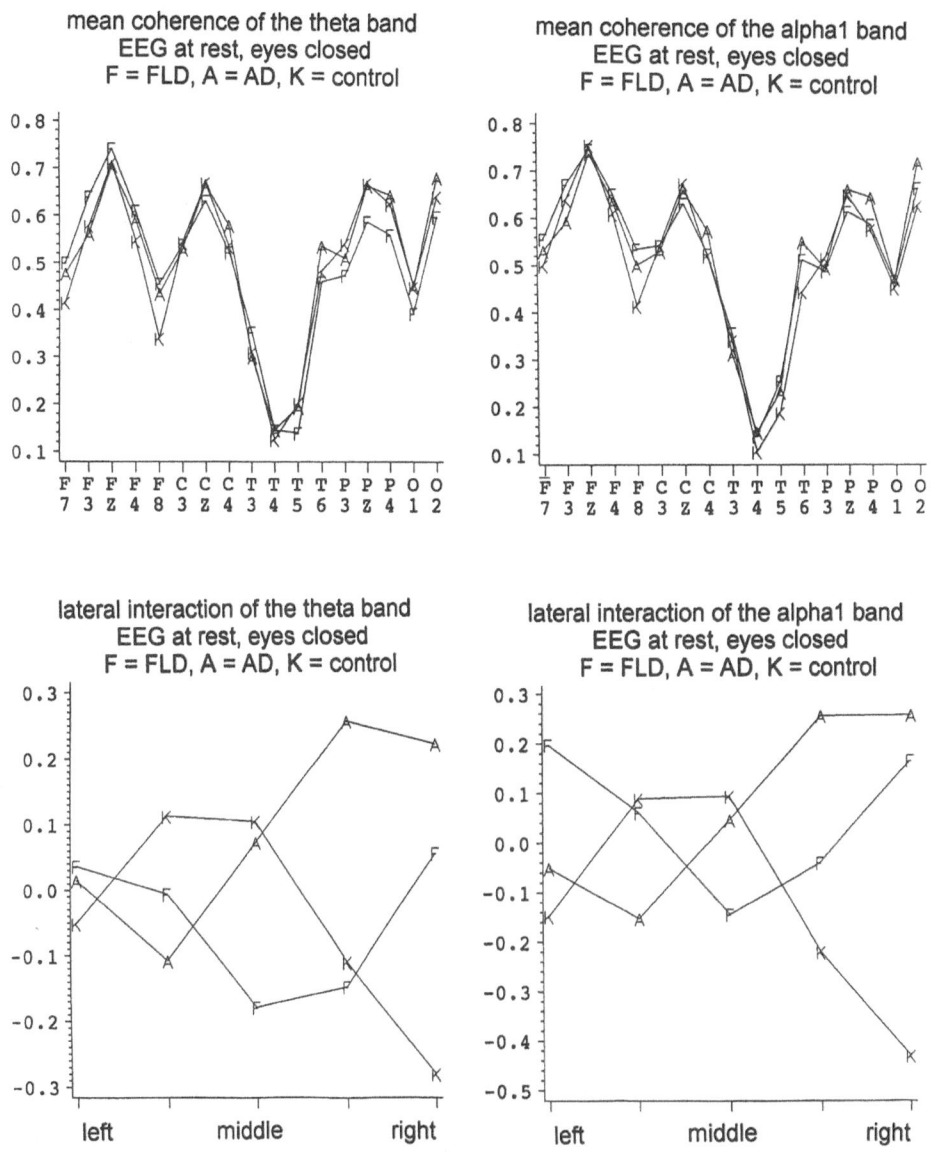

Fig. 2. Means for coherences

Table 3. Topographical ANOVA for Grassberger-Procaccia dimension

	Eyes closed	Eyes open
Diag	.10	.09
Diag*Sagit	.41	.95
Diag*Lat	.42	.08

P-values from repeated measures ANOVA for Grassberger-Procaccia dimensions in conditions EEG at rest with eyes closed and open. "Diag" is the main effect (Control vs. FLD vs. AD)

coherences were standardized before plotting in order to enlarge group differences graphically. Lateral interactions were plotted by averaging left, middle and right electrodes respectively in the lower half of Fig. 2. Though only two frequency bands are shown for reasons of brevity, results in Fig. 2 may be integrated by stating a "U-curve" for FLD, a "zig-zag-curve" for AD and an "inverted U-curve" for controls.

Grassberger-Procaccia dimension

The fractal dimension according to the Grassberger-Procaccia method served as an index of dimensional complexity for each EEG location. In a recent paper we have shown (Besthorn et al., 1995), that AD patients had lower scores. According to Table 3, there were no significant results from topographical ANOVA. The absolute decrease of fractal dimension in AD (see Fig. 3) was similar to Besthorn et al. (1995), where these group differences between controls and AD had been significant due to a larger sample size.

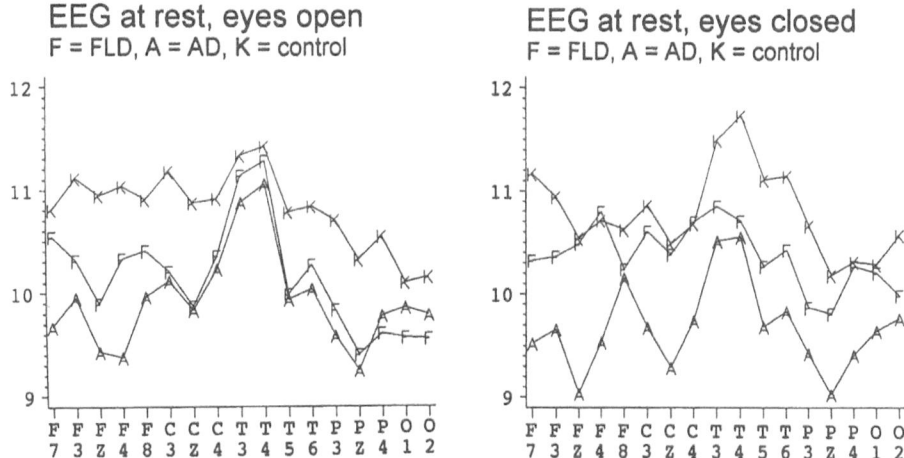

Fig. 3. Means for Grassberger-Procaccia dimension

Dvorak dimension

The Dvorak dimension estimates dimensional complexity from all EEG channels as a multivariate input, and therefore has no topographical information. Since there were no multiple electrodes, no topographical ANOVA was undertaken and each pair of groups was tested by U-tests. As shown in Table 4, only one of 6 tests was significant, in spite of large group differences (see Fig. 4). FLD and AD patients had lower dimensions than controls. Group differences of the Dvorak dimension were larger than group differences of the Grassberger-Procaccia dimensions. The Dvorak dimension was numerically smaller than the Grassberger-Procaccia dimension since it is modelling a "global brain attractor". In the case of the Grassberger-Procaccia dimension, locally active attractors add some complexity to the global attractor and thus Grassberger-Procaccia dimensions with their single electrode dimensions were numerically higher.

Table 4. U-Tests for Dvorak dimension

	Eyes closed	Eyes open
FLD — Control	.03	.12
FLD — AD	.73	.55
Control — AD	.15	.06

P-values from U-tests on group differences

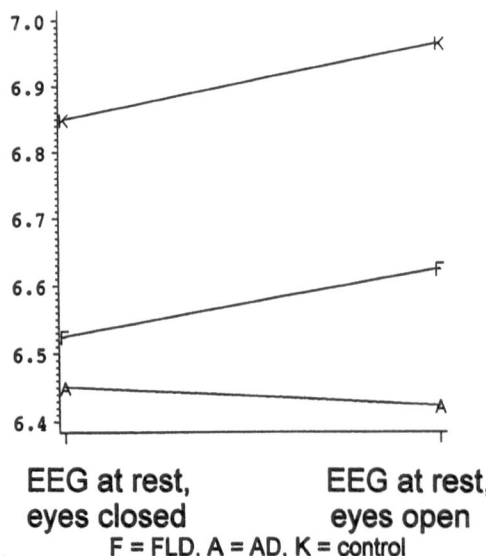

F = FLD, A = AD, K = control

Fig. 4. Means for Dvorak dimension

Table 5. Discriminant analysis

		classified into		
		controls	AD	FLD
true	controls	9	1	4
	AD	1	12	1
	FLD	5	2	7

66% of the subjects were classified correctly, while a random classification would yield 33%

Discriminant analysis

A simulation may show, that discriminant analysis gives exceedingly good classifications, if too many predictors are used: Classifying 100 cases in two groups of equal size yields 58% correct decisions using 10 randomly generated variables, 85% correct decisions using 50 variables and 100% using 100 variables. The reason is, that random variables generate random correlations with the classification criterion and by chance one or more of these correlations may be substantial. Thus the number of predictors should be small compared to the number of cases (Lachenbruch, 1975) in order to reveal robust effects.

Since the problem of too many predictors is of special relevance to EEG studies with several EEG electrodes, parameters and frequency bands, we used principal components analysis (PCA) in order to compress groups of variables into artificial factors. Three groups of variables were chosen. Bandpower variables of the theta band from frontal EEG locations were submitted to PCA. The first component comprising the greatest common variance of these variables was kept as the first predictor. The second predictor was obtained from a PCA on parietal and occipital alpha and beta power, and the third predictor resulted from PCA on frontal Grassberger-Procaccia dimensions. The selection of variable groups to be compressed was heuristically driven by the above reported results. A discriminant analysis using jackknifing was computed with these three predictors. The classification results are given in Table 5.

Discussion

According to our results, the increased theta band power in FLD was significantly higher than in controls as supposed other authors (Stigsby et al., 1981), but it was not as high as in AD. This result is interpreted in terms of the theta band being related to dementing processes. In contrast to FLD patients, AD patients had higher delta power than controls. Higher frequency bands showed a topographical interaction for FLD. In frontal leads FLD patients had patterns that were comparable to AD patients, and in anterior leads they were similar to normal controls. AD patients had lower alpha and beta power than controls. This interaction may be related to the location of the main area of brain atrophy in FLD.

In coherence analyses, which were not undertaken in previous papers, FLD showed consistently patterns that were distinguishable from AD and also from controls: FLD had a "U-curve", while AD had a "zig-zag-curve" and controls were characterized by an "inverted U-curve". Though an interpretation of these results in terms of regional atrophies is intriguing, coherence parameters were best suited to separate FLD from controls as well as FLD from AD patients. We have shown in a recent paper using a larger sample (Besthorn et al., 1994) that AD patients have lower coherences than controls in the theta, alpha and beta band. A similar main effect could not be demonstrated in FLD, where only the topographical interactions were significant.

Fractal dimension or dimensional complexity (Pritchard et al., 1991) was examined by the Grassberger-Procaccia dimension and the Dvorak dimension. Recent studies (Besthorn et al., 1995; Pritchard et al., 1994) on decreased dimensions in AD were fully supported, and a decrease of the fractal dimension has now been demonstrated in FLD. The interpretation of decreasing fractal dimensions as an index of complexity is compatible with a decreased complexity of cognitive processes in different types of dementia (Pritchard et al., 1994; Lutzenberger et al., 1992) due to neuronal degeneration (DeKosky and Scheff, 1990; Förstl et al., 1992).

Discriminant analysis based on a selection of quantitative EEG parameters classified individuals from the AD, FLD and control group with considerable success. This underscores the validity of the data analyses presented. The electrophysiological similarities between the FLD and controls groups are documented by the misclassifications between these groups, which — contrary to the results with AD — were not infrequent. The clinical differential diagnosis between different forms of degenerative dementia is to some extent arbitrary and Alzheimer-type neuropathological changes with frontal onset are clinically indistinguishable from FLD (Baldwin and Förstl, 1993). Therefore, an admixture of atypical cases in the FLD group cannot be ruled out with final certainty. This limitation needs to be considered in the interpretation of our discriminant analysis. The prognostic importance and specifity of our analyses is currently under prospective evaluation.

Acknowledgements

This study was supported by the Deutsche Forschungsgemeinschaft, SFB 258, project K2 (Förstl/Beyreuther) and SAP AG Walldorf/Baden.

References

Baldwin B, Förstl H (1993) "Pick's disease" — 101 years on: still there, but in need of reform. Br J Psychiatry 163: 100–104

Besthorn C (1992) Improving algorithms for Grassberger-Procaccia dimension calculations using Euclidian norms. EEG chaos newsletter 3: 21–24

Besthorn C, Förstl H, Geiger-Kabisch C, Sattel H, Gasser T, Schreiter-Gasser U (1994) EEG coherences in Alzheimer disease. Electroencephalogr Clin Neurophysiol 90: 242–245

Besthorn C, Sattel H, Geiger-Kabisch C, Zerfaβ R, Förstl H (1995) Parameters of EEG fractal dimension in Alzheimer's disease. Electroencephalogr Clin Neurophysiol 95: 84–89

Bullock TW, McClune MC (1989) Lateral coherence of the electrocorticogram: a new measure of brain synchrony. Electroencephalogr Clin Neurophysiol 73: 479–488

Brenner RP, Reynolds CF, Ulrich RF (1988) Diagnostic efficacy of computerized spectral versus visual EEG analysis in elderly normal, demented and depressed subjects. Electroencephalogr Clin Neurophysiol 69: 110–117

Caputo JG, Malraison B, Atten P (1986) Determination of attractor dimensions and entropy for various flows: an experi-mentalists viewpoint. In: Mayer-Kress G (ed) Dimension and entropies in chaotic systems. Springer, New York

Coben LA, Chi D, Snyder AZ, Storandt M (1990) Replication of a study of frequency analysis of the resting awake EEG in mild probable Alzheimer disease. Electroencephalogr Clin Neurophysiol 75: 148–154

DeKosky ST, Scheff SW (1990) Synapse loss in frontal cortex biopsies in Alzheimer's disease: correlation with cognitive severity. Ann Neurol 27: 457–464

Dvorak I (1990) Takens versus multichannel reconstruction in EEG correlation exponent estimates. Phys Lett A 151: 225–233

Fenton, GW (1986) Electroenphysiology of Alzheimer's disease. Br Med Bull 62: 29–33

Folstein MF, Folstein SE, McHugh PR (1975) "Mini-Mental-State": a practical method for grading the cognitive state of patients for the clinician. J Psychiatr Res 12: 189–198

Förstl H, Burns A, Levy R, Cairns N, Luthert P, Lantos, P (1992) Neurologic signs in Alzheimer's disease. Arch Neurol 49: 1038–1042

Förstl H, Besthorn C, Geiger-Kabisch C, Sattel H, Schreiter-Gasser U (1993) Psychotic features and the course of Alzheimer's disease: relationship to cognitive, electroencephalographic and computerized tomography findings. Acta Psychiatr Scand 87: 395–399

Förstl H, Besthorn C, Hentschel F, Geiger-Kabisch C, Sattel H, Schreiter-Gasser U (1996) Frontal lobe degeneration and Alzheimer's disease: a controlled study on clinical findings, volumetric brain changes and quantitative electroencephalogry data. Dementia 7: 27–34

Frank GW, Lookman T, Nerenberg MAH (1990) Recovering the attractor: a review of chaotic time series analysis. Can J Phys 68: 711–718

Gasser T, Bächer P, Möcks J (1982) Transformation toward the normal distribution of broad band spectral parameters of the EEG. Electroencephalogr Clin Neurophysiol 53: 119–124

Gasser T, Jennen-Steinmetz C, Verleger R (1985) EEG coherence at rest and during a visual task in two groups of children. Electroencephalogr Clin Neurophysiol 67: 151–158

Giannitrapani D, Collins J (1988) EEG differentiation between Alzheimer's and non-Alzheimer's dementias. In: Giannitrapani D, Murri R (eds) The EEG of mental activities. Karger, Basel, pp 26–41

Grassberger P, Procaccia I (1983) Measuring the strangeness of strange attractors. Physica D 9: 189–208

Gustafson L, Nilsson L (1982) Differential diagnosis of presenile dementia on clinical grounds. Acta Psychiatr Scand 65: 194–209

Hooijer C, Jonker C, Posthuma J, Visser SL (1990) Reliability, validity and follow-up of the EEG in senile dementia: sequelae of sequential measurement. Electroencephalogr Clin Neurophysiol 76: 400–412

Hughes CP, Berg L, Danziger WL, Coben LA, Martin RL (1982) A new clinical scale for the staging of dementia. Br J Psychiatry 140: 566–572

Jansen, BH (1992) "Is it?" and "so what?" — a critical review of EEG chaos. In: Duke DW, Pritchard WS (eds) Measuring chaos in the human brain. World Scientific, Singapure

Katznelson RD (1981) EEG recording, electrode placement, and aspects of generator localization. In: Nunez PL (ed) Electrical fields of the brain. Oxford University Press, New York, pp 176–213

Lachenbruch PA (1975) Discriminant analysis. Hafner, New York

Lutzenberger W, Birbaumer N, Flor H, Rockstroh B, Elbert T (1992) Dimensional analysis of the human EEG and intelligence. Neurosci Lett 143: 10–14

Matousek M, Petersèn I (1973) Frequency analysis of the EEG in normal children (1–15 years) and in normal adolescents (16–21 years). In: Kellaway P, Peterson I (eds) Automation of clinical electroencephalography. Raven, New York, pp 75–102

McKhann G, Drachmann D, Folstein M, Katzman R, Price D, Stadlan EM (1984) Clinical diagnosis of Alzheimer's disease: report of the NINCDS-ADRDA Work Group under the auspices of Department of Health and Human Services Task Force on Alzheimer's Disease. Neurology 34: 939–944

Möcks J, Gasser T (1984) How to select epochs of the EEG at rest for quantitative analysis. Electroencephalogr Clin Neurophysiol 58: 89–92

Möcks J, Gasser T, Sroka L (1989) Approaches to correcting EOG artifacts. J Psychophysiol 3: 21–26

Neary D, Snowden JS, Northen B, Goulding P (1988) Dementia of frontal lobe type. J Neurol Neurosurg Psychiatry 51: 353–361

Nunez P (1991) Comments on the paper by Miller, Lutzenberger, Elbert. J Psychophysiol 5: 279–280

O'Donnel RD, Berkhout J, Adey RW (1974) Contamination of scalp EEG spectrum during contraction of cranio-facial muscles. Electroencephalogr Clin Neurophysiol 37: 145–151

Peitgen HO, Jürgens H, Saupe D (1992) Chaos and fractals. New frontiers of science. Springer, New York

Penttilä M, Partanen JV, Soininen H, Riekkinen PJ (1985) Quantitative analysis of occipital EEG in different stages of Alzheimer's disease. Electroencephalogr Clin Neurophysiol 60: 1–6

Pritchard WS, Duke DW, Coburn KL (1991) Altered EEG dynamical responsivity associated with normal aging and propable Alzheimer's disease. Dementia 2: 102–105

Pritchard WS, Duke DW (1992) Dimensional analysis of no-task human EEG using the Grassberger Procaccia method. Psychophysiology 29: 182–192

Pritchard WS, Duke DW, Coburn KL, Moore NC, Tucker KA, Jann MW, Hostetler RM (1994) EEG based, neural-net predictive classification of Alzheimer's disease versus control subjects is augmented by non-linear EEG measures. Electroencephalogr Clin Neurophysiol 91: 118–130

Röschke J, Aldenhoff J (1991) The dimensionality of human's electroencephalogram during sleep. Biol Cybernet 64: 307–313

Schellberg D, Besthorn C, Pfleger W, Gasser T (1993) Emotional activation and topographic EEG band power. J Psychophysiol 7: 24–33

Soininen H, Partanen J, Laulumaa V, Helkala EL, Laakso M Riekkinen PJ (1991) Longitudinal EEG spectral analysis in early stage of Alzheimers disease. Electroencephalogr Clin Neurophysiol 72: 290–297

Stigsby B, Johannesson G, Ingvar DM (1981) Regional EEG analysis and regional cerebral blood flow in Alzheimer's and Pick's disease. Electroencephalogr Clin Neurophysiol 51: 537–547

Szelies B, Mielke R, Herholz K, Heiss WD (1994) Quantitative topographical EEG compared to FDG PET for classification of vascular and degenerative dementia. Electroencephalogr Clin Neurophysiol 91: 131–139

Takens F (1981) Detecting strange attractors in turbulence. In: Rand DA, Young LS
    (eds) Lecture notes in mathematics, vol 898. Springer, New York
Theiler J (1991) Some comments on the correlation dimension of $1/f^{**}\alpha$ noise. Phys Lett
    A 155: 480–493

Authors' address: Dr. C. Besthorn, Zentralinstitut für Seelische Gesundheit, P.O.B.
12 21 20, D-68159 Mannheim, Federal Republic of Germany.

J Neural Transm (1996) [Suppl] 47: 183–191

Vascular dementia: perfusional and metabolic disturbances and effects of therapy

R. Mielke, J. Kessler, B. Szelies, K. Herholz, K. Wienhard,
and **W.-D. Heiss**

Max-Planck-Institut für Neurologische Forschung und Universitätsklinik für
Neurologie, Köln, Federal Republic of Germany

Summary. Positron emission tomography (PET) has elucidated basic patho-physiological mechanism that produce the cognitive decline in vascular dementia (VD). The typical pattern of glucose metabolism seen in VD with scattered areas of focal cortical and subcortical hypometabolism differs from that in AD with marked hypometabolism affecting the association areas. The total volume of metabolically inactive tissue is significantly related to severity of dementia. Rather than the quantity of tissue destruction, the critical effect may be the quantity of cortical hypometabolism caused by subcortically induced disconnection. Studies with HMPAO SPECT have shown focal deficits in VD and AD patients that are comparable to those seen with FDG PET. In mildly demented patients performance for the classification AD versus VD is much better by PET because it might be more sensitive for imaging small functional pathological changes. A longitudinal analysis of rCMRGl in VD showed that the progression of dementia can be delayed by the adenosine uptake blocker propentofylline and that neuropsychological and metabolic changes are closely related.

Introduction

Due to advances in neuroimaging vascular dementia (VD) is increasingly diagnosed as an important cause of cognitive impairment in the elderly. Based on different diagnostic criteria the frequency of VD ranged from 4.5 to 39% within the total group of organic brain diseases with dementia as leading symptom (Kase, 1991). Populatio — based studies have shown a very high prevalence of 47% above 85 years of age, while only 44% were attributable to Alzheimer's disease (AD) (Skoog et al., 1993). Although these data give evidence that VD is the second most common cause of dementia, the patho-physiological mechanisms that produce the cognitive decline are not completely enlightened. Yet, in contrast to AD, dementia due to cerebrovascular disease seems to be potentially treatable or a preventable condition if an early diagnosis by modern neuroimaging technics can be made.

Focal cerebral lesions caused by blood flow disturbances can induce cognitive impairment by at least two mechanisms: multiple ischemic lesions in sometimes neurologically silent regions reduce the amount of gray matter necessary for higher cognitive functions. The early neuropathological studies by Tomlinson et al. (1968, 1970) suggested that the infarct size is important in vascular dementia and emphasized that infarct volume must exceed a not precisely defined threshold of 80 to 150 cm³. However, these postmortem studies could not clarify a relationship between the total volume of brain infarction and degree of cognitive decline. Rarely, small singular infarcts of critical locations can cause dementia syndrome, such as thalamic dementia.

Vascular dementia is usually defined according to the International Classification of Diseases (ICD 10) of the World Health Organization (1991). The term multi-infarct dementia represents here one subentity with preferential cortical infarctions. Clinically, multi-infarct dementia is often diagnosed based on rating scales, for example the Hachinski score (Hachinski et al., 1975) that only formalises neurological examination. Similar to the NINCDS-ADRDA (National Institute of Neurological and Communicative Disorder in Stroke-Alzheimer's disease and Related Disorders Association) criteria for the clinical diagnosis of Alzheimer's disease (McKhann et al., 1984), Roman et al. (1993) recently reported the NINDS-AIREN (National Institute of Neurological Disorder and Stroke-Association Internationale pour la Recherche et l'Enseignement en Neurosciences) criteria for the diagnosis of vascular dementia. These criteria included neuroimaging data for the diagnostic classification. While CT and MRI scan show morphological alterations such as infarcts and brain atrophy at advanced stages of the disease positron emission tomography (PET) is currently the only reliable method affording three-dimensional measurement of cortical energy metabolism in dementia, that is closely related to neuropsychological function.

Results of positron emission tomography

In VD-patients PET of F-18-fluoro-2-deoxy-D-glucose (FDG) can clearly differentiate scattered areas of focal cortical and subcortical hypometabolism that differs from the typical metabolic pattern seen in AD with marked hypometabolism affecting the association areas (Benson et al., 1983; Kuhl et

---➤

Fig. 1. Transaxial slices of regional cerebral glucose metabolism (upper row) and regional cerebral blood flow (lower row) images in VD and AD at two levels in comparison to a normal control demonstrating coupling of metabolism and flow. Patients presented similar severity of dementia. The PET of the 66 year old AD patient shows the typical pattern with pronounced bilateral decrease in metabolism and flow, particularly in the parieto-temporal and frontal associative cortex with relative recessing of the primary sensory and sensorimotor areas. In VD the PET images of a 68 year old patient show scattered areas of focal cortical hypometabolism and impairmant of flow
Fig. 4. a,b Transaxial slices of FDG PET (a) and HMPAO SPECT in the same AD patient (upper row) and VD patient. Severity of dementia is mild (MMSE 23). FDG PET allows better differentiation between AD and VD

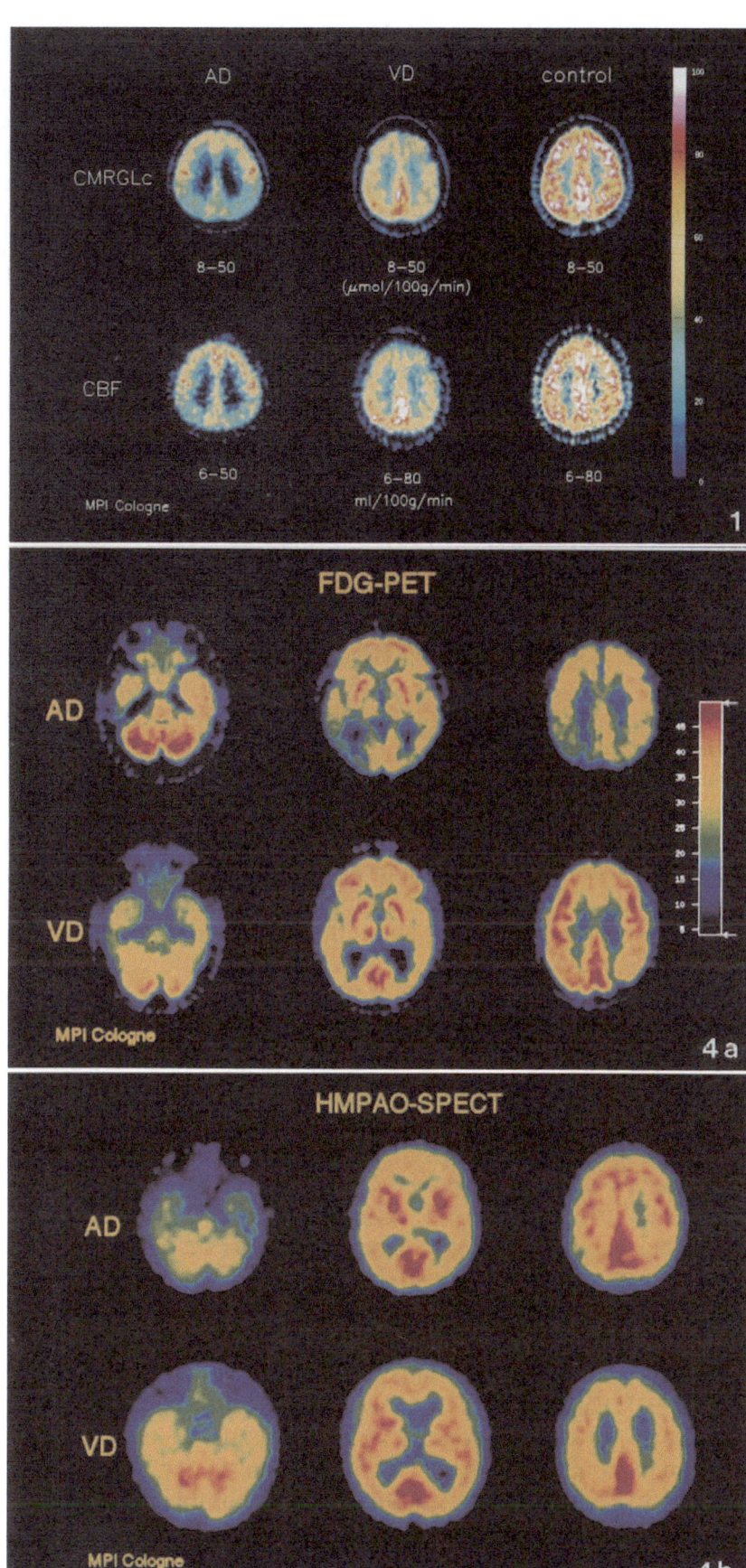

CMRGLc

AD   VD   control

8–50   8–50   8–50
(µmol/100g/min)

CBF

6–50   6–80   6–80
ml/100g/min

MPI Cologne

1

FDG-PET

AD

VD

MPI Cologne

4 a

HMPAO-SPECT

AD

VD

MPI Cologne

4 b

al., 1983). In another study (Mielke et al., 1992), in VD we observed in many areas (middle frontal cortex, temporo-parietal cortex, basal ganglia, cerebellum and brainstem) a significant reduction of regional cerebral glucose metabolism (rCMRGl) in comparison to normals. In subcortical areas and primary sensorimotor cortex, this hypometabolism was slightly more marked than in AD, while the association areas were less affected than in AD, albeit there was no significant difference in rCMRGL between VD and AD. The general pattern, however, was different: A metabolic ratio (rCMRGl of association areas divided by rCMRGl of primary areas, basal ganglia, cerebellum and brainstem), mainly reflecting the contrast between association areas and subcortical regions, was significantly lower in AD than in VD. These findings are consistent with earlier studies on this topic (Herholz et al., 1990; Kuhl et al., 1985). In a retrospective study, Herholz et al. (1990) found lower values of this ratio in AD patients than in patients with VD. Kuhl et al. (1983) reported a significantly lower parietal to cerebellar ratio in AD than in MID patients. Thus, we could not identify a single region that could discriminate between VD and AD, but we found the composite pattern, as expressed in the metabolic ratio, significantly different. The PET images (Fig. 1) demonstrate typical findings in vascular and primary degenerative dementia in two patients with identical severity of dementia as expressed by the Mini-Mental score (MMSE; Folstein et al., 1975). For this metabolic ratio, which reflects the pattern of metabolic pathology in AD, a significant effect of the dementia severity tested by MMSE as a covariate (p < 0.001) and of the diagnostic group (p < 0.01) was found. The different regression lines of the metabolic ratio on MMSE scores in VD and AD are illustrated in Fig. 2. They show that the metabolic ratio was generally higher in VD than AD. In addition, there was a parallel decline of the metabolic ratio with increasing dementia severity in both groups suggesting equal ability to discriminate VD and AD in early and advanced stages of the disease. The volume of regions that were significantly hypometabolic (rCMRGl less than lower 95% prediction limit of the control population) were calculated in comparison to the rCMRGL of normals. It reflects the metabolically altered tissue and did not differ between VD and AD: 76.1 cm^3 in VD and 79.7 cm^3 in AD. The ANCOVA showed a significant relation between MMSE and the volume of affected regions (p < 0.001) but no effect of the diagnostic classification in VD and AD. Thus, the relation between the hypometabolic volume and dementia severity was similar in VD and AD. It indicates that the degree of cognitive dysfunction depends rather on the extent of the metabolic impairment than on the pathogenetic basis of VD or AD. Considering that the VD patients in this study had mainly leukoaraiosis and small subcortical infarcts, it indicates, furthermore, that even small infarcts in combination with leukoaraiosis may contribute to cognitive decline. This is in some contrast to the findings of Tomlinson et al. (1968) who stressed that VD must be due to multiple vascular lesions destroying a critical volume of brain tissue. Rather than the total volume of infarction, the overall volume of functional tissue loss is more important, since it also includes the effects of incompletely infarcted tissue and morphologically intact but deafferented cortex. Hypometabolism in such

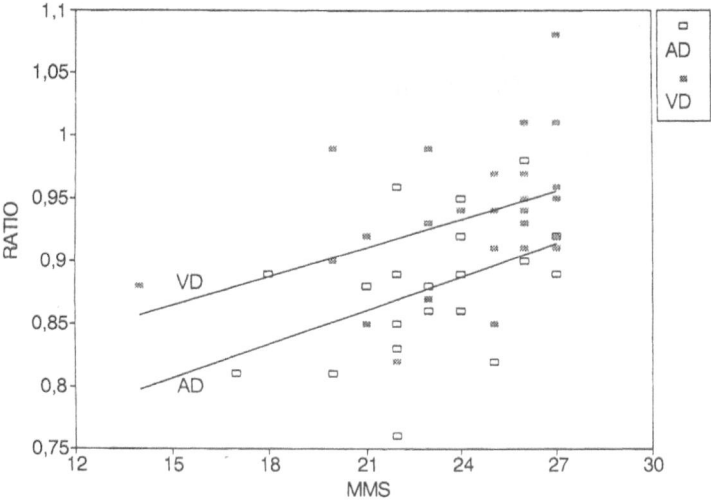

Fig. 2. Regression lines of the metabolic ratio on MMSE in VD-patients and AD-patients

functionally disconnected regions is a common finding in FDG PET (Kuhl et al., 1980; Heiss et al., 1983). Furthermore, the volume of metabolically impaired brain tissue of the VD patients in the present study (76.1 cm³) may be roughly comparable with the volume of 100 cm³ found by Tomlinson et al. (1968).

Comparison of FDG PET and HMPAO SPECT

Single photon emission tomography (SPECT) is another neuroimaging technology yielding some information on selected physiological variables, in dementia especially on cerebral perfusion. Due to the widespread use of single photon emitters, such as ⁹⁹ᵐTc in nuclear medicine departments, SPECT is a more widely available method. Studies with SPECT have shown focal deficits in AD and VD patients that are comparable to those seen with FDG PET (Gemmel et al., 1988; Podreka et al., 1987; Sacquegna et al., 1988). However, in mildly demented patients there are discrepant reports (Gemmel et al., 1987; Neary et al., 1987; Weinstein et al., 1991) concerning sensitivity and specificity of SPECT. The most important differentialdiagnosis to VD is primary degenerative dementia. Therefore, it seems useful to proove the diagnostic accuracy of FDG-PET and SPECT in seperating these two major dementia types. For this purpose, first SPECT of Tc-99m-hexamethylpropylene amine oxime (HMPAO) and afterwards FDG-PET was performed under identical resting conditions within three hours in 12 patients with VD and in 20 patients with probable AD (Mielke et al., 1994). This was possible due to a radiation energy of ⁹⁹ᵐTc below the discrimination threshold of the PET scanner. The functional pattern of both scans was condensed to a ratio of regional values of association areas divided by regional values of regions typically less affected by AD (primary cortical areas, basal ganglia and cerebellum). The comparison of regional perfusion data obtained from HMPAO SPECT with metabolic data from PET was justified by previous studies that demonstrated preserved coupling of blood flow and oxygen consumption or glucose metabolism (Frackowiak et al., 1981; Gibbs et al., 1986; Mielke, 1994). Although it has been reported for brain tissue suffering from ischemic injury that postischemic perfusion can be severely deranged (Heiss et al., 1992), these changes are usually restricted to the acute and subacute phase of ischemia. The latter could be excluded as only VD patients without any recent ischemic infarction entered this study. For the ratio that represents the contrast between most affected association regions and less affected primary and subcortical regions, with both functional imaging methods VD patients had significantly higher values in comparison to the AD group (FDG-PET: p < 0.001; HMPAO-SPECT: p < 0.05). Qualitatively, this has been reported for SPECT in several studies based on visual inspection (Gemmel et al., 1987, 1988, 1990; Podreka et al., 1987; Weinstein et al., 1991). The metabolic ratio was correlated with dementia severity (r = 0.64, p < 0.01) confirming earlier findings on this topic (Mielke et al., 1992), whereas there was no such relationship between the MMSE and the pattern obtained by SPECT due to a larger variance of data. Comparing specifity and sensitivity of the metabolic and perfusion ratio by receiver operating characteristic (ROC) curves, performance for the classification VD versus AD was much better by PET. The diagnostic accuracy was calculated as the percentage area under the ROC curve. For FDG PET it was 89.6% and for HMPAO SPECT 67.1% (p < 0.001) (Fig. 3). This is in accordance with the results of Messa et al. (1994), who found even for a high-resolution SPECT system a lower sensitivity than for PET in the differentiation of AD pathology. Comparing mildly (MMSE >20) and moderately (MMSE ≤20) demented patients separately, diagnostic accuracy was clearly superior for FDG PET, that showed even in patients with mild cognitive impairment reliable results: diagnostic accuracy for MMSE

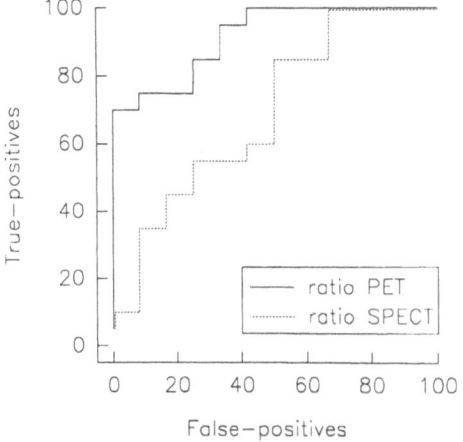

Fig. 3. ROC curves of discrimination between AD and VD patients by FDG PET and HMPAO SPECT

>20: FDG PET 87.2%, HMPAO SPECT 62.9% (p < 0.001); diagnostic accuracy for MMSE ≤20: FDG PET 100%, HMPAO SPECT 80.1% (p < 0.001) (Mielke et al., 1995). These results show that for the differential diagnosis between AD and VD in mildly demented cases HMPAO SPECT is of little value. This is due to a lower contrast of SPECT images possibly together with the lower radiation energy of ^{99m}Tc. Both may be responsible for a reduced power to detect regional perfusion variations in VD while FDG PET might be more sensitive for imaging small functional pathological changes.

Longitudinal analysis of rCMRGl

Cross sectional studies have shown that rCMRGl is closely related to neuropsychological function and to the severity of dementia as, for example measured by the MMSE. However, the cross sectional approach does not reflect the individual progression of metabolic disturbances. Under clinical and therapeutic aspects, the relationship between longitudinal changes of rCMRGl and progression of dementia is of particular relevance. Therefore, disease progression and effects of therapeutic intervention by propentofylline, a xanthine derivative with neuroprotective and blood flow improving properties (DeLeo et al., 1987), were measured in a longitudinal analysis in 25 VD patients. In relative metabolic data there was a significant improvement between groups for the propentofylline treated patients in the left motor cortex (p < 0.01) and basal ganglia (p < 0.05). The increase of relative values in the left motor cortex was significant in the propentofylline group (p < 0.05), while in the placebo group there was a significant deterioration in the frontal association cortex (p < 0.05). Neuropsychologically, visual information processing as tested with the fragmented picture task (Kessler et al., 1993), was improved in the propentofylline-group and a trend towards a slowing of the progression of cognitive deterioration in patients with VD was observed (Heiss et al., 1995). Changes in thalamic metabolism were closely related to auditory verbal memory performance (r = 0.58; p < 0.01) and changes in frontal metabolism to the digit symbol task (r = 0.47; p < 0.05) which involves motor behavior and planning and finally, there was a significant correlation between change of metabolism in the temporoparietal association cortex and recognition (r = −0.5; p < 0.05). Thus, the results of this longitudinal analysis showed that neuropsychological and metabolic changes are closely related in VD, as also previously shown in primary degenerative dementia (Mielke et al., 1994), and reflect the clinical course.

References

Benson DF, Kuhl DE, Hawkins RA, Phelps ME, Cummings JL, Tsai SY (1981) The fluorodeoxyglucose 18F scan in Alzheimer's disease and multiinfarct dementia. Arch Neurol 40: 711–714

DeLeo J, Toth L, Schubert P, Rudolphi K, Kreutzberg GW (1987) Ischemia-induced neuronal cell death, calcium accumulation, and glial response in the hippocampus of the mongolian gerbil and protection by propentofylline (HWA 285). J Cereb Blood Flow Metab 7: 745–751

Folstein MF, Folstein SE, McHugh PR (1975) Mini-mental State: a practical method for grading the cognitive status of patients for the clinician. J Psychiatr Res 12: 189–198

Frackowiak RSJ, Pozzilli C, Legg NJ, du Boulay GH, Marshall J, Lenzi GL, Jones T (1981) Regional cerebral oxygen supply and utilization in dementia. Brain 104: 753–778

Gemmel HG, Sharp PF, Besson JAO, Crawford JR, Ebmeier KP, Davidson J, Smith FW (1987) Differential diagnosis in dementia using cerebral blood flow agent TC-99m HM-PAO: a SPECT study. J Comput Assist Tomogr 11: 398–402

Gemmell HG, Sharp PF, Besson JAO, Ebmeier KP, Smith FW (1988) A comparison of TC-99m HM-PAO and I-123 IMP cerebral SPECT images in Alzheimer's disease and multi-infarct dementia. Eur J Nucl Med 14: 463–466

Gemmel HG, Evans NTS, Besson JAO, Roeda D, Davidson J, Dodd MG, Sharp PF, Smith FW, Crawford JR, Newton RH, Kulkarni V, Mallard JR (1990) Regional cerebral blood flow imaging: a quantitative comparison of Technetium-99m-HMPAO SPECT with $C^{15}O_2$ PET. J Nucl Med 31: 1595–1600

Gibbs JM, Frackowiak RSJ, Legg NJ (1986) Regional cerebral blood flow and oxygen metabolism in dementia due to vascular disease. Gerontology 32 [Suppl 1]: 84–86

Hachinski VC, Iliff LD, Zilhka E, DuBoulay GH, McAllister VL, Marshall J, Russell RWR, Symon L (1975) Cerebral blood flow in dementia. Arch Neurol 32: 632–637

Heiss WD, Ilsen HW, Wagner R, Pawlik G, Wienhard K, Eriksson L (1983) Remote functional depression of glucose metabolism in stroke and its alteration by activating drugs. In: Heiss WD, Phelps ME (eds) Positron emission tomography of the brain. Springer, Berlin Heidelberg New York Tokyo, pp 162–168

Heiss WD, Huber M, Fink GR, Herholz K, Pietrzyk U, Wagner R, Wienhard K (1992) Progressive derangement of periinfarct viable tissue in ischemic stroke. J Cereb Blood Flow Metab 12: 193–203

Heiss WD, Mielke R, Kessler J, Ghaemi M, Szelies B, Kittner B, Herholz K, Pietrzyk U (1995) Longitudinal study of propentofyllin in vascular dementia. J Cereb Blood Flow Metab 15: 106

Herholz K, Adams R, Kessler J, Szelies B, Grond M, Heiss WD (1990) Criteria for the diagnosis of Alzheimer's disease with positron emission tomography. Dementia 1: 156–164

Kase CS (1991) Epidemiology of multi-infarct dementia. Alzheimer Dis Assoc Disord 5: 71–76

Kessler J, Schaaf A, Mielke R (1993) Fragmentierter Bildertest – ein Wahrnehmungs-und Gedächtnistest. Hogrefe, Göttingen Bern Toronto Seattle

Kuhl DE, Phelps ME, Kowell AP, Metter EJ, Selin C, Winter J (1980) Effects of stroke on local cerebral metabolism and perfusion: mapping by emission computed tomography of 18FDG and 13NH3. Ann Neurol 8: 47–60

Kuhl DE, Metter EJ, Riege WH, Hawkins RA, Mazziotta JC, Phelps DE, Kling AS (1983) Local cerebral glucose utilization in elderly patients with depression, multiple infarct dementia, and Alzheimer's disease. J Cereb Blood Flow Metab 3: 494–495

Kuhl D, Metter E, Benson F, Ashford JW, Riege WH, Fujikawa DG, Markham CH, Mazziotta JC, Maltese A, Dorsey DA (1985) Similarities of cerebral glucose metabolism in Alzheimer's and Parkinson's dementia. J Cereb Blood Flow Metab 5: 169–170

McKhann G, Drachman D, Folstein M, Katzman R, Price D, Stadlan EM (1984) Clinical diagnosis of Alzheimer's disease: report of the NINCDS-ADRDA work group under the auspices of Department of Health and Human Services Task Force on Alzheimer's disease. Neurology 19: 939–944

Messa C, Perani D, Lucignani G, Zenorini A, Zito F, Rizzo G, Grassi F, Del Sole A, Franceschi M, Gilardi MC, Fazio F (1994) High-resolution technetium-99m-HMPAO SPECT in patients with probable Alzheimer's disease: comparison with fluorine-18-FDG PET. J Nucl Med 35: 210–216

Mielke R (1994) Pathophysiologie und Diagnostik von vaskulären Demenzen — Untersuchungen zur Hirndurchblutung und zum Hirnstoffwechsel. Thesis, Köln

Mielke R, Herholz K, Grond M, Kessler J, Heiss WD (1992) Severity of vascular dementia is related to volume of metabolically impaired tissue. Arch Neurol 49: 909–913

Mielke R, Pietrzyk U, Jacobs A, Fink GR, Ichimiya A, Kessler J, Herholz K, Heiss WD (1994) HMPAO SPECT and FDG PET in Alzheimer's disease and vascular dementia: comparison of perfusion and metabolic pattern. Eur J Nucl Med 21: 1052–1060

Mielke R, Herholz K, Grond M, Kessler J, Heiss WD (1994) Clinical deterioration in probable Alzheimer's disease correlates with progressive metabolic impairment of association areas. Dementia 5: 36–41

Mielke R, Jacobs A, Kessler J, Pietrzyk U, Herholz K, Heiss WD (1995) Diagnostic accuracy of FDG PET and HMPAO SPECT for the differentiation between Alzheimer's disease and vascular dementia depends on severity of disease. J Neurol 241: 35

Neary D, Snowdon JS, Shields RA, Burjan AWI, Northen B, Macdermott N, Prescott MC, Testa HJ (1987) Single photon emission tomography using [99]mTc-HM-PAO in the investigation of dementia. J Neurol Neurosurg Psychiatry 50: 1101–1109

Podreka I, Suess E, Goldenberg G, Steiner M, Brücke T, Müller CH, Lang W, Neirinckx RD, Deecke L (1987) Initial experience with Technetium-99m HM-PAO brain SPECT. J Nucl Med 28: 1657–1666

Roman GC, Tatemichi TK, Erkinjuntti T, Cummings JL, Masdeu JC, Garcia JH, Amaducci L, Orgogozzo JM, Brun A, Hofman A, Moody DM, O'Brien MD, Yamaguchi T, Grafman J, Drayer BP, Bennett DA, Fisher M, Ogata J, Kokmen E, Bermejo F, Wolf PA, Gorelick PB, Bick KL, Pajeau AK, Bell MA, DeCarli C, Culebras A, Korczyn AD, Bogousslavsky J, Hartmann A, Scheinberg P (1993) Vascular dementia: diagnostic criteria for research studies. Neurology 43: 250–260

Sacquegna T, DeCarolis P, Daidone R, Dondi M (1988) Single-photon emission tomography with technetium Tc 99m hexamethylpropylene amine oxime in Binswanger's disease. Arch Neurol 45: 603–604

Skoog I, Nilsson L, Palmertz B, Andreasson LA, Svanborg A (1993) A population-based study of dementia in 86-year-olds. N Engl J Med 328: 153–158

Tomlinson BE, Blessed G, Roth M (1968) Observations on the brains of non-demented old people. J Neurol Sci 7: 331–356

Tomlinson BE, Blessed G, Roth M (1970) Observations on the brains of demented old people. J Neurol Sci 11: 205–242

Weinstein HC, Haan J, van Royen EO, Derix MMA, Lanser JBK, van der Zant F, Dunnewold RJW, van Kroonenburgh MJPG, Pauwels EKJ, van der Velde EA, Hijdra A, Buruma OJS (1991) SPECT in the diagnosis of Alzheimer's disease and multi-infarct dementia. Clin Neurol Neurosurg 93: 39–43

Weltgesundheitsorganisation (1991) Dilling H, Mombour W, Schmidt MH (eds) Internationale Klassifikation psychischer Störungen ICD 10 Kp V (F). Klinisch-diagnostische Leitlinien. Huber, Bern

Authors' address: W.-D. Heiss, M.D., Max-Planck-Institut für Neurologische Forschung, Gleueler Strasse 50, D-50931 Köln, Federal Republic of Germany.

J Neural Transm (1996) [Suppl] 47: 193–203
© Springer-Verlag 1996

The spectrum of depressive pseudo-dementia

P. Fischer

Department of General Psychiatry, University Hospital for Psychiatry,
Vienna, Austria

Summary. Depressive disorder causes cognitive symptoms. In the case of severe cognitive symptoms or when psychometric procedures measure cognitive decline in the range of dementia, depressed patients may be diagnosed as Depressive Pseudo-Dementia (DPD). There is no data that depressive disorder can cause dementia without coexisting depressive symptoms. The latter symptoms are frequently overseen because cognitive symptoms are equated with organic brain disease. There are typical neuropsychological features of cognitive decline in depressive disorders, like psychomotor retardation and the slow-start phenomenon.

Most patients referred to as DPD, suffer from depression-induced cognitive symptoms outside the range of dementia, but complain of memory disturbance and inability to think or concentrate. The diagnosis of DPD draws attention to a problem in the diagnosis of psychiatric disorders in the elderly: Old people suffering from depression are at particular risk of beeing labelled as demented. The most important step to diagnose depression causing dementia is the search for signs and symtoms of affective disorder even after having found cognitive symptoms.

Introduction

Depressive Pseudo-Dementia (DPD) is a term which mixes various levels of psychiatric terminology. "Depressive" is indicating "depressive disorder" and "dementia" is indicating that a "syndrome of dementia" is observed. Clinicians use the diagnosis of DPD with various meaning (Kiloh, 1961; Shraberg, 1978; Wells, 1979; Good, 1981; McAllister and Price, 1982; Reifler et al., 1982; McAllister, 1983; Arie, 1983; Bulbena and Berrios, 1986; Rabins, 1988; Förstl, 1991; Emery and Oxman, 1992). Diagnostic criteria are lacking and definitions vary (McAllister, 1983). While some scientists recommend abandoning this term (Reifler, 1982; Zimmer and Lauter, 1984), it nevertheless belongs to the standard vocabulary of most psychiatrists and gerontopsychiatrists. The frequent comeback of the impossible term DPD, for instance in the DSM-IV, points to the usefulness of the term in clinical practice, which draws attention to a problem in the diagnosis of psychiatric disorders in the elderly: Old people suffering from depression are at particular risk of being labelled as demented. It is very important for the patient to detect depressive disorder, because it is a treatable condition and otherwise could lead to suicide or chronic care.

The history of the term "pseudo-dementia"

Wernicke gave the diagnosis of pseudo-dementia to patients with a syndrome of dementia caused by neurotic crisis (Ganser state). At this time dementia was defined as the most severe and irreversible form of the organic brain syndrome. "Pseudo" at this time pointed to the fact that a severe syndrome of cognitive inability might be reversible.

Sixty years later the term "Pseudo-Dementia" was the title of a paper by Kiloh (1961), who described 10 patients, 3 of whom "initially mimicked the picture of dementia" but turned out to suffer from endogenous depression. Kiloh described some more patients with hysterical pseudo-dementia in the sense of Wernicke. Indicators of depressive illness in Kiloh's patients were a) past psychiatric history, b) abrupt onset and c) therapeutic response to antidepressant therapy. Since 1980 (DSM-III) dementia means a reversible or irreversible clinical syndrome of various severity, but caused by organic brain disorder and caused neither by affective disorder nor by schizophrenia. "pseudo" now indicated "not caused by organic brain disease but by functional disorder".

The myth of depressive pseudo-dementia

A wide spectrum of cases are labeled DPD (Table 1). In the strict sense, DPD means patients with purley cognitive disability without depressive symptoms, who nevertheless suffer from depressive disorder and not from organic brain disease. I have never investigated such a patient nor have I found any in the wide literature of DPD. There are some cases where the description of depressive symptoms is lacking, but in all case descriptions, where affective and behavioral symptoms are given, the patients with DPD suffered from cognitive *and* depressive symptoms. Thus, I believe that there are no cases with depressive disorder who present with severe cognitive disturbance but without depressive symptoms. The existence of these patients is a myth.

The most important step to diagnose depression causing dementia is the search for signs and symptoms of affective disorder: a history and family history of affective disorder, a (sub)acute onset, depressed mood, poor appetite and weight loss, delusions of self-blame, or delusions of hopelessness, or delusions of physical ill health (cancer, Alzheimer disease) suggest that the particular patient is suffering a treatable condition (Rabins et al., 1984).

Table 1. The spectrum of depressive pseudodementias

	Description		Nosology		
	depressive syndrom	dementia syndrom	depressive disorder	dementia disorder	Frequency
Dementia syndrome of depressive disorder without depressive syndrom	−	+	+	−	myth
Dementia syndrome of depressive disorder with depressive syndrom	+	+	+	−	rare
"Melancholia cum delirio"	+	?	+	−	rare
Depressive syndrome in dementia disorder (dementia persisting after successful antidepressant therapy)	+	+	+	+	frequent
Depressive syndrome in dementia disorder (without dementia after successful antidepressant therapy)	+	+	+	+	rare
"Depressive pseudodementia" (i.e.: depressive syndrom which is misinterpreted as dementia)	+	−	+	−	frequent

Depressive pseudo-dementia: the psychometric diagnosis

Symptoms and disorders

Psychopathological symptoms can be roughly classified into cognitive and non-cognitive symptoms. Typical cognitive symptoms are impairment of long-term memory, aphasia or disturbed attention. Typical non-cognitive symptoms are depressed mood, anxiety, or flat affect. A typical syndrome of dementia consists not only cognitive symptoms but also includes mood and sleep disturbances or anxiety (DSM-IV). Thus, the organic disorder causes cognitive and non-cognitive symptoms. The other way round depressive disorder causes non-cognitive symptoms (depressed mood, diminished interest, loss of pleasure, . . .) and cognitive symptoms. The DSM-IV mentions "diminished ability to think or concentrate, memory complaints, and distractibility".

Cognitive symptoms in depressive disorder

Kraepelin (1896) already described that depression can interfere with cognitive function. The DSM-IV defines DPD descriptively by "cognitive impairments due to major depressive episode". More than 50% of patients with major depressive episodes suffer from cognitive symptoms in the fields of concentration, psychomotor speed and memory, which improve following antidepressive therapy. About 70% of elderly depressed patients suffer from cognitive symptoms in psychometric terms and do not only complain of cognitive symptoms. The biological substrates are still unknown. The severity of cognitive symptoms in depressive disorder depends on a) severity of depression, b) age and c) cerebral comorbidity. Using standardized psychometric procedures especially with time-limited tests or speed tests a high proportion of clearly depressed patients will exhibit scores below the dementia cut-off. Frequently published tests are the Digit-Symbol-Test of the Wechsler Adult Intelligence Scale or the Trail-Making-Test of Reitan (Austin et al., 1992). Other typical power tests which usually show deficits early in the course of Alzheimer's disease remain unimpaired in depressive disorder. This is, for instance, the case with the Token-Test (DeRenzi and Vignolo, 1962).

In elderly depressed populations, using rigid testing procedures, about 50% of depressed elderly will show MMSE scores lower than 24 (international dementia cut-off) before antidepressant treatment and normal scores (higher than 27) after successful treatment (Pearlson et al., 1989; Alexopoulos et al., 1993). MMSE in depressed in-patients of a geriatric hospital in Vienna showed differences between various investigators. Investigators who were familiar to the patient measured higher scores than neutral psychologists. The percentage of elderly depressed diagnosed as "dementia syndrome of depression" depends on the mode of testing. The term "dementia syndrome of depressive disorder" simulates a clear diagnostic entity which is not reliable.

Psychometric testing in depressive disorder

There are a lot of problems in the psychometric investigation of both elderly patients and depressed patients (Table 2). The elderly show age-dependent psychomotor retardation, and this is even more pronounced in depression. The elderly is unfamiliar with tests but usually works with high motivation. The finding of cognitive deficits in depressed patients is not attributable to motivational factors (Richards and Ruff, 1989). The depressed patient at any age suffers from some degree of psychomotor slowing, but also exhibits concentrational deficits, higher cognitive interference, and anticipates his/her failure in tests. While some work showed the diminished effortful processing of depressed patients, other neuropsychologists showed the different time-course of effortful processing during depression. Normally there is a shift from controlled, effortful processing in the beginning of a task towards more

Table 2. Problems in the psychometric investigation of depressed patients and elderly subjects

Elderly	Depressed
slowing down	psychomotor retardation
anticipation of failure	anticipation of failure
unfamiliar with tests	afraid of tests
auditory problems	concentrational deficit
visual problems	motivational deficit (?)
education	anticholinergic side effects
age-associated memory impairment	slow start phenomenon

automatic, superficial processing later in the task (Brand et al., 1992). Some depressed patients show the socalled slow-start phenomenon; their effortful processing reaches a later peak. Therefore, depressed patients are especially impaired in the beginning of psychometric tests, i.e. in the first learning trial (Blau and Ober, 1988). While tests can measure scores in the range of dementia, detailed observation and psychopathology can help in the detection of DPD as the mimickry of true dementia. I believe that cognitive symptoms in depression can usually be differentiated from dementia on clinical grounds alone. One argument in this direction is that there is usually a difference between psychometric test scores and activities of daily living in patients with pseudo-dementia. Another argument is that changes in standardized testing procedures induce enormous improvement of depressed patients. This is illustrated by case 1.

The "dementia syndrome of depressive disorder"

Case 1: This 65 years old male patient was admitted to our department because of "organic depression". He scored 23 on the Mini-Mental-State-Examination (MMSE) and showed concentrational deficits and a profound memory deficit. The patient declined in the Fuld-Object-Memory-Evaluation (FOME: 10 items in 5 trials using the selective reminding procedure: Fig. 1) after having recalled 2 items in the first and 3 items in the second inquiring. Two days later the FOME was repeated with different items. This second testing was carried out without the time limit of 60 seconds per inquiry. After 7 minutes the patient had correctly recalled all 10 items of the FOME and again did so after the second distractor-condition. Thus, according to our test criteria for the diagnosis of dementia the patient suffered from a "dementia syndrome" which vanished in pure power-testing. Cognitive symptoms disappeared after ECT and prophylactic antidepressant therapy with paroxetine led to the first manic episode in the patient's life.

During a period of two years (June 1992–June 1994) we saw 19 cases who were admitted suspicious of dementia but were diagnosed and treated as pure affective disorder. Four of these 19 cases fulfilled our neuropsychological cut-off criteria for a syndrom of dementia but also suffered from severe depressive episode and lost their depressive and cognitive symptoms following ECT and/or antidepressive pharmacotherapy. In every case the observations during testing made one suspect the patient of suffering from depressive disorder.

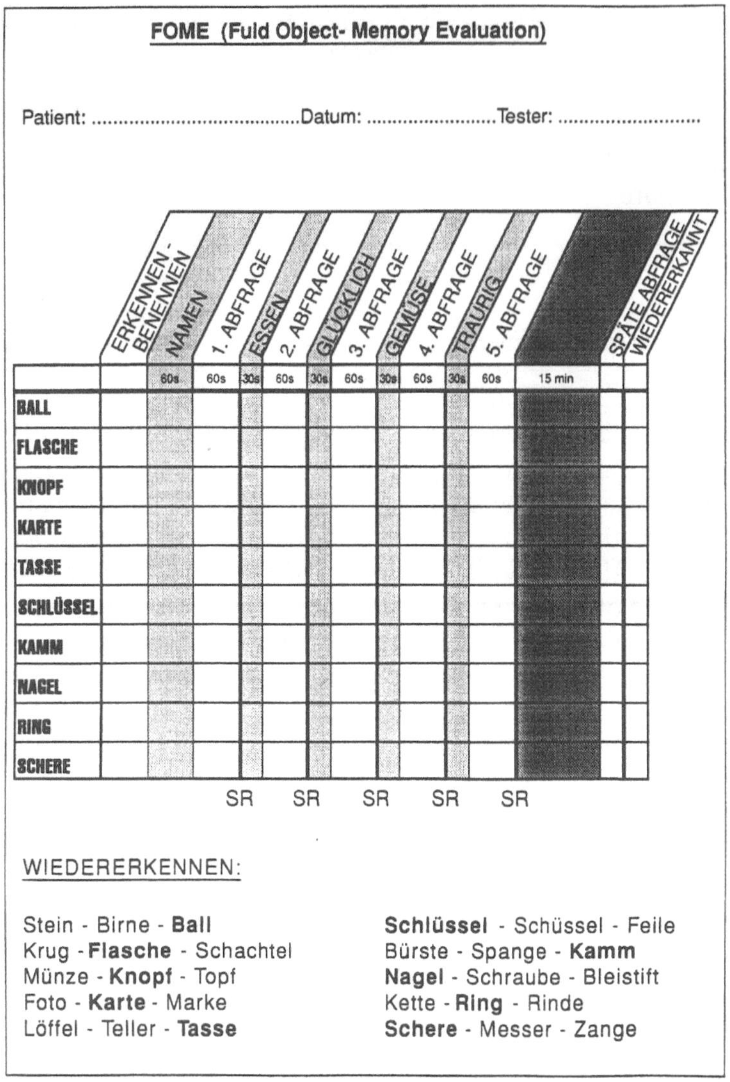

FOME (Fuld Object- Memory Evaluation)

Patient: ....Datum: ....Tester: ....

	ERKENNEN-BENENNEN / NAMEN	1. ABFRAGE	ESSEN / 2. ABFRAGE	GLÜCKLICH / 3. ABFRAGE	GEMÜSE / 4. ABFRAGE	TRAURIG / 5. ABFRAGE		SPÄTE ABFRAGE	WIEDERERKANNT
	60s	60s	30s	60s	30s	60s	30s	60s	30s	60s	15 min		
BALL													
FLASCHE													
KNOPF													
KARTE													
TASSE													
SCHLÜSSEL													
KAMM													
NAGEL													
RING													
SCHERE													
		SR		SR		SR		SR		SR			

WIEDERERKENNEN:

Stein - Birne - **Ball**   **Schlüssel** - Schüssel - Feile
Krug - **Flasche** - Schachtel   Bürste - Spange - **Kamm**
Münze - **Knopf** - Topf   **Nagel** - Schraube - Bleistift
Foto - **Karte** - Marke   Kette - **Ring** - Rinde
Löffel - Teller - **Tasse**   **Schere** - Messer - Zange

Fig. 1. German version of the Fuld Object Memory Evaluation

Psychomotor retardation and slow-start phenomenon interfered especially with memory testing in these patients.

Some more patients showed specific cognitive dysfunction outside the range of dementia and also showed psychomotor retardation, or distractibility indicating cognitive symptoms in depressive disorder. Only one out of these depressed patients showed psychomotor speed in the range of controls.

Melancholia cum delirio

Some severely depressed patients can no longer cooperate in testing but claim that they are demented. They call themselves "disturbed" and frequently answer by "I don't know"-answers. They usually don't show psychomotor retardation but are agitated and are not capable of cooperating with detailed cognitive assessment. They mimic the picture of delirium rather than that of dementia. The old term "melancholia cum delirio" suits well to this group of patients, which is also called DPD in the literature. "Mélancholie avec délire" was firstly described by Pinel in 1798. Case 2 gives an example for this type of DPD.

Case 2: An 88-year-old woman from the Maimonides-centre, a Jewish geriatric unit in Vienna, had suffered more than 25 depressive and some hypomanic episodes during her life and came to admittance in a state of "melancholia cum delirio" like described above. There was no doubt about her depressive disorder, but most colleagues who were lacking information on the history of the particular patient interpreted the delirious symptomatology as triggered by some age-associated organic factor. Antidepressant therapy with fluoxetine made her euthymic and she left the hospital. She is now, 4 years later, in an euthymic state and scores 41 in the FOME and 30 on the MMSE. Nevertheless she only remembers the discharge from our department and no details of the severe depressive episode including the 3 weeks treatment at our department, that means she suffered retrograde amnesia for her depressive episode.

To my knowledge, this observation of retrograde amnesia in depression, which is not a unique one (see also case 3) is not described in the recent literature. Eugen Bleuler already mentioned it when he wrote that depressed patients store information but forget "to lock it up".

The typical patient with depressive pseudo-dementia

Thirty percent of the patients who are admitted to our out-patient clinic "suspicious of dementia" suffer from depression which is misinterpreted as dementia by the practicioner or even by the neurologist. Usually these patients complain of memory impairment and frequently are afraid of or delusionally sure of suffering from Alzheimer's disease. Memory complaints in elderly psychiatric patients are correlated with severity of depression and are not correlated with severity of cognitive decline (Pettinati et al., 1985). In some instances, persons who complained about memory loss actually functioned better than those who did not (Kahn et al., 1975).

Psychometric testing shows no or only small cognitive deficits in most of these patients. For education of these patients and their doctors the term DPD is not exact but very useful. These syndromes mimic dementia, are influenced by expectation of cognitive disease in the elderly, have a subjective basis but do not survive psychometric investigation. Most patients in the literature, e.g. all 10 patients described by Wells in 1979, were not demented in psychometric terms (age 33–69) but showed mild cognitive symptoms. Case 3 illustrates such a patient.

Case 3: A 58-year-old professor of philosophy was transferred to the memory clinic by a neurologist, who had treated the patient for 8 months because of Alzheimer's disease. The patient looked disturbed, anxious and rather agitated. He complained of being unable to think, that he frequently lacked the correct vocabulary in his lectures, and that he was unable to prepare his lectures any more. He wanted to commit suicide when the diagnosis of Alzheimer's disease was found to be correct.

He told a nice story which may have influenced the neurologist in diagnosing a dementing disorder. Some weeks after .the start of sleep disturbance the patient suffered from giddiness and visited his otorhinolaryngologist. The next day he did not find his car. He searched for it together with his wife. The next day after another extensive search through the streets near his house the patient reported his car stolen to the police. Two weeks later the patient and his wife bought another new car. One month later, while the patient was still depressed, the wife visited the otorhinolaryngologist because of otic pains and found the "stolen" car in front of the office. Though confronted with this fact, the patient still cannot remember that he had driven with his old car to the doctor and had returned home by subway. This event obviously influenced the neurologist in his diagnosis of Alzheimer's disease. Further exploration showed that the patient was easily distractible and showed a lot of depressive symptoms including loss of pleasure, insomnia, loss of energy, loss of appetite and weight loss, morning pessimism, depressed mood, etc. Psychometric testing showed no deficit in word finding (subtest naming of the Aachener-Aphasie-Test: 120/120), memory (Fuld Object memory test: 45/50) without psychomotor slowing and correct answers in test of concentrational abilities. MMSE was 28 (memory 1/3). The first episode of depression was treated with paroxetine and full remission occured within 3 weeks.

Combinations of dementing disorder with depressive disorder

This category of patients is frequently seen at our memory clinic, but is rarely called DPD. It is the typical Alzheimer's disease patient who early in his/her disease also develops depression. Depression is a frequent feature in Alzheimer's disease (Fischer et al., 1990). Dementia can present as depression with relatively little cognitive impairment (Reding et al., 1985). To our experience, every early Alzheimer patient shows deficits in logical memory and episodic memory. In a small minority of cases dementia vanishes following antidepressant therapy and comes out later again. Nevertheless, memory deficits usually indicate the organic comorbidity. These patients with "Depressive Pseudo-Pseudo-Dementia" were described by Kral's (1982) longitudinal study of 22 patients with DPD, the greater percentage of whom became demented. Other samples at other institutions showed a better prognosis of DPD patients years (Sachdev et al., 1990; Rabins et al., 1984; Alexopoulos et al., 1993). The majority of Alzheimer patients with depression lose their depressive syndrome following antidepressant therapy but are still demented after successful antidepressant therapy.

We investigated 6 depressed in-patients of a geriatric care unit with MMSE scores between 19 and 26, who showed no progression of their mild cognitive symptoms during a period of 1 to 4 years. Depressive symptoms improved following antidepressive therapy with clomipramine. The neuropathological post-mortem diagnosis was Alzheimer's disease according to 3 different diagnostic algorithms in all cases. The lack of progression is not contradicting a diagnosis of Alzheimer's disease (McKhann et al., 1984). All 6 patients exhibited significant memory deficits and showed not only psychomotor retardation but also bradyphrenia.

Other pseudo-dementias

At our Memory Clinic we also see a significant proportion of cases with neurotic Pseudo-Dementia. Frequently these cases mimic dementia very closely and show no features of depressive disorder (Kiloh, 1961; Nott and Fleminger, 1975; Bendefeldt et al., 1976; McEvoy and Wells, 1979; Wells, 1979; Good, 1981). It is the symbolic meaning of the symptom and the family structure which make these cases suspicious. Organic investigations show normal CCT, MRT, SPECT and EEG in spite of severe cognitive dysfunction. The lowest MMSE score in such a patient at our memory clinic was 3 (!). The functioning in everyday life usually did not correlate with the massive psychometric break down. The picture did not always fit to the so-called Ganser state and the symptom of "Vorbeireden" was frequently lacking. This diagnosis is alway uncertain and the course and outcome of psychotherapy decides the diagnosis.

Conclusions

Taken together, DPD is not a homogenous syndrome but a wide spectrum of cases are summarized under this diagnostic label. Depressive disorder causes cognitive symptoms. It is perhaps the age of the particular patient which makes the finding of cognitive symptoms indicative of beginning dementing illness. There is no data that depressive disorder can cause dementia without coexisting depressive symptoms. The latter symptoms are frequently overlooked because cognitive symptoms are equated with organic brain disease. Although cognitive impairment is the hallmark of the organic syndromes, it is not diagnostic of organicity.

In the case of severe cognitive symptoms or in the case that psychometric procedures measure cognitive decline in the range of dementia, depressed patients may be diagnosed as DPD. They all suffer from typical depressive symptoms, too. Psychometric testing favours dementia scores in depressed patients by various factors. There are typical neuropsychological features of cognitive decline in depressive disorder like psychomotor retardation and the slow-start phenomenon. A subgroup of patients with psychomotor agitation and complaints of cognitive disturbance are not testable and mimic the clinical picture of delirium rather than that of depression. We call them "melancholia cum delirio".

Most patients who are called DPD suffer from depression-induced cognitive symptoms outside the range of dementia, but complain of memory disturbance and inability to think or concentrate. There are some rare patients with incipient Alzheimer's disease and major depressive episode who improve intellectually following antidepressive therapy. In these cases the diagnosis of Depressive Pseudo-Dementia has to be corrected following long-term observation.

Old people suffering from depression are at particular risk of being labelled as demented. The most important step to diagnose depression causing dementia is the search for signs and symptoms of affective disorder even after having found cognitive symptoms.

References

Alexopoulos GS, Meyers BS, Young RC, Mattis S, Kakuma T (1993) The course of geriatric depression with "reversible dementia": a controlled study. Am J Psychiatry 150: 1693–1699

American Psychiatric Association (1980) Diagnostic and statistical manual of mental disorders, 3rd edn. APA, Washington DC

American Psychiatric Association (1994) Diagnostic and statistical manual of mental disorders, 4th edn. APA, Washington DC

Arie T (1983) Pseudodementia. Br Med J 286: 1301–1302

Austin MP, Ross M, Murray C, O'Carroll RE, Ebmeier KP, Goodwin GM (1992) Cognitive function in major depression. J Affect Disord 25: 21–30

Bendefeldt F, Miller LL, Ludwig AM (1976) Cognitive performance in conversion hysteria. Arch Gen Psychiatry 33: 1250–1254

Blau E, Ober BA (1988) The effect of depression on verbal memory in older adults. J Clin Exp Neuropsychol 10: 81

Bleuler E (1916) Lehrbuch der Psychiatrie. Springer, Berlin

Brand AN, Jolles J, Gispen-de-Wied C (1992) Recall and recognition memory deficits in depression. J Affect Disord 25: 77–86

Bulbena A, Berrios GE (1986) Pseudodementia: facts and figures. Br J Psychiatry 148: 87–94

DeRenzi E, Vignolo LA (1962) The Token test: a sensitive test to detect receptive disturbances in aphasics. Brain 85: 665–678

Emery VO, Oxman TE (1992) Update on the dementia spectrum of depression. Am J Psychiatry 149: 305–317

Fischer P, Simanyi M, Danielczyk W (1990) Depression in dementia of Alzheimer type and multi-infarct dementia. Am J Psychiatry 147: 1484–1487

Folstein MF, Folstein SE, McHugh PR (1975) "Mini-Mental State": a practical method for grading the cognitive state of patients for the clinician. J Psychiatr Res 12: 189–198

Fuld PA (1980) Guaranteed stimulus-processing in the evaluation of memory and learning. Cortex 16: 255–271

Förstl H (1991) Das Demenzsyndrom der Depression. Neuropsychiatrie 5: 23–25

Good MI (1981) Pseudodementia and physical findings masking significant psychopathology. Am J Psychiatry 136: 811–814

Huber W, Poeck K, Weninger D, Willmes K (1982) Aachener Aphasie Test. Hogrefe, Göttingen

Kahn RL, Zarit SH, Hilbert NM, Niederehe G (1975) Memory complaint and impairment in the aged. The effect of depression and altered brain function. Arch Gen Psychiatry 32: 1569–1573

Kiloh LG (1961) Pseudo-dementia. Acta Psychiatr Scand 37: 336–351

Kraepelin E (1896) Lehrbuch der Psychiatrie. Barth, Leipzig

Kral VA (1982) Depressive Pseudodemenz und senile Demenz vom Alzheimertyp. Nervenarzt 53: 284–286

McAllister TW, Price TRP (1982) Severe depressive pseudodementia with and without dementia. Am J Psychiatry 139: 626–629

McAllister TW (1983) Overview: pseudodementia. Am J Psychiatry 140: 528–533

McEvoy JP, Wells CE (1979) Case studies in neuropsychiatry II. Conversion pseudodementia. J Clin Psychiatry 40: 447–449

McKhann G, Drachman D, Folstein M, Katzman R, Price D, Stadlan EM (1984) Clinical diagnosis of Alzheimer's disease: report of the NINCDS-ADRDA Work Group under auspices of Department of Health and Human Services Task Force on Alzheimer's disease. Neurology 34: 939–944

Nott PN, Fleminger JJ (1975) Presenile dementia: the difficulties of early diagnosis. Acta Psychiatr Scand 51: 210–217

Pearlson GD, Rabins PV, Kim WS, Speedie LJ, Moberg PJ, Burns A, Bascom MJ (1989) Structural brain CT changes and cognitive deficits in elderly depressives with and without reversible dementia ("pseudodementia"). Psychol Med 19: 573–584

Pettinati HM, Brown M, Mathisen KS (1985) Memory complaints in depressed geriatric inpatients. Ann NY Acad Sci 444: 528–530

Pinel P (1798) Nosographie philosophique. Salpêtrière, Paris

Rabins PV, Merchant A, Nestadt G (1984) Criteria for diagnosing reversible dementia caused by depression: validation by 2-year follow-up. Br J Psychiatry 144: 488–492

Rabins PV (1988) Does reversible dementia exist and is it reversible? Arch Intern Med 148: 1905

Reding M, Haycox J, Blass J (1985) Depression in patients referred to a dementia clinic. A three-year prospective study. Arch Neurol 4: 894–896

Reifler BV (1982) Arguments for abandoning the term pseudodementia. J Am Geriatr Soc 30: 665–668

Reifler BV, Larson E, Hanley R (1982) Coexistence of cognitive impairment and depression in geriatric outpatients. Am J Psychiatry 139: 623–626

Richards PM, Ruff RM (1989) Motivational effects on neuropsychological functioning: comparison of depressed versus nondepressed individuals. J Consult Clin Psychol 57: 396–402

Sachdev PS, Smith JS, Angus-Lepan H, Rodriguez P (1990) Pseudodementia twelve years on. Neurol Neurosurg Psychiatry 53: 254–259

Shraberg D (1978) The myth of pseudodementia: depression and the aging brain. Am J Psychiatry 135: 601–603

Wells CE (1979) Pseudodementia. Am J Psychiatry 136: 895–900

Zimmer R, Lauter H (1984) Zum Problem der depressiven Pseudodemenz. Z Gerontol 17: 109–112

Author's address: Doz. Dr. P. Fischer, Klinische Abteilung für Allgemeinpsychiatrie, Universitätsklinik für Psychiatrie, Währinger Gürtel 18-20, A-1090 Wien, Austria.

J Neural Transm (1996) [Suppl] 47: 205–218
© Springer-Verlag 1996

Molecular biology of APO E alleles in Alzheimer's and non-Alzheimer's dementias

C. M. Morris, H. M. Massey, R. Benjamin, A. Leake, C. Broadbent,
M. Griffiths, H. Lamb, A. Brown, P. G. Ince, S. Tyrer, P. Thompson,
I. G. McKeith, J. A. Edwardson, R. H. Perry, and E. K. Perry

MRC Neurochemical Pathology Unit and Department of Neuropathology, Newcastle
General Hospital, Westgate Road, Newcastle upon Tyne, Tyne and Wear,
United Kingdom

Summary. Current research into the aetiology of the dementias is focused upon genetic factors which give rise to the disease process. Recently the Apolipoprotein E gene (APO E) and in particular the ε4 allele has been shown to be a risk factor for late onset Alzheimer's disease (AD) where there is an increased frequency of the ε4 allele. The ε4 allele has also been shown to reduce the age at onset of dementia in AD in a dose dependant manner, with the ε2 allele having an opposing effect.

We have genotyped a large series of clinically and neuropathologically confirmed cases of AD and found the expected increase in the Apolipoprotein ε4 allele frequency when compared to a control population. Similarly, in Lewy Body Dementia (LBD) an increased ε4 frequency is also found though a normal ε2 frequency exists, unlike in AD where the ε2 frequency is reduced. No changes in APO E allele frequencies were found in presenile AD, Parkinson's disease with or without dementia, or in Down's syndrome. No association was found between any of the APO E alleles and the histopathological indices of AD, cortical senile plaques and neurofibrillary tangles, in any disease category. Neurochemical indicators of AD, loss of choline acetyltransferase activity was also unaffected by APO E genotype.

Whilst their appears to be a strong association between the APO E allele and AD and also in LBD, other related neurodegenerative disorders associated with dementia do not show such a linkage. Changes in the ε2 allele frequency may indicate a genetic difference between AD and LBD. The ε4 allele does not appear to influence the burden of AD type pathology and this is particularly relevant given the relative lack of NFT in LBD indicating that factors other than SP or NFT may govern the onset of dementia.

Introduction

The aetiology of Alzheimer's disease (AD) appears to be complex involving both genetic and epigenetic/environmental factors. Whilst the majority of presenile cases of AD appear to involve genetic factors as a primary cause, either as mutations in the newly identified S182 protein (Sherrington et al., 1995) or E5-1 genes (Rogaev et al., 1995), or in the Amyloid Precursor Protein (APP; Goate et al., 1991; Murrel et al., 1991), late onset AD may be a more heterogeneous disorder with genetic factors, though playing an influential role, being readily modified by epigenetic factors. The main genetic factor influencing late onset AD would appear to be the Apolipoprotein E gene (APO E) on chromosome 19, with the ε4 allele of APO E being associated with an increased risk of developing AD and the ε2 allele having a protective effect (Corder et al., 1994).

The APO E gene on chromosome 19 spans approximately 4kb with 4 exons encoding a mature protein of 299 amino acids. This product, Apolipoprotein E (APO E), is one of the main lipid transporting proteins found in the serum (see Mahley and Rall,1989 for review), and is involved in the transport of triglycerides and cholesterol in the form of very low- (VLDL), or low density lipoproteins (LDL). Three allelic forms of APO E are generally identified, APO E ε3, APO E ε4, and APO E ε2, which are found at frequencies of approximately 77%, 15%, and 8% respectively, in most populations. The commonest allele of APO E, ε3, has arginine at residue 158 and cysteine at residue 112, in the ε2 form, the arginine at position 158 is replaced by cysteine, and in ε4 the cysteine residue at 112 is replaced by arginine, due to single base changes in the gene in both cases.

In 1993 several groups demonstrated the association of the APO E ε4 allele with late onset sporadic and familial AD (Corder et al., 1993; Saunders et al., 1993; Poirer et al., 1993). This finding has been confirmed by numerous other groups world wide (Yoshizawa et al., 1994; Lannfelt et al., 1994; Dai et al., 1994; Lucotte et al., 1994; Locke et al., 1995; Martins et al., 1995; Nalbantoglu et al., 1994; Sorbi et al., 1994). In AD there is a significant increase in the frequency of the ε4 allele compared to the control population with a concomitant reduction in the frequency of the ε2 allele. The ε2 allele has been suggested to show a protective effect in preventing AD with individuals possessing this allele generally living longer and developing AD at a later age (Corder et al., 1994). The association of the ε4 allele with AD is coupled to the finding that the ε4 allele shows a dose dependant reduction in the age at onset of dementia, with ε4 homozygotes showing an earlier age at onset (i.e. 75yrs) of dementia than ε4 heterozygotes (i.e. 80yrs), and cases of AD without the ε4 allele showing a much later age of onset (i.e. 85yrs) (Corder et al., 1993; Saunders et al., 1993).

A biological basis for this effect has been suggested on the basis of interactions of Apo E with the major proteins of AD, the β-amyloid peptide of senile plaques (SP) and cerebrovascular amyloid, and Tau in neurofibrillary tangles (NFT). Apo E has been shown to bind to β-amyloid and induce the formation of monofibrils (Castaño et al., 1995; Strittmatter et al., 1993a; Sanan et al., 1994; Wisniewski et al., 1994), with Apo E showing isoform specific differences in binding (Ma et al., 1994). Apo E ε4 shows highest affinity for β-amyloid, with Apo E ε3 having intermediate, and Apo E ε2 having lowest affinity (Ma et al., 1994). This ability to form fibrils from β-amyloid monomers has been suggested to cause accelerated β-amyloid deposition, though it may be the marginally reduced ability of Apo E ε4 to prevent β-amyloid nucleation rather than a direct promoting effect per se (Evans et al., 1995). These differences in Apo E binding to β-amyloid have led to the suggestion that there is a dose dependant increase in β-amyloid deposition with the APO E ε4 allele (Strittmatter et al., 1994b; Rebeck et al., 1993; Schmechel et al., 1993; Ohm et al., 1995).

Apo E also shows some binding to Tau with the common ε3 isoform able to bind to Tau and prevent it's phosphorylation, though ε3 appears unable to bind to already hyperphosphorylated Tau. (Strittmatter et al., 1994a). Apo E ε4 appears unable to bind to Tau and this is suggested to give rise to the formation of NFT in AD (Strittmatter et al., 1994b; Ohm et al., 1995). Similar findings of Apo E ε4 "promoting" hyperphosphorylation have also been shown with the microtubule protein MAP-2c (Huang et al., 1994).

Variable results have been associated with early onset familial and sporadic AD and the ε4 allele. Certain studies have shown a positive association with early onset AD (Dai et al., 1994; van Duijn et al., 1994) with familial cases showing higher frequencies than non-familial cases (van Duijn et al., 1994) and also an association with the ε2 allele which reduced survival (van Duijn et al., 1995). Other studies have not shown early onset AD to be associated with the ε4 allele in sporadic cases (Locke et al., 1995; Sorbi et al., 1994), or in chromosome 14 linked families (Van Broeckhoven et al., 1994).

Lewy body dementia (LBD) (Gibb et al., 1989; Hansen et al., 1990; Lennox et al., 1989; Perry et al., 1990) represents a significant proportion of dementia cases in the elderly with up to 20% of cases being ascribed to this in some studies (Perry et al., 1990). Clinically, LBD is characterised by presentation with acute confusion or clouding of consciousness, and psychotic symptoms, often taking the form of auditory or visual hallucinations (McKeith et al., 1992). Extrapyramidal symptoms are often found late in the disease course though Parkinson's disease is often not a presenting feature. Certain neuropathological similarities exist between AD and LBD with both showing the presence of senile plaques at similar densities in the neocortex, neurofibrillary tangles are however absent or scarce in LBD (Perry et al., 1990). LBD is also characterised by the presence of widespread Lewy bodies throughout the neo- and archi-cortex and the presence of Lewy bodies and cell loss in subcortical nuclei, particularly the substantia nigra.

Because of the association of the ε4 allele with AD, and the presence of β-amyloid in other related disorders such as LBD and Down's syndrome, several groups have reported genotyping studies. In LBD (Bétard et al., 1994; Galasko et al., 1994; Harrington et al., 1994; Benjamin et al., 1994; Pickering-Brown et al., 1994; Lippa et al., 1995), the ε4 allele frequency is elevated in a manner analagous to that found in AD. In vascular dementia (Bétard et al., 1994; Kawamata et al., 1994), Parkinson's disease (Benjamin et al., 1994; Koller et al., 1995; Marder et al., 1994), alcoholic dementia (Muramatsu et al., 1994) and Down's syndrome (Royston et al., 1994; Martins et al., 1995; Wisniewski et al., 1995) no apparent association was observed with APO E ε4 suggesting that the ε4 allele specifically affects β-amyloidosis with a late onset, not associated with APP abnormalities.

As part of our studies on the clinical and pathological determinants of AD we have APO E genotyped a large series of AD cases and controls, and determined the effect of the different APO E alleles on neuropathological and neurochemical parameters. The frequency of the different APO E alleles has also been compared in Lewy body dementia (LBD), Parkinson's disease (PD) with and without evidence of dementia, and in pre-senile cases of AD, and in Down's syndrome.

Methods

Genomic DNA was isolated from frozen brain tissue using standard proteinase K digestion followed by Phenol/Chloroform extraction. Amplification of the APO E gene containing the allelic sites was performed by a modification of the method of Wenham and colleagues (Wenham et al., 1991; Hixon and Vernier, 1990). PCR primers used in the amplification were: forward; 5'-TCCAAGGAGCTGCAGGCGGCGCA-3', reverse; 5'-ACAGAATTCGCCCCGGCCTGGTACACTGCCA-3'. The reactions were performed in a final volume of 50 μl standard buffer containing 15 pmol of each primer, 1.0 U Taq polymerase (Boehringer, UK), 10% DMSO, 200 μM each deoxy-nucleotide, and 200 ng of DNA. Reaction conditions were an initial denaturation at 95°C for 5 minutes followed by 40 cycles of annealing at 65°C for 30 seconds, extension at 70°C for 1.5 minutes, and denaturation at 94°C for 30 seconds. The resultant amplification products were then digested overnight at 37°C with 2.5 U of Cfo I enzyme (Boehringer, UK) in the buffer supplied. Following digestion, the PCR products were electrophoresed through a composite 3% Nu Sieve/ 1% standard agarose (Flowgen, UK) gel, and the bands visualised using ethidium bromide fluorescence. Digestion of the PCR product (227 bp) with Cfo I results in the production of from 5 to 7 bands depending on the allele present. The presence of the ε2 allele is shown by the presence of an 81 bp band, the presence of the ε3 allele by 91 bp band and a 48 bp band, and the presence of the ε4 allele by a 72 bp band.

Neuropathological investigations of the cases was performed on formalin fixed paraffin embedded material. Senile plaques were demonstrated using the von Braunmühl silver impregnation method which demonstrates compact and neuritic SP but not diffuse amyloid deposits. Neurofibrillary tangles were demonstrated using a modified Palmgren's silver method. The presence of archi- and neocortical and brainstem Lewy bodies was demonstrated using haematoxylin and eosin staining and anti-ubiquitin immunocytochemistry.

Mean neocortical SP and NFT counts were determined by counting 5 fields in each section from each of the four cortical lobes, and averaging the resultant count/mm2 for each lobe . The average count for the four lobes as a whole was then taken as the mean plaque count for the neocortex as a whole.

Choline acetyltransferase (ChAT) activity in the brains of selected cases was determined on frozen unfixed tissue in the hippocampus or parietal cortex by the method of Fonnum (Fonnum, 1975) by previously described methods (Perry et al., 1992).

Statistical analysis of allele frequencies was by the Chi-square test and all other parameters by the Mann-Whitney U-test.

Results

In the current series of late onset AD cases, the APO E ε4 allele showed a significant increase compared to the control population (see Table 1), with a

Table 1. Apolipoprotein E allele frequencies in Alzheimer's disease and related neurodegenerative diseases

	APO E allele frequency[¶]		
	ε2	ε3	ε4
Control (99)	0.08	0.77	0.22
EOAD (17)	0.06	0.61	0.33
SDAT (64)	0.03[†]	0.51	0.46*
LBD (42)	0.08[‡]	0.54	0.38*
PD (11)	0.05	0.77	0.18
PD+D (12)	0.04	0.75	0.21
Down's (28)	0.04	0.68	0.29

EOAD early onset AD; *SDAT* late onset/senile dementia of the Alzheimer type; *LBD* Lewy body dementia; *PD* Parkinson's disease; *PD+D* Parkinson's disease with dementia; *Down's* Down's syndrome. [¶]Allele frequencies sum to 1.00 ± 0.01 depending on rounding error. Numbers in parenthesis indicate the number of cases genotyped. *Significantly different from the control population ($p < 0.05$, Chi Square test). [†]$p < 0.10 > 0.05$, Chi Square test. [‡]Significantly different from the SDAT population ($p < 0.05$, Chi Square test)

concomitant reduction in the frequencies of the ε2 and ε3 alleles (though not significantly). Early onset AD cases showed no apparent change in any of the allele frequencies compared to the control group. The LBD group, similar to the late onset AD group, also showed an elevated ε4 allele frequency compared to the control population, but unlike the late onset AD group, showed no reduction in the ε2 allele frequency. Compared with the late onset AD group, the ε2 allele frequency was significantly elevated in LBD (Table 1). No apparent changes in allelic frequencies were observed between the PD groups or the Down's syndrome group and the control population (Table 1).

Calculated odds ratios for the affected groups showed the ε4 allele to be a significant risk factor for the development of late onset AD (O.R. = 2.82; 95% CI = 1.68–4.71) and LBD (O.R. = 2.50; 95% CI = 1.36–4.58). The ε2 allele showed a protective effect in late onset AD (O.R. = 0.34; CI = 0.11–1.1) though not in LBD (O.R. = 1.18; 95% CI = 0.45–3.08).

Analysis of the data for effect of genotype on cortical AD neuropathology revealed no significant changes in any of the groups studied for any parameter (see Table 2 for example). APO E ε4 showed no dose dependant increase in either SP or NFT in early or late onset AD, LBD, PD with or without dementia, or in Down's syndrome. The protective ε2 allele did not show any reduction in neuropathology in any of the disease states (data not shown). Comparisons made between the late onset AD group and the LBD group showed the expected reduction in cortical NFT densities in LBD (Table 2).

210   C. M. Morris et al.

Table 2. Effect of APO E ε4 allele dosage on cortical senile plaque and neurofibrillary tangle densities in late onset AD and LBD

	APO E ε4 allele dosage		
	2ε4	1ε4	0ε4
SDAT-SP/mm^2	15.7 ± 7.1 (9)	15.3 ± 3.3 (20)	13.0 ± 2.6 (12)
LBD-SP/mm^2	11.8 ± 1.4 (3)	15.5 ± 3.2 (15)	18.8 ± 3.7 (9)
SDAT-NFT/mm^2	14.1 ± 5.7 (12)	12.7 ± 4.2 (18)	12.0 ± 5.8 (12)
LBD-NFT/mm^2	4.3 ± 2.4 (3)*	0.2 ± 0.7 (14)*	0.2 ± 1.9 (9)*

Data are medians ± SEM of mean cortical SP and NFT densities in four neocortical regions. Numbers in parenthesis indicate the number of cases studied. *SDAT* late onset AD; *LBD* Lewy Body Dementia. *Significantly different from SDAT group (p < 0.01, Mann Whitney U-test)

Table 3. Effect of apolipoprotein E ε4 allele dosage on choline acetyltransferase activity in late onset AD, Lewy body dementia, and in controls

	APO E ε4 allele dosage		
	2ε4	1ε4	0ε4
SDAT nmol/mgP[†]	4.3 ± 0.4 (5)	3.4 ± 1.3 (6)	5.5 ± 1.3 (6)
Cont nmol/mgP[†]	—	13.4 ± 1.0 (4)	15.4 ± 1.2 (17)
LBD nmol/mgP[‡]	—	7.9 ± 1.4 (4)	5.3 ± 1.1 (5)

Data are medians ± SEM of (n) cases in units of nmol/mg protein/hr. [†]Choline Acetyl Transferase activity was determined in the hippocampus in late onset AD (SDAT) cases and in normal controls (Cont). [‡]Choline acetyltransferase activity was determined in the parietal cortex of cases of Lewy body dementia (LBD). Numbers in parenthesis indicate the number of cases studied

In late onset AD and in LBD where an association with the ε4 allele was shown, ChAT activity was assessed in the most severely affected areas, namely the hippocampus in late onset AD and also in control cases, and in parietal cortex in LBD. In no group did APO E ε4 show any dose related effect (see Table 3).

Discussion

The present study shows a significantly increased frequency of the apolipoprotein E ε4 allele in patients with sporadic late-onset AD (senile dementia of the Alzheimer type). This confirms the results of similar studies in American, European and Japanese populations (Corder et al., 1993; Saunders et al., 1993; Poirer et al., 1993; Yoshizawa et al., 1994; Lannfelt et al., 1994; Dai et al., 1994; Lucotte et al., 1994; Locke et al., 1995; Martins et al., 1995; Nalbantoglu et al., 1994; Sorbi et al., 1994) suggesting that the APO E ε4 allele is one of the major determinants of AD in the elderly. The APO E ε4 frequency of 0.49 in this SDAT population is higher than the APO E ε4 frequencies reported previously. A possible explanation for this is that all the cases chosen for this study had to fulfil strict clinical and neuropathological criteria and hence the diagnosis of AD was not in doubt. Other studies have often relied on clinical diagnosis with no neuropathological confirmation, which may result in a reduced frequency.

The odds ratio for the APO E ε4 allele (a measure of the relative risk of developing AD) of 2.82 in this late onset AD population implies that there is an almost 3-fold risk of AD in APO E ε4 positive individuals compared to ε4 negative individuals. The stratified odds ratio for APO E ε4 heterozygotes alone was not significant in this population (1.91, 95% CI 0.75–4.83). It was not possible to calculate the odds ratio for APO E ε4 homozygotes in this population because of an absence of APO E ε4/ε4 individuals in the corresponding control group. The results, however, suggest that the presence of a single ε4 allele may not always be sufficient on its own to increase the risk of AD, but when two ε4 alleles are present the risk of AD is considerably enhanced (100% of ε4/ε4 individuals in this SDAT population had AD compared to 52% of ε4 heterozygotes and 22% of those without the ε4 allele). Therefore while the ε4 allele is a risk factor for AD it is far from being a diagnostic indicator or a predictor of disease (Corder et al., 1995).

The apparent absence of an association between APO E ε4 and early-onset AD (Saunders et al., 1993; Lannfelt et al., 1994; Van Broeckhoven et al., 1994) was confirmed by this study although this is not the case in other studies which have indicated a positive association (see Dai et al., 1994; van Duijn et al., 1994). Two of the cases in this series were APO E ε4/4 and had onset before the age of 65 which suggests that in some instances, cases who are homozygous for ε4 may present as early onset AD. Given that the majority of ε4 homozygotes actually present as late onset AD it would be of interest to determine if there are any other factors which cause early onset of symptoms in some individuals. Recent work has identified a synergistic effect between head trauma and APO E (Mayeux et al., 1995; Nicholl et al., 1995) and the possibility that such factors or other genes (Kamboh et al., 1995) may play a role in some cases of AD is certainly possible.

The specificity of APO E ε4 as a risk factor for late onset AD was evaluated by comparing the APO E ε4 frequencies in LBD, Down's syndrome and PD with the ε4 frequency in the late onset AD and control group (Table 1). The increased frequency of APO E ε4 in LBD supports the hypothesis that APO E ε4 may be a general risk factor for β-amyloid associated neurodegeneration with both disease states showing similar ε4 allele frequencies. The presence of a normal APO E ε2 allele frequency in LBD may however suggest some minor genetic differences between LBD and late onset AD. In this series of cases the number of ε4/4 cases was reduced compared to AD (12% vs. 30% respectively) with an increased number of ε2 positive cases in LBD compared to AD (17% vs. 6% respectively). The presence of the ε2 allele in relatively few LBD cases however suggests that the APO E status may not be the sole determinant in LBD. Genetic determinants other than ε2 which may differentiate between LBD and late onset AD are currently being investigated.

Recent studies (Saunders et al., 1993; Pickering-Brown et al., 1994; Royston et al., 1994; Martins et al., 1995; Wisniewski et al., 1995) have failed to show an increased ε4 frequency in Down's syndrome patients, and the present results would appear to confirm this. The Down's syndrome patients in this study are of an older age profile (mean of 52 years) and the majority were clinically demented with neuropathological evidence of AD-type pathology. The major genetic determinant of AD in these cases would therefore appear to be the presence of three copies of the APP gene.

Both demented and non-demented Parkinsonian patients showed no significant increase in APO E ε4 frequency, compared to age-matched controls, suggesting that the biological basis of dementia in PD differs from that found in AD and LBD and is not linked to APO E (Benjamin et al., 1994; Koller et al., 1995; Marder et al., 1994). This rationale is supported by the lack of any quantitative difference in AD-type pathology between demented and non-demented Parkinsonian patients and the low levels of SP and NFT found in these cases compared to AD cases (Perry et al., unpublished). The substrate for dementia in PD may therefore be more related to subcortical pathology and resulting changes in cortical neurochemistry than in cortical neuropathology per se.

A more complex relationship appears to exist between APO E ε4 gene dosage and quantitative measures of senile plaques and neurofibrillary tangles. Previous studies (Strittmatter et al., 1994b; Rebeck et al., 1993; Schmechel et al., 1993; Berr et al., 1994; Ohm et al., 1995; Hansen et al., 1994) have shown a dose related increase in β-amyloid SP and/or NFT counts with the number of ε4 alleles which would suggest a direct biochemical role for ε4. The current results and others (Soininen et al., 1995) argue against a direct biochemical role for the Apo E ε4 isoform in SP or NFT formation.

One possibility which would maintain Apo E biochemistry as being central to late onset AD but which would allow for it having little or no effect on pathology is that Apo E may initiate the biochemical cascade but thereafter the process is self-sustaining (Roses, 1994a,b). β-amyloid may initially deposit on an Apo E framework but following this, β-amyloid would self assemble to form SP (Morris et al., in press).

The cases of late onset AD in the present study had a duration of illness in excess of 5 years which would suggest that any disease process would be well advanced. If, as is thought, a threshold of pathology is required before onset of symptoms, and SP and NFT only accumulate slowly (Mann et al., 1988; MacKenzie, 1994), no change in SP or NFT counts would be expected between different APO E genotypes. The present results would seem to support this.

Apo E has been suggested to have interactions with normal tau, with ε3 and possibly ε2 stabilising normal tau and ε4 unable to do so (Strittmatter et al., 1994a,b). The presence of Apo E in NFT as demonstrated by immunocytochemistry would appear to support this suggestion (Han et al., 1994; Namba et al., 1991; Kida et al., 1995). However, the absence of a consistent relationship between ε4 allele number and NFT densities, and the similar ε4 allele frequencies between late onset AD and LBD, the latter which is characterised by negligible NFT formation, is evidence against this hypothesis. It is possible that whilst Apo E may be found in neurones as a result of receptor mediated uptake (Han et al., 1994), it does not reach a compartment where it can directly interact with tau. The in vitro studies which demonstrate Apo E and tau interaction (Strittmatter et al., 1994a,b) may not take place in vivo.

The significantly different ε4 frequencies between LBD and Parkinsonian patient groups, both of which are characterised by Lewy body formation, would suggest that APO E ε4 does not play a role in the formation of Lewy bodies. These results in PD and LBD have recently been confirmed by other groups (Marder et al., 1994; St Clair et al., 1994; Koller et al., 1995). These results would seem to suggest that the formation of Lewy bodies is not affected by APO E and that other factors may be involved.

Central cholinergic activity appears to relate to cognitive decline in AD (Perry et al., 1978) and it appears that APO E genotype also has an effect upon cognitive function in AD cases (Feskens et al., 1994; Ganguli et al., 1995; Helkala et al., 1995; Lehtoverta et al., 1995; Nitsch et al., 1995). Few studies have so far addressed the possibility that APO E genotype may also affect the neurochemistry of AD though one study suggests that the dosage of the ε4 allele can reduce central ChAT activity (Soininen et al., 1995). The reduction in cholinergic activity was, however, found to be related to the age of the cases studied suggesting that such changes may not be apparent in age matched cases. The current study (Table 3) would appear to support this possibility since no change was identified in ChAT activity with ε4 dosage in aged normals, late onset AD, or in LBD.

The APO E ε4 allele appears to represent a significant risk factor for late onset dementia such as AD and LBD involving β-amyloid deposition (Roses, 1994a). APO E status does not however appear to influence other related disorders such as early onset AD, Down's syndrome, or PD. The suggestion that APO E might modulate SP formation, whilst not supported by the present study, may still be possible through the amyloid promoting activity of Apo E protein (Castaño et al., 1995; Strittmatter et al., 1993a; Sanan et al., 1994; Wisniewski et al., 1994). APO E ε4 does not, however, appear to influence NFT formation on the basis of results from AD or LBD and its suggested biochemical role in NFT formation therefore needs to be re-evaluated. Future studies should be directed towards expanding current research on APO E genetics and biochemistry to determine the importance of this significant disease determinant.

References

Benjamin R, Leake A, Edwardson JA, McKeith IG, Ince PG, Perry RH, Morris CM (1994) Apolipoprotein E genes in Lewy body and Parkinson's disease. Lancet 343: 1565

214   C. M. Morris et al.

Berr C, Hauw J-J, Delaère P, Duyckaerts C, Amouyel P (1994) Apolipoprotein E allele
    ε4 is linked to increased deposition of the amyloid β-peptide (A-β) in cases with or
    without Alzheimer's disease. Neurosci Lett 178: 221–224
Bètard C, Robitaille Y, Gee M, Tiberghien D, Larrivée D, Roy P, Mortimer JA,
    Gauvreau D (1994) Apo E allele frequencies in Alzheimer's disease and vascular
    dementia. NeuroReport 5: 1893–1896
Castaño EM, Prelli F, Wisniewski T, Golabek A, Kumar RA, Soto C, Frangione B (1995)
    Fibrillogenesis in Alzheimer's disease of the amyloid β peptides and apolipoprotein
    E. Biochem J 306: 599–604
Corder E, Basun H, Lannfelt L, Viitanen M, Winblad B (1995) Apolipoprotein E-ε4 gene
    dose. Lancet 346: 967–968
Corder EH, Saunders AM, Strittmatter WJ, Schmechel DE, Gaskell PC, Small GW,
    Roses AD, Haines JL, Pericak-Vance MA (1993) Gene dose of apolipoprotein E
    type 4 allele and the risk of Alzheimer's disease in late onset families. Science 261:
    921–923
Corder EH, Saunders AM, Strittmatter WJ, Schmechel DE, Gaskell PC, Rinnuler JB,
    Locke PA, Conneally PM, Schmader KE, Small GW, Roses AD, Haines JL, Pericak-
    Vance MA (1994) Protective effect of apolipoprotein E type 2 allele for late onset
    Alzheimer's disease. Nature Genet 7: 180–184
Dai XY, Nanko S, Hattori M, Fukuda R, Nagata K, Isse K, Ueki A, Kazamatsuri H (1994)
    Association of apolipoprotein E4 with sporadic Alzheimer's disease is more pro-
    nounced in early onset type. Neurosci Lett 175: 74–76
Evans KC, Berger EP, Cho C-G, Weisgraber KH, Lansbury PT Jr (1995) Apolipoprotein
    E is a kinetic but not a thermodynamic inhibitor of amyloid formation: implications
    for the pathogenesis and treatment of Alzheimer disease. Proc Natl Acad Sci USA
    92: 763–767
Feskens EJM, Havekes LM, Kalmijn S, de Knijff P, Launer LJ, Kromhout D (1994)
    Apolipoprotein ε4 allele and cognitive decline in elderly men. Br Med J 309: 1202–
    1206
Fonnum F (1975) A rapid radiochemical method for the determination of choline
    acetyltransferase. J Neurochem 24: 407–409
Galasko D, Saitoh T, Xia Y, Thal LJ, Katzman R, Hill LR, Hansen L (1994) The
    apolipoprotein E allele ε4 is over represented in patients with the Lewy body variant
    of Alzheimer's disease. Neurology 44: 1950–1951
Ganguli M, Cauley JA, De Kosky ST, Kamboh MI (1995) Dementia among elderly
    apolipoprotein E type 4/4 homozygotes: a prospective study. Genet Epidemiol 12:
    309–311
Goate AM, Chartier-Harlin MC, Mullan M, Brown J, Crawford F, Fidani L, Giuffra L,
    Haynes A, Irving N, James L, Mant R, Newton P, Rooke K, Roques P, Talbot C,
    Pericak-Vance MA, Roses AD, Williamson R, Rossor M, Owen M, Hardy J (1991)
    Segregation of a missense mutation in the amyloid precursor protein gene with
    familial Alzheimer's disease. Nature 349: 704–706
Han S-H, Hulette C, Saunders AM, Einstein G, Pericak-Vance M, Strittmatter WJ, Roses
    AD, Schmechel DE (1994) Apolipoprotein E is present in hippocampal neurones
    without neurofibrillary tangles in Alzheimer's disease and in age-matched controls.
    Exp Neurol 128: 13–26
Hansen LA, Galasko D, Samuel W, Xia Y, Chen X, Saitoh T (1994) Apolipoprotein-E ε-
    4 is associated with increased neurofibrillary pathology in the Lewy body variant of
    Alzheimer's disease. Neurosci Lett 182: 63–65
Harrington CR, Louwagie J, Rossau R, Vanmechelen E, Perry RH, Perry EK, Xuereb
    JH, Roth M, Wischik CM (1994) Influence of apolipoprotein E genotype on senile
    dementia of the Alzheimer and Lewy body types. Significance for etiological theories
    of Alzheimer's disease. Am J Pathol 145: 1472–1484
Helkala E-L, Koivisto K, Hänninen T, Vanhanen M, Kervinen K, Kuusisto J, Mykkänen
    L, Kesäniemi YA, Laakso M, Riekkinen P Sr (1995) The association of

apolipoprotein E polymorphism with memory: a population based study. Neurosci Lett 191: 141–144

Hixon JE, Vernier DT (1990) Restriction isotyping of human apolipoprotein E by gene amplification and cleavage with HhaI. J Lipid Res 31: 545–548

Huang DY, Goedert M, Jakes R, Weisgraber KH, Garner CC, Saunders AM, Pericak-Vance MA, Schmechel DE, Roses AD, Strittmatter WJ (1994) Isoform-specific interactions of apolipoprotein E with the microtubule-associated protein MAP 2c: implications for Alzheimer's disease. Neurosci Lett 182: 55–58

Kamboh MI, Sanghera DK, Ferrell RE, DeKosky ST (1995) APO E 4-associated Alzheimer's disease risk is modified by α1-antichymotrypsin polymorphism. Nature Genet 10: 486–488

Kawamata J, Tanaka S, Shimohama S, Ueda K, Kimura J (1994) Apolipoprotein E polymorphism in Japanese patients with Alzheimer's disease or vascular dementia. J Neurol Neurosurg Psychiatry 57: 1414–1416

Kida E, Choi-Miura N-H, Wisniewski KE (1995) Deposition of apolipoproteins E and J in senile plaques is topographically determined in both Alzheimer's disease and Down's syndrome. Brain Res 685: 211–216

Koller WC, Glatt SL, Hubble JP, Paolo A, Tröster AI, Handler MS, Horvat RT, Martin C, Schmidt K, Karst A, Wijsman EM, Yu C-E, Schellenberg GD (1995) Apolipoprotein E genotypes in Parkinson's disease with and without dementia. Ann Neurol 37: 242–245

Lannfelt L, Lilius L, Nastase M, Viitanen M, Fratiglioni L, Eggertsen G, Berglund L, Angelin B, Linder J, Winblad B, Basun H (1994) Lack of association between apolipoprotein E allele ε4 and sporadic Alzheimer's disease. Neurosci Lett 169: 175–178

La Du MJ, Falduto MT, Manelli AM, Reardon CA, Getz GS, Frail DE (1994) Isoform-specific binding of apolipoprotein E to β-amyloid. J Biol Chem 269: 23403–23406

Lehtovirta M, Laakso MP, Soininen H, Helisalmi S, Mannermaa A, Helkala E-L, Partanen K, Ryynänen M, Vainio P, Hartikainen P, Riekkinen PJ Sr (1995) Volumes of hippocampus amygdala and frontal lobe in Alzheimer patients with different apolipoprotein E genotypes. Neuroscience 67: 65–72

Lippa CF, Smith TW, Saunders AM, Crook R, Pulaski-Salo D, Davies P, Hardy J, Roses AD, Dickson D (1995) Apolipoprotein E genotype and Lewy body disease. Neurology 45: 97–103

Locke PA, Conneally PM, Tanzi RE, Gusella JF, Haines JL (1995) Apolipoprotein E4 allele and Alzheimer disease: examination of allelic association and effect on age at onset in both early- and late-onset cases. Genet Epidemiol 12: 83–92

Lucotte G, Visvikis B, Leininger-Müler B, Berriche DS, Réveilleau S, Couderc R, Babron MC, Aguillon D, Siest G (1994) Association of apolipoprotein E allele ε4 with late onset sporadic Alzheimer's disease. Am J Med Genet 54: 286–288

Ma J, Yee A, Brewer B, Jr, Das S, Potter H (1994) Amyloid-associated proteins α-1 antichymotrypsin and apolipoprotein E promote assembly of Alzheimer β-protein into filaments. Nature 372: 92–94

MacKenzie IRA (1994) Senile plaques do not progressively accumulate with age. Acta Neuropathol 87: 520–525

Mahley RW, Rall SC Jr (1989) Type III hyperlipoproteinaemia (dysbetalipoproteinaemia): the role of apolipoprotein E in normal and abnormal lipoprotein metabolism. In: Scriver CR, Beaudet AL, Sly WS, Valle D (eds) The metabolic basis of inherited disease, 6th edn. McGraw-Hill, New York, pp 1195–1213

Mann DMA, Marcyniuk B, Yates PO, Neary D, Snowden JS (1988) The progression of the pathological changes of Alzheimer's disease in frontal and temporal neocortex examined both at biopsy and at autopsy. Neuropathol Appl Neurobiol 14: 177–195

Marder K, Maestre G, Cote L, Mejia H, Alfaro B, Halim A, Tang M, Tycko B, Mayeux R (1994) The apolipoprotein ε4 allele in Parkinson's disease with and without dementia. Neurology 44: 1330–1331

216   C. M. Morris et al.

Martins RN, Clarnette R, Fisher C, Broe GA, Brooks WS, Montgomery P, Gandy SE (1995) Apo E genotypes in Australia: roles in early and late onset Alzheimer's disease and Down's syndrome. NeuroReport 6: 1513–1516

Mayeux R, Ottman R, Maestre G, Ngai C, Tang M-X, Ginsberg H, Chun M, Tycko B, Shelanski M (1995) Synergistic effects of traumatic head injury and apolipoprotein-ε4 in patients with Alzheimer's disease. Neurology 45: 555–557

McKeith IG, Perry RH, Fairbairn AF, Jabeen S, Perry EK (1992) Operational criteria for senile dementia of the Lewy body type (SDLT). Psychol Med 22: 911–922

Muramatsu T, Higuchi S, Arai H, Sasaki H, Yamada K, Hayashida M, Trojanowski JQ (1994) Apolipoprotein E ε4 allele distribution in alcoholic dementia and in Alzheimer's disease in Japan. Ann Neurol 36: 797–799

Murrel J, Farlow M, Ghetti B, Benson MD (1991) A mutation in the amyloid precursor protein associated with heriditary Alzheimer's disease. Science 254: 97–99

Nalbantoglu J, Gilfix BM, Bertrand P, Robitaille Y, Gauthier S, Rosenblatt DS, Poirer JS (1994) Predictive value of apolipoprotein E genotyping in Alzheimer's disease: results of an autopsy series and an analysis of several combined studies. Ann Neurol 36: 889–895

Namba Y, Tomonaga M, Kawasaki H, Otomo E, Ikeda K (1991) Apolipoprotein E immunoreactivity in cerebral amyloid deposits and neurofibrillary tangles in Alzheimer's disease and kuru plaque amyloid in Creutzfeldt-Jakob disease. Brain Res 541: 163–166

Nicoll JAR, Roberts GW, Graham DI (1995) Apolipoprotein E ε4 allele is associated with deposition of amyloid β-protein following head injury. Nature Med 1: 135–137

Nitsch RM, Rebeck GW, Deng M, Richardson I, Tennis M, Schenk DB, Vigo-Pelfrey C, Lieberburg I, Wurtman RJ, Hyman BT, Growdon JH (1995) Cerebrospinal fluid levels of amyloid β-protein in Alzheimer's disease: inverse correlation with severity of dementia and effect of apolipoprotein E genotype. Ann Neurol 37: 512–518

Ohm TG, Kirca M, Bohl J, Scharnagl H, Groß W, März W (1995) Apolipoprotein E polymorphism influences not only cerebral senile plaque load but also Alzheimer-type neurofibrillary tangle formation. Neuroscience 66: 583–587

Perry EK, Tomlinson BE, Blessed G, Bergmann K, Gibson PH, Perry RH (1978) Correlation of cholinergic abnormalities with senile plaques and mental test scores in senile dementia. Br Med J 2: 1457–1459

Perry EK, Johnson M, Kerwin JM, Piggott MA, Court JA, Shaw PJ, Ince PG, Brown A, Perry RH (1992) Convergent cholinergic activities in ageing and Alzheimer's disease. Neurobiol Aging 13: 393–400

Perry RH, Irving D, Blessed G, Fairbairn A, Perry EK (1990) Senile dementia of the Lewy body type: a clinically and neuropathologically distinct form of Lewy body dementia in the elderly. J Neurol Sci 95: 119–139

Pickering-Brown SM, Mann DMA, Bourke JP, Roberts DA, Balderson D, Burns A, Byrne J, Owen F (1994) Apolipoprotein E4 and Alzheimer's disease pathology in Lewy body disease and in other β-amyloid-forming diseases. Lancet 343: 1155

Poirer J, Davignon J, Bouthillier D, Kogan S, Bertrand D, Gauthier S (1993) Apolipoprotein E polymorphism and Alzheimer's disease. Lancet 342: 697–699

Rebeck GW, Reiter JS, Strickland DK, Hyman BT (1993) Apolipoprotein E in sporadic Alzheimer's disease: allelic variation and receptor interactions. Neuron 11: 575–580

Roses AD (1994a) Apolipoprotein E affects the rate of Alzheimer's disease expression: β-amyloid burden is a secondary consequence dependant on Apo E genotype and duration of disease. J Neuropathol Exp Neurol 53: 429–437

Roses AD, (1994b) Apolipoprotein E is a relevant susceptibility gene that affects rate of expression of Alzheimer's disease. Neurobiol Aging 15: S165–S167

Roses AD (1995) Apolipoprotein E genotyping in the differential diagnoses not prediction, of Alzheimer's disease. Ann Neurol 38: 6–14

Royston MC, Mann D, Pickering-Brown S, Owen F, Perry R, Raghavan R, Khin-Nu C, Tyrer S, Day K, Crook R, Hardy J, Roberts GW (1994) Apolipoprotein E ε2 allele promotes longevity and protects patients with Down's syndrome from dementia. NeuroReport 5: 2583–2585

Sanan DA, Weisgraber KH, Russel SJ, Mahley RW, Huang D, Saunders A, Schmechel D, Wisniewski T, Frangione B, Roses AD, Strittmatter WJ (1994) Apolipoprotein E associates with β-amyloid peptide of Alzheimer's disease to form novel monofibris. Isoform Apo E4 associates more efficiently than Apo E3. J Clin Invest 94: 860–869

Saunders AM, Strittmatter WJ, Schmechel D, St George Hyslop PH, Pericak-Vance MA, Joo SH, Rosi BL, Gusella JF, Crapper-MacLachlan DR, Alberts MJ, Hulette C, Crain B, Goldgaber D, Roses AD (1993) Association of apolipoprotein E allele ε4 with late-onset familial and sporadic Alzheimer's disease. Neurology 43: 1467–1472

Schmechel DE, Saunders AM, Strittmatter WJ, Crain B, Hulette CM, Joo SH, Pericak-Vance MA, Goldgaber D, Roses AD (1993) Increased amyloid β-peptide deposition as a consequence of apolipoprotein E genotype in late onset Alzheimer's disease. Proc Natl Acad Sci USA 90: 9649–9653

Sherrington R, Rogaev EI, Liang Y, Rogaeva EA, Levesque G, Ikeda M, Chi H, Lin G, Holman K, Tsuda T, Mar L, Foncin J-F, Bruni AC, Montesi MP, Sorbi S, Rainero I, Pinessi L, Nee L, Chumakov I, Pollen D, Brookes A, Sanseau P, Polinsky RJ, Wasco W, Da Silva HAR, Haines JL, Pericak-Vance MA, Tanzi RE, Roses AD, Fraser PE, Rommens JM, St George-Hyslop PH (1995) Cloning of a gene bearing missense mutations in early onset familial Alzheimer's disease. Nature 375: 754–760

Soininen H, Kosunen O, Helisalmi S, Mannermaa A, Paljärvi L, Talasniemi S, Ryynänen M, Riekkinen P Sr (1995) A severe loss of choline acetyltransferase in the frontal cortex of Alzheimer patients carrying apolipoprotein ε4 allele. Neurosci Lett 187: 79–82

Sorbi S, Nacmias B, Forleo P, Latorraca S, Gobbini I, Bracco L, Piacentini S, Amaducci L (1994) Apo E allele frequencies in Italian sporadic and familial Alzheimer's disease. Neurosci Lett 177: 100–102

St Clair D, Norrman J, Perry R, Yates C, Wilcock G, Brookes A (1994) Apolipoprotein E ε4 allele frequency in patients with Lewy body dementia, Alzheimer's disease and age-matched controls. Neurosci Lett 176: 45–46

Strittmatter WJ, Saunders AM, Schmechel D, Pericak-Vance AM, Enghild J, Salvesen GS, Roses AD (1993a) Apolipoprotein E: high avidity binding to β-amyloid and increased frequency of type ε4 allele in late-onset familial Alzheimer's disease. Proc Natl Acad Sci USA 90: 1977–1981

Strittmatter WJ, Weisgraber KM, Huang DY, Dong L-M, Salvesen GS, Pericak-Vance AM, Schmechel D, Saunders AM, Goldgaber D, Roses AD (1993b) Binding of human apolipoprotein E to synthetic amyloid β peptide: isoform specific effects and implications for late onset Alzheimer's disease. Proc Natl Acad Sci USA 90: 8098–8102

Strittmatter WJ, Saunders AM, Goedert M, Weisgraber KM, Dong L-M, Jakes R, Huang DY, Pericak-Vance AM, Schmechel D, Roses AD (1994a) Isoform specific interactions of apolipoprotein E with microtubule-associated protein tau: implications for Alzheimer's disease. Proc Natl Acad Sci USA 91: 11183–11186

Strittmatter W, Weisgraber KH, Goedert M, Saunders AM, Huang D, Corder EH, Dong LM, Jakes R, Alberts MJ, Gilbert JR, Han SH, Hulette C, Einstein G, Schmechel DE, Pericak-Vance MA, Roses A (1994) Hypothesis: microtubule instability and paired helical filament formation in Alzheimer's disease brain are related to apolipoprotein E genotype. Exp Neurol 125: 163–171

van Broeckhoven C, Backhovens H, Cruts M, Martin JJ, Crook R, Houlden H, Hardy J (1994) APOE genotype does not modulate age of onset in families with chromosome 14 encoded Alzheimer's disease. Neurosci Lett 169: 179–180

van Duijn CM, de Knijff P, Cruts M, Wehnert A, Havekes LM, Hofman A, Van Broeckhoven C (1994) Apolipoprotein E4 allele in a population-based study of early-onset Alzheimer's disease. Nature Genet 7: 74–78·

van Duijn CM, de Knijff P, Wehnert A, De Voecht J, Bronzova JB, Havekes LM, Hofman A, Van Broeckhoven C (1995) The apolipoprotein E ε2 allele is associated with an increased risk of early-onset Alzheimer's disease and a reduced survival. Ann Neurol 37: 605–610

Wenham PR, Price WH, Blundell G (1991) Apolipoprotein E genotyping by one-stage PCR. Lancet 337: 1158–1159

Wisniewski T, Castano EM, Golabek A, Vogel T, Frangione B (1994) Acceleration of Alzheimer's fibril formation by apolipoprotein E in vitro. Am J Pathol 145: 1030–1035

Yoshizawa T, Yamakawa-Kobayashi K, Komatsuzaki Y, Arinami T, Oguni E, Mizusawa H, Shoji S, Hamaguchi H (1994) Dose-dependant association of Apolipoprotein E allele ε4 with late onset sporadic Alzheimer's disease. Ann Neurol 36: 656–659

Authors' address: Dr. C. M. Morris, MRC Neurochemical Pathology Unit and Department of Neuropathology, Newcastle General Hospital, Westgate Road, Newcastle upon Tyne, Tyne and Wear, NE4 6BE, United Kingdom.

J Neural Transm (1996) [Suppl] 47: 219–229

Transmissible cerebral amyloidosis

P. Brown

Laboratory of CNS Studies, National Institute of Neurological Disorders and Stroke,
National Institutes of Health, Bethesda, Md, USA

Summary. Transmissible cerebral amyloidosis occurs in three forms — sporadic, iatrogenic, and familial. Clinical and epidemiological aspects of sporadic disease are briefly described, followed by an up-to-date review of the increasing numbers and varieties of iatrogenic and mutation-positive familial cases.

Introduction

Creutzfeldt-Jakob disease (CJD) in both its sporadic and familial forms was first recognized in Germany in the 1920's (Creutzfeldt, 1920; Jakob, 1923; Kirschbaum, 1924). The exclusively familial Gerstmann-Sträussler-Scheinker syndrome (GSS) was recognized in Austria, also in the 1920's (Gerstmann, 1928); epidemic Kuru was discovered in New Guinea in the 1950's (Gajdusek and Zigas, 1957), and Fatal Familial Insomnia (FFI) was described in Italy in the 1980's (Lugaresi et al., 1986). The first published reports of iatrogenic CJD occurred in the 1970's (Bernoulli et al., 1977; Duffy et al., 1974). With the exception of Kuru, which has remained confined to New Guinea and is rapidly becoming extinct, each of these diseases has since been found to have a world-wide distribution, and all belong to the same pathophysiologic family that we have chosen to call transmissible cerebral amyloidosis (TCA).

Sporadic disease

Cases of sporadic CJD account for approximately 90% of all patients with TCA, and occur in a totally random time and space distribution at the rate of about one case per million people per year. No sporadic case clustering or any other evidence for an exogenous source of infection has ever been convincingly demonstrated (Raubertas et al., 1989; Wientjens et al., 1996), leaving us with the disquieting idea that sporadic CJD results from a stochastic *de novo* generation of amyloid protein, a kind of cerebral "spontaneous combustion" occurring without reference to any outside influence.

The clinical features of sporadic CJD are presented in Figs. 1 and 2, and Table 1 (Brown et al., 1994). These features are by now too well known to be rehearsed in detail, and consist of an onset in late middle age, peaking at 60–65 years, a clinical presentation that typically includes some form of mental deterioration, either alone or in combination with cerebellar or visual signs, an evolution that may highlight pathologic involvement of any one of several different neuronal systems (neocortical, cerebellar, visual, pyramidal, or extrapyramidal), but which usually includes a subacute progression into dementia that is associated with myoclonus and electroencephalographic (EEG) periodicity. The median duration of illness is about four months, although the approximately 10% of cases of long duration raise the mean to 7 months.

However, many individual case reports attest to the spectral richness of sporadic disease, which may depart from the norm in any given patient to an extraordinary degree: one patient may have major bulbar or pseudobulbar signs, another an amyotrophic lateral sclerosis syndrome, still others an illness dominated by visual deterioration with ocular palsies, peripheral neuropathies or paretic signs. Thus, despite the majority of mainstream cases that have allowed us to define the typical illness, sporadic CJD can imitate a

Table 1. Clinical characteristics of 232 experimentally transmitted sporadic cases of Creutzfeldt-Jakob disease

Symptoms/signs	Percentage of patients with symptoms or signs		
	At onset	On first exam	During course
Mental deterioration	69	85	100
Memory loss	48	66	100
Behavioral abnormalities	29	40	57
Higher cortical functions	16	36	73
Cerebellar	33	56	71
Visual/oculomotor	19	32	42
Vertigo/dizziness	13	15	19
Headache	11	11	18
Sensory	6	7	11
Involuntary movements	4	18	91
Myoclonus	1	9	78
Other (incl. tremor)	3	12	36
Pyramidal	2	15	62
Extra-pyramidal	0.5	9	56
Lower motor neuron	0.5	3	12
Seizures	0	2	19
Pseudobulbar	0.5	1	7
Periodic EEG*	0	0	60
Triphasic 1 cycle/sec	0	0	48
Burst suppression	0	0	14

*EEG electroencephalogram; the figures shown are lower than in published small series of repeatedly studied patients

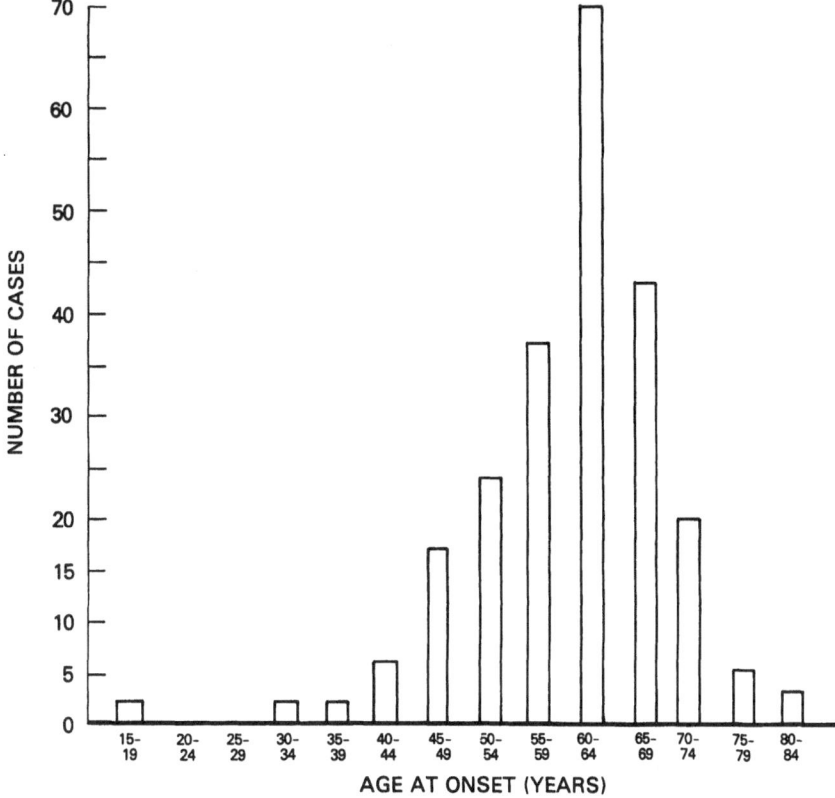

Fig. 1. Distribution of the ages at onset of illness in 232 experimentally transmitted cases of sporadic Creutzfeldt-Jakob disease (CJD)

wide variety of diseases, including CNS tumors, vascular accidents, and metabolic derangements, as well as a host of other neurodegenerative disorders, most notably Alzheimer's disease (AD) which occasionally cannot be distinguished from CJD short of autopsy examination. The point is worth belaboring, because claims of uniquely distinctive clinical features associated with different familial illnesses tend to be deaf to their echos in the general population of sporadic CJD patients.

Iatrogenic disease

In 1974 and again in 1977, isolated instances of iatrogenic CJD were reported; the first in a patient who had received a corneal graft (Duffy et al., 1974), and the second in two patients who had been subjected to stereotactic electroencephalography (Bernoulli et al., 1977). The presumption was that the graft, taken from a patient later found to have died of CJD, and the EEG instruments, which had earlier been used on a CJD patient with intractable epilepsy, were contaminated with the infectious agent. In the case of the EEG electrodes, the presumption was proven, as one of the electrodes was later

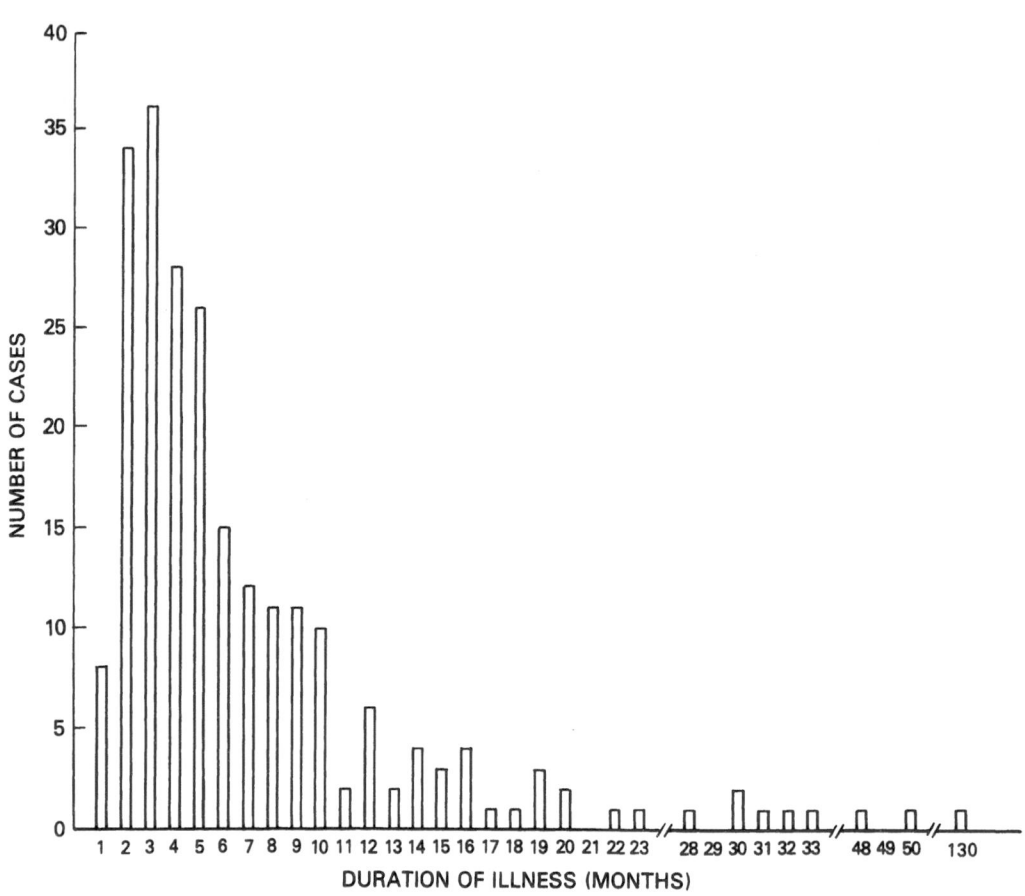

Fig. 2. Distribution of the durations of illness in 230 transmitted cases of sporadic CJD
(duration was unknown for 2 cases in Fig. 1)

experimentally implanted into the brain of a chimpanzee and duly transmitted
disease after an 18-month incubation period similar to that of the patients
themselves (Brown, 1994). Retrospective studies uncovered a few earlier
cases having probably resulted from contaminated neurosurgical instruments
(Foncin et al., 1980; Masters et al., 1979; Will and Matthews, 1982), but the
iatrogenic stew did not really begin to bubble until 1985, with the advent of
iatrogenic disease in young hypopituitary patients treated with cadaveric-
derived native human growth hormone (Brown et al., 1985).

The current tally of such cases stands at 65, mostly limited to patients
residing in the United States, England, and France, although cases have also
occurred in Brazil and New Zealand from hormone prepared in the United
States (Brown, 1996). The calculated risk of acquiring the disease is rather
different in the three countries, and is inversely related to the average incubation period elapsing between treatment and the onset of CJD (Table 2), a
conjunction that suggests the level of contamination had differed from country to country, being least in the United States, and greatest in France (the
higher the level of contamination, the greater the risk of disease, and the

shorter the incubation period). Two cases that occurred in the United States deserve special mention: one case died of intercurrent pneumonia before any symptoms of CJD had appeared, and only on review of the autopsy was it appreciated that typical changes of CJD were present in the hypothalamus; the other case had a minimum incubation period of 35 years between the end of treatment and the onset of CJD, and gives us pause in counseling patients who ask whether enough time has passed for them to stop worrying about ever getting the disease.

While our attention was focused on this evolving outbreak of CJD-infected growth hormone patients, unanticipated trouble came from another direction — the use of cadaveric dura mater grafts in neurosurgery. The first case of iatrogenic CJD from this source was reported in 1987 (Thadani et al., 1988) and during the past few years had increased to a total of 24 patients, almost all of whom received grafts collected and processed by a single company during the period 1981 through 1985. Until this time, the company had used irradiation to sterilize the dural patches, which was not adequate to inactivate the agent of CJD, but since then the company has added an exposure to 1N NaOH, which is a far more effective decontaminating procedure.

The interval between infection and disease, as well as the clinical presentation of CJD apparently depend heavily on the route of infection in different types of iatrogenic disease (Table 3). With direct intracerebral or ocular nerve infection (neurosurgical instruments or corneal grafts), incubation times are measured in months, and the onset of illness is indistinguishable from that of sporadic cases of CJD; with cerebral surface infection (dura mater grafts) incubation times vary widely from months to years, and the onset of illness may occasionally resemble sporadic disease, but are in most cases predominantly cerebellar; after peripheral routes of infection (pituitary hormone therapy), incubation times are sometimes prolonged for decades, and the onset of illness is uniformly cerebellar (Brown, 1996).

The important question of genetic resistance (or susceptibility) to exogenous infection has now been investigated in a sufficiently large number of cases for us to be confident of the results. In all forms of iatrogenic disease, whatever the route of infection, homozygosity at polymorphic codon 129 of the gene that encodes the amyloid protein (PrP) is far more frequent in

Table 2. Comparative risks and mean incubation periods of Creutzfeldt-Jakob disease (CJD) following treatment with cadaveric human growth hormone grouped according to country in which hormone was prepared

Country	Number of patients	Treated population	Risk of CJD	Mean incubation period (years)
United States[1]	15	8,600	0.2%	17 ($\pm$6)
United Kingdom	15	1,750	0.9%	12 ($\pm$3)
France	35	1,700	2.1%	9 ($\pm$11)

[1] Includes one Brazilian patient and one New Zealand patient who received hormone prepared in the United States

Table 3. Iatrogenic cases of Creutzfeldt-Jakob disease grouped according to the mode of infection (route of entry of the infectious agent into the brain)

Mode of infection	Number of patients	Agent entry into brain	Mean incubation period (range)	Clinical presentation
Corneal transplant	2	Optic nerve	17 mos (16, 18)	Dementia/Cereb
Stereotactic EEG	2	Intra-cerebral	18 mos (16, 20)	Dementia/Cereb
Neurosurgery	4	Intra-cerebral	20 mos (15–28)	Vis/Dem/Cereb
Dura mater graft	24	Cerebral surface	5.5 yrs (1.5–12)	Cereb (Vis/Dem)
Gonadotrophin	4	Hematogenous	13 yrs (12–16)	Cerebellar
Growth hormone	65	Hematogenous	12 yrs (5–30)	Cerebellar

iatrogenic cases of CJD than in the general population (Brown et al., 1994; Collinge et al., 1991; Deslys et al., 1994). The pathogenetic basis for this effect remains obscure, but has been proposed to involve a process in which similarly configured protein molecules associate to form dimers, polymers and chain-polymer fibrils.

Familial disease

In the rapidly expanding category of familial disease we move from genetic susceptibility to genetic causality. Familial disease accounts for approximately 10% of all cases of TCA, and all cases in which an adequate family history has been recorded have one of nearly 20 different mutations so far discovered in the amyloid protein gene (Fig. 3) (Goldfarb and Brown, 1994). This gene is located in humans on the short arm of chromosome 20, and encodes a membrane-bound glycoprotein of as yet unknown function that in individuals with TCA is rather mysteriously converted to an insoluble isoform with a propensity to form amyloid fibrils.

The first mutation was reported in 1989, consisting of a 144 base-pair insert in the upstream region of octapeptide coding repeats between codons 51 and 91 of the translated portion of the gene (Owen et al., 1989). Since this original discovery, several further insert mutations have been described having lengths of between 96 and 216 base pairs (encoding between 4 and 9 octapeptide repeat sequences), as well as 24 base pair deletions (encoding single octapeptide repeats), all of which are located in the same region of the gene. Most of these mutations have been confined to one or at most two families, and the resulting disease has been distinguished by an unusually early age at onset (on average, in the mid-30's), long duration (often extending four or more years), and clinical and neuropathologic features that can range from the typical picture of CJD to an undifferentiated dementing illness with little or no spongiform change at autopsy. However, it is important to remember that in every family so far described, no matter how atypical the disease in most members, there is always at least one member whose illness enough resembles typical CJD to be able to suspect the diagnosis clinically.

The second mutation to be discovered was a point mutation at codon 102 in a family with GSS (Hsiao et al., 1989), which has now been linked to the disease in numerous other unrelated families, including Gerstmann's original Austrian family (Kretzschmar et al., 1991). Most members of each family show the classical phenotype of GSS, although a recently deceased member of Gerstmann's family had an illness more suggestive of CJD than GSS (Hainfellner et al., 1995). Other mutations producing a GSS-type of disease with comparatively long durations of illness and the presence of multicentric PrP-positive plaques occur as point mutations at codons 105, 117, 145, 198, and 217, and as a 192 base-pair insert mutation in the region of octapeptide coding repeats. The insert mutation produced typical GSS in all but one family member, who had an illness that was indistinguishable from sporadic CJD (Goldfarb et al., 1992); however, each of the point mutations produced phenotypes that depart somewhat from the classical codon 102 phenotype: codon 105 produces an element of spastic paraparesis (Kitamoto et al., 1993); codon 117 may have a prominent pseudo-bulbar component (Tranchant et al., 1991), and codons 145, 198 and 217 show clinico-neuropathological pictures that combine the features of both GSS and AD (Dlouhy et al., 1992; Hsiao et al., 1992; Kitamoto et al., 1993).

Apart from the codon 102 point mutation, each of the different GSS mutations, like insert mutations, has been found in only one or two families. In contrast, a point mutation at codon 200 that produces a typical CJD-like syndrome is by far the most common mutation that has yet been linked to familial TCA, and is responsible not only for the disease in dozens of apparently unrelated individual families living in various parts of the world, but also for CJD case clusters in Slovakia, Israel, and Chile (Brown, 1994). More recently, mutations at codon 180, 208, and 210 have been identified in

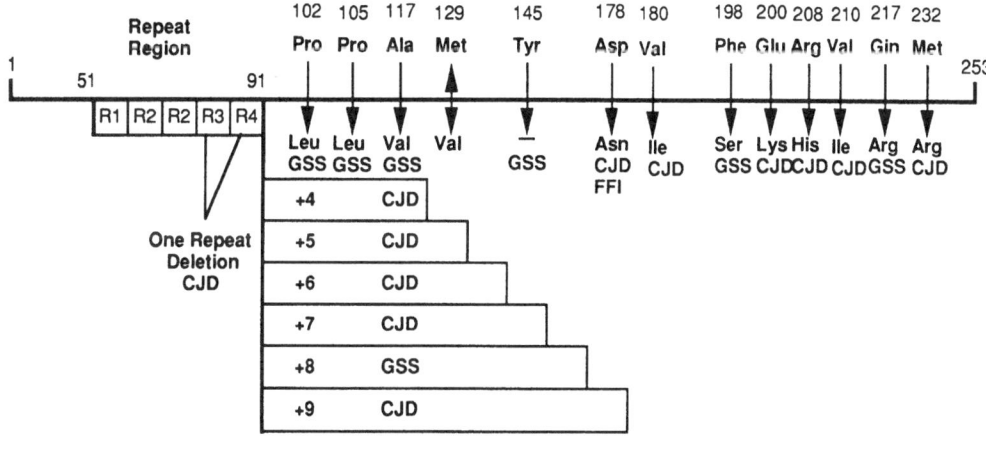

Fig. 3. Schematic illustration of mutations associated with familial forms of transmissible cerebral amyloidosis. Polymorphic codon 129 is not in itself pathogenic but does influence phenotypic features of disease

European, American, and Japanese patients that also reproduce the clinical and neuropathological features of typical sporadic CJD (Hitoshi et al., 1993; Mastrianni et al., 1995; Pocchiari et al., 1993).

Finally, a mutation at codon 178 has been found to have the intriguing property of producing either of two different phenotypes, depending on the genotype of the normally polymorphic codon 129 (Goldfarb et al., 1992). When the 178 mutant allele encodes valine at codon 129, the disease in most particulars resembles CJD, but when the mutant allele encodes methionine at codon 129, the disease takes on a decidedly thalamic flavor, and has been distinguished by the name Fatal Familial Insomnia (FFI). The separation is not absolute, however, because some affected members of FFI families do not experience insomnia, and conversely, a small proportion of patients with sporadic CJD, and at least one family with a mutation at codon 200, have displayed prominent sleep disorders or other autonomic dysfunctions (Brown et al., 1994; Chapman et al., 1996).

Although we can see a tendency for "upstream" mutations to produce GSS, and for "downstream" mutations to produce CJD, there is really no clear-cut localization of mutational phenotypes to particular areas of the gene. The more important matter is that without exception, all pathogenic mutations code for predicted non-β protein domains. We know that synthetic peptides duplicating these regions may undergo in vitro transformation into β-sheet fibrils, and that mixtures for normal and mutant peptides are more fibrillogenic than either peptide alone (Goldfarb et al., 1993). It seems highly likely, therefore, that such mixtures encoded in vivo by the normal and mutant alleles of mutation-carrying individuals similarly facilitate β-sheet formation and thereby generate the insoluble protein fibrils that eventually accumulate as neurone-damaging amyloid.

Conclusion

Sporadic CJD remains by far the most important and least understood form of TCA, accounting for some 90% of cases, and has so far resisted all efforts at identifying either an environmental or endogenous cause. Iatrogenic CJD is presently undergoing intensive experimental and epidemiological scrutiny, with results that encourage us to hope we are nearing the end of outbreaks attending modern day medical achievements, and providing knowledge that will enable us to foresee and thereby avoid most, if not all, future incidents. Familial disease has yielded up most of its etiologic mysteries to molecular genetics, and may well be the first to succumb to therapeutic strategies based upon advances in the field of genetic engineering.

References

Bernoulli C, Siegfried J, Baumgartner G, Regli F, Rabinowics T, Gajdusek DC, Gibbs CJ Jr (1977) Danger of accidental person-to-person transmission of Creutzfeldt-Jakob disease by surgery. Lancet i: 478–479

Brown P (1994) Transmissible human spongiform encephalopathy (infectious cerebral amyloidosis): Creutzfeldt-Jakob disease, Gertmann-Sträussler-Scheinker syndrome, and kuru. In: Calne D (ed) Neurodegenerative disease. Saunders, Philadelphia, pp 839–876

Brown P (1996) Environmental causes of human spongiform encephalopathy. In: Baker H, Ridley R (eds) Prion diseases. Humana Press, Totowa, NJ, pp 139–154

Brown P, Gajdusek DC, Gibbs CJJ, Asher DM (1985) Potential epidemic of Creutzfeldt-Jakob disease from human growth hormone therapy. N Engl J Med 313: 728–31

Brown P, Gibbs C Jr, Rodgers-Johnson P, Asher D, Sulima M, Bacote A, Goldfarb L, Gajdusek D (1994) Human spongiform encephalopathy: the National Institutes of Health series of 300 cases of experimentally transmitted disease. Ann Neurol 35: 513–529

Brown P, Goldfarb L, Cervenáková L, McCombie W, Scalici C, Masullo C, Graupera G, Ligan J, Gajdusek D (1994) Iatrogenic Creutzfeldt-Jakob disease: an example of the interplay between ancient genes and modern medicine. Neurology 44: 291–293

Chapman J, Arlazoroff A, Cervenáková L, Goldfarb L, Neufeld M, Werber E, Brown P, Gajdusek D, Korczyn A (1996) Fatal familial insomnia in a case of familial Creutzfeldt-Jakob disease with the codon 200[Lys] mutation. Neurology 46: 758–761

Collinge J, Palmer MS, Dryden AJ (1991) Genetic predisposition to iatrogenic Creutzfeldt-Jakob disease. Lancet 337: 1441–1442

Creutzfeldt HG (1920) Über eine eigenartige herdförmige Erkrankung des Zentralnervensystems. Z Ges Neurol Psychiat 57: 1–18

Deslys J, Marcé D, Dormont D (1994) Similar genetic susceptibility in iatrogenic and sporadic Creutzfelt-Jakob disease. J Gen Virol 75: 23–27

Dlouhy SF, Hsiao K, Farlow MR, Foroud T, Conneally PM, Johnson P, Prusiner SB, Hodes ME, Ghetti B (1992) Linkage of the Indiana kindred of Gerstmann-Sträussler-Scheinker disease to theprion protein gene. Nature Genet 1: 64–67

Duffy P, Wolf J, Collins G, DeVoe AG, Streeten B, Cowen D (1974) Possible person-to-person transmission of Creutzfeldt-Jakob disease. N Engl J Med 290: 692

Foncin J, Gaches J, Cathala F, El Sherif E, Le Beau J (1980) Transmission iatrogène interhumaine possible de maladie de Creutzfeldt-Jakob avec atteinte des grains du cervelet. Rev Neurol (Paris) 136: 280

Gajdusek DC, Zigas V (1957) Degenerative disease of the central nervous system in New Guinea: epidemic occurrence of "kuru" in the native population. N Engl J Med 257: 974–978

Gerstmann J (1928) Über ein noch nicht beschriebenes Reflexphänomen bei einer Erkrankung des zerebellaren Systems. Wien Med Wochenschr 78: 906–908

Goldfarb L, Brown P (1994) The transmissible spongiform encephalopathies. Ann Rev Med 46: 57–65

Goldfarb LG, Brown P, Vrbovská A, Baron H, McCombie WR, Cathala F, Gibbs CJ Jr, Gajdusek DC (1992) An insert mutation in the chromosome 20 amyloid precursor gene in a Gerstmann-Sträussler-Scheinker family. J Neurol Sci 111: 189–194

Goldfarb LG, Petersen RB, Tabaton M, Brown P, LeBlanc AC, Montagna P, Cortelli P, Julien J, Vital C, Pendelbury WW, Haltia M, Wills PR, Hauw JJ, McKeever PE, Monari L, Schrank B, Swergold GD, Autilio-Gambetti L, Gajdusek DC, Lugaresi E, Gambetti P (1992) Fatal familial insomnia and familial Creutzfeldt-Jakob disease: disease phenotype determined by a DNA polymorphism. Science 258: 806–808

Goldfarb LG, Brown P, Haltia M, Ghiso J, Frangione B, Gajdusek DC (1993) Synthetic peptides corresponding to different mutated regions of the amyloid gene in familial Creutzfeldt-Jakob disease show enhanced in vitro formation of morphologically distinct amyloid fibrils. Proc Natl Acad Sci (USA) 90: 4451–4454

Hainfellner J, Brantner-Inthaler S, Cervenáková L, Brown P, Kitamoto T, Tateishi J, Diringer H, Liberski P, Regele H, Feucht M, Mayr N, Wessely P, Summer K,

Seitelberger F, Budka H (1995) The original Gerstmann-Sträussler-Scheinker family of Austria: divergent clinicopathological phenotypes but constant PrP genotype. Brain Pathol 11: 201–213

Hitoshi S, Nagura H, Yamanouchi H, Kitzmoto T (1993) Double mutations at codon 180 and codon 232 of the PRNP gene in an apparently sporadic case of Creutzfeldt-Jakob disease. J Neurol Sci 120: 208–212

Hsiao K, Baker HF, Crow TJ, Poulter M, Owen F, Terwilliger JD, Westaway D, Ott J, Prusiner SB (1989) Linkage of a prion protein missense variant to Gerstmann-Sträussler syndrome. Nature 338: 342–245

Hsiao KK, Dlouhy SR, Farlow MR, Cass C, Da Costa M, Conneally PM, Hodes ME, Ghetti B, Prusiner SB (1992) Mutant prion proteins in Gerstmann-Sträussler-Scheinker disease with neurofibrillary tangles. Nature Genet 1: 68–71

Jakob A (1923) Spastische Pseudosklerose. In: Foerster O, Wilmanns K (eds) Monographien aus dem Gesamtgebiete der Neurologie und Psychiatrie. Springer, Berlin, pp 215–245

Kirschbaum W (1924) Zwei eigenartige Erkrankungen des Zentralnervensystems nach Art der spastischen Pseudosklerose (Jakob). Z Ges Neurol Psychiat 92: 175–202

Kitamoto T, Amano N, Terao Y, Nakazato Y, Isshiki T, Mizutani T, Tateishi J (1993) A new inherited prion disease (PrP-P105L mutation) showing spastic paraparesis. Ann Neurol 34: 808–813

Kitamoto T, Iizuka R, Tateishi J (1993) An amber mutation of prion protein in Gerstmann-Sträussler-syndrome with mutant PrP plaques. Biochem Biophys Res Commun 192: 525–531

Kretzschmar HA, Honold G, Seitelberger F, Feucht M, Wessely P, Mehraein P, Budka H (1991) Prion protein mutation in family first reported by Gerstmann, Sträussler, and Scheinker. Lancet 337: 1160

Lugaresi E, Medori R, Montagna P, Baruzzi A, Cortelli P, Lugaresi A, Tinuper P, Zucconni M, Gambetti P (1986) Fatal familial insomnia and dysautonomia with selective degeneration of thalamic nuclei. N Engl J Med 315: 997–1003

Masters CL, Harris JO, Gajdusek DC, Gibbs CJ Jr, Bernoulli C, Asher DM (1979) Creutzfeldt-Jakob disease: patterns of world wide occurrence and the significance of familial and sporadic clustering. Ann Neurol 5: 177–188

Mastrianni JA, Iannicola C, Myers R, Prusiner SB (1995) Identification of a new mutation of the prion protein gene at codon 208 in a patient with Creutzfeldt-Jakob disease (Abstract). Ann Neurol 45 [Suppl 4]: A201

Owen F, Poulter M, Lofthouse R, Collinge J, Crow TJ, Risby D, Baker HF, Ridley RM, Hsiao K, Prusiner SB (1989) Insertion in prion protein gene in familial Creutzfeldt-Jakob disease. Lancet i: 51–52

Pocchiari M, Salvatore M, Cutruzzolá F, Genuardi M, Allocatelli CT, Masullo C, Macchi G, Aléma G, Galgani S, Xi YG, Petraroli R, Silverstrini MC, Brunori M (1993) A new point mutation of the prion protein gene in Creutzfeldt-Jakob disease. Ann Neurol 34: 802–807

Raubertas R, Brown P, Cathala F, Brown I (1989) The question of clustering of Creutzfeldt-Jakob disease. Am J Epidemiol 129: 146–154

Thadani V, Penar PL, Partington J, Kalb R, Janssen R, Schonberger LB, Rabkin CA, Prichard JW (1988) Creutzfeldt-Jakob disease probably acquired from a cadaveric dura mater graft. J Neurosurg 69: 766–769

Tranchant C, Doh-Ura K, Steinmetz G, Chevalier Y, Kitamoto T, Tateishi J, Warter JM (1991) Mutation du codon 117 du gène du prion dans une maladie de Gerstmann-Sträussler-Scheinker. Rev Neurol (Paris) 147: 274–278

Wientjens D, Davinipour Z, Hofman A, Kondo K, Matthews B, Will R, van Duijn C (1996) Risk factors for Creutzfeldt-Jakob disease: a re-analysis of case-control studies. Neurology (in press)

Will RG, Matthews WB (1982) Evidence for case-to-case transmission of Creutzfeldt-Jakob disease. J Neurol Neurosurg Psychiatry 45: 235–238

Author's address: Dr. P. Brown, Building 36, Room 5B21, National Institutes of Health, Bethesda, Maryland 20892, U.S.A.

J Neural Transm (1996) [Suppl] 47: 231–246

Human prion diseases

J. W. Ironside

Neuropathology Laboratory, Department of Pathology, The University of Edinburgh,
Western General Hospital, Edinburgh, United Kingdom

Summary. The classical prion diseases in man comprise Creutzfeldt-Jakob disease (CJD), Kuru and Gerstmann-Sträussler-Scheinker syndrome (GSS). Recent advances in the biochemistry and the molecular biology of the transmissible agents responsible for these human spongiform encephalopathies have prompted renewed interest in their clinical and pathological features. A broadening spectrum of human prion diseases has now been identified including novel entities such as Fatal Familial Insomnia and variants of CJD and GSS characterised by specific abnormalities in the human prion protein (PrP) gene on chromosome 20. Accumulation of PrP in the central nervous system is a characteristic feature of all these disorders, although the relationship between PrP localisation, classical neuropathology, clinical features and genotype still requires clarification. A national surveillance project for CJD was established in 1990 in the United Kingdom in order to assess the possible implications of bovine spongiform encephalopathy for human health. The identification of an apparently new variant of CJD in young patients in UK raises the possibility of such a link; further studies are required to assess the significance of this observation.

Introduction

The classical human prion diseases which were recognised in the earlier years of this century comprise Creutzfeldt-Jakob disease (CJD) (Creutzfeldt, 1920; Jakob, 1921), Gerstmann-Sträussler-Scheinker syndrome (GSS) (Gerstmann et al., 1936) and Kuru (Gajdusek and Vigas, 1957). These diseases were first identified on the basis of distinctive clinical features and characteristic neuropathology. The principal neuropathological features of these conditions — spongiform change, neuronal loss, astrocytosis and amyloid plaque formation (Bastian, 1991; Bell and Ironside, 1993a) — were noted to resemble those in the brains of sheep affected with scrapie, a naturally occurring transmissible disease with a widespread distribution. Recognition of these similarities led to the successful attempts to transmit these human diseases to experimental animals (Gajdusek et al., 1966; Gibbs et al., 1968; Masters et al., 1981). Since then, the enormous increase in our knowledge of the biochemistry and molecular biology of the transmissible agents responsible for this group of diseases (Prusiner, 1994) has prompted renewed interest in the neuropathology of these disorders. In addition to the classical neuropathological features of spongiform change, neuronal loss, astrocytosis and amyloid plaque formation, these disorders are characterised by an accumulation of prion protein (PrP) in the central nervous system (Prusiner, 1994). Extensive studies on experimental scrapie have identified PrP as a major component of the infectious agent, but as yet no nucleic acid component has unequivocally been demonstrated in either the human or animal spongiform encephalopathies. The demonstration that PrP accumulates in the brain in these disorders has led to the use of the term prion disease rather than spongiform encephalopathy, which is appropriate in that spongiform change is not a major finding in all cases, particularly in GSS and Kuru.

PrP biochemistry and molecular genetics

The identification of PrP as a major component of the transmissible agent in spongiform encephalopathies has been accompanied by increasing knowledge of the biochemistry and molecular biology of the protein and its gene. In man, the PrP gene is located on the short arm of the chromosome 20, with the entire open reading frame residing within a single exon, as in other species (Prusiner, 1994). The gene product in its normal (or cellular) isoform is a rapidly synthesized and degraded cell membrane glycoprotein 33–35 kD which is expressed at high levels in adult neurones and is thought to play a role in synaptic function. This glycoprotein is also expressed in several other adult tissues, including skeletal muscle, heart and lung where its functions are unknown. The disease-associated isoform of PrP has a molecular weight of 27–30 kD and is derived by limited proteolysis from an abnormal isoform of its larger precursor (Prusiner, 1994). The biochemical differences between the cellular and disease-associated isoforms of PrP have allowed the development of various strategies to identify the abnormal protein in tissue homogenates and sections using antibodies to PrP (Bell and Ironside, 1993a; Hayward et al., 1994).

PrP accumulation in the human prion diseases appears to be confined to the central nervous system. PrP accumulation outside the central nervous system has been reported in the uncommon skeletal muscle disorder inclusion body myositis (Askanas et al., 1993), where another cell surface glycoprotein, the Aβ protein, also accumulates (Askanas et al., 1992). The cellular mechanisms behind this accumulation are unknown and this disorder does not exhibit any other clinical or neuropathological features suggestive of human prion disease. It is of interest to note that transgenic mice over-expressing wild-type PrP develop a myopathy with structural features similar to those found in inclusion body myositis (Westaway et al., 1994). Further investigations are in progress to establish the significance of these findings and their relationship to the human disease.

Table 1. Current classification of human prion diseases: all are transmissible

— Creutzfeldt-Jakob disease	Sporadic Familial Iatrogenic
— Gerstmann-Sträussler-Scheinker disease	Classical Variants with neurofibrillary tangles
— Kuru	
— Fatal familial insomnia	
— Atypical prion dementia*	

*transmission not yet reported

The broadening spectrum of human prion diseases

Human prion diseases occur in several forms (Table 1), the commonest of which is sporadic CJD. This rare disease has a relatively constant world-wide instance of around one case/million population/year (Will, 1991). CJD also occurs as a familial disorder, accounting for around 10–15% of all cases of CJD (Baker and Ridley, 1992). Investigations of the PrP gene on chromosome 20 in this group of patients have demonstrated a wide range of genetic abnormalities, including point mutations, insert sequences and deletions (Baker and Ridley, 1992; Goldfarb et al., 1994). Not all mutations in the PrP gene appear to be pathogenic and in many cases the phenotypic expression is not constant. CJD may also occur as a result of accidental iatrogenic transmission of the infective agent; this rare event has been recorded after a variety of medical and surgical procedures (Brown et al., 1992). The largest group of iatrogenic CJD cases is in recipients of human cadaveric pituitary hormones, including growth hormone and gonadotrophins, where peripheral injection of the transmissible agent has resulted in characteristic clinical and pathological features which are distinct from those of sporadic CJD (Frasier and Foley, 1994).

The ability to identify the disease-associated isoform of PrP within brain tissue has allowed detailed studies on the site of accumulation of PrP within the central nervous system in the classical human prion diseases, and has also allowed other disorders to be classified as prion diseases on the basis of accumulation of this abnormal protein in the brain. Perhaps the best example of this is fatal familial insomnia, an inherited disease in which spongiform change is a variable and inconstant feature, but the disorder is characterised by an accumulation of prion protein in the region of the thalamus and by a specific PrP genotype (Medori et al., 1992; Gambetti et al., 1993). Progressive subcortical gliosis is a rare and rather poorly characterised disorder which appears to be associated with an accumulation of PrP within the brain, but the relationship between this disorder and other human prion diseases awaits clarification (Petersen et al., 1995). Attempts to demonstrate accumulation of PrP in other rare forms of human dementia have generally proven unsuccessful (Jendroska et al., 1994).

Clinicopathological features of human prion disease

Creutzfeldt-Jakob disease

Sporadic

Sporadic CJD occurs in a world-wide distribution with a relatively uniform instance of around 1/million population/year. The mean age of onset is around 60 years, but a wide age range has been described from 14–83 years (Bastian, 1991). In most patients CJD presents as a rapidly progressive dementia with a clinical course lasting around 8 months, although a significant minority of cases have a longer history with a survival of 2 years or more following diagnosis (Will, 1991). A wide range of neurological abnormalities have been described, but the commonest features include a subacute dementia with pyramidal and extrapyramidal signs (Bastian, 1991). Myoclonus is present at varying stages of illness in 90% of patients and seizures may occur in a minority of cases. Electroencephalogram investigations show a characteristic periodic discharge in most patients at some stage in the illness, although this abnormality is not entirely specific for CJD (Will, 1991). Clinical criteria for the diagnosis of sporadic CJD have been established and provide a useful framework for the probability of CJD in a patient with a subacute dementia (Budka et al., 1995).

The classical neuropathological features in sporadic CJD include spongiform change, neuronal loss and astrocytosis with PrP plaques present in around 15% of cases (Bell and Ironside, 1993a). Spongiform change is characteristically present in the cerebral cortex (Fig. 1a), but the severity and the distribution of this abnormality varies enormously from case to case (Masters and Richardson, 1978). The basal ganglia (Fig. 1b), thalamus, cerebellum (Fig. 1c) and brain stem may also be involved by spongiform change to a variable extent. Neuronal loss and astrocytosis are most evident in cases of long duration, which frequently exhibit severe cortical atrophy (Bastian, 1991). PrP plaques are most evident in the cerebellum where a "kuru" type morphology is most characteristic (Fig. 1d). PrP immunocytochemistry reveals a widespread distribution of the abnormal protein in a variety of patterns including perivacuolar, synaptic (Fig. 2a), perineuronal, plaque (Fig. 1d) and tract staining (Kitamoto et al., 1992; Bell and Ironside, 1993a; Hayward et al., 1994). The significance of these various staining patterns is poorly understood at present. These abnormalities may also be recognised in brain biopsies performed on patients with suspected CJD, although the extreme variability of the cortical lesions in this disease should be borne in mind when interpreting these specimens. Neuropathological criteria for the diagnosis of CJD and related disorders have recently been established and provide a helpful benchmark for the laboratory investigation of this group of diseases (Budka et al., 1995). Other reported neuropathological changes in human prion diseases are listed in Table 2.

Studies of PrP genotype in sporadic CJD have indicated that most patients do not have a mutation deletion or insertion in the gene (Baker and

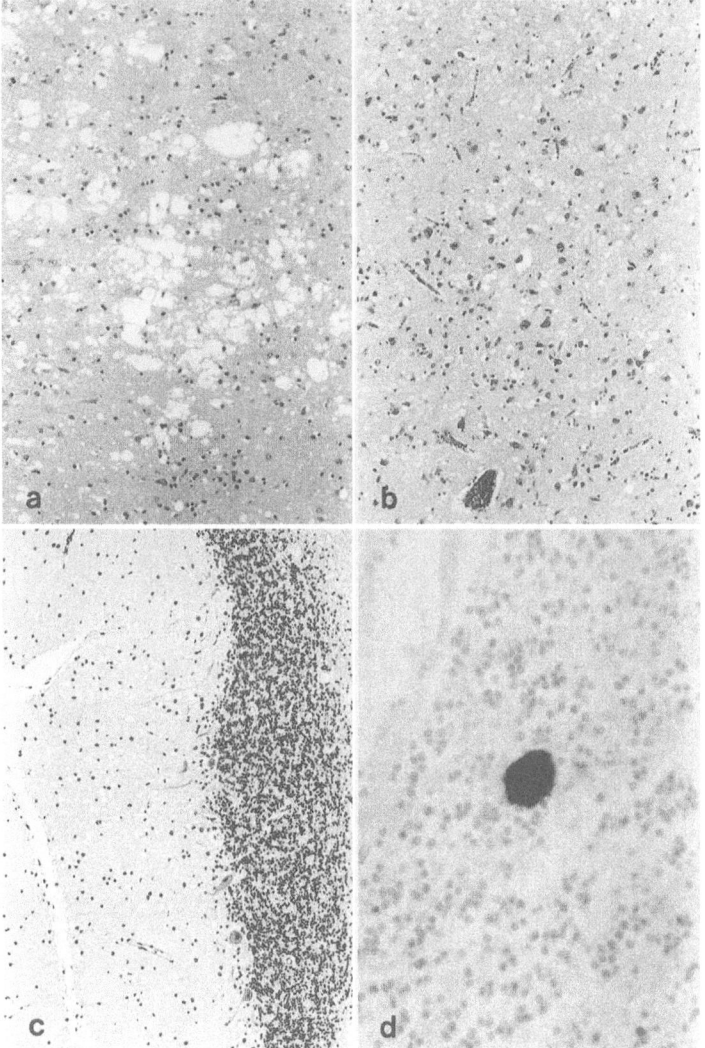

Fig. 1. **a** Confluent spongiform change in the cerebral cortex with multiple irregular clear vacuoles which have coalesced to form larger cystic spaces. Haematoxylin and eosin ×160. **b** Spongiform change in the basal ganglia shows a microvacuolar pattern with multiple small vacuoles scattered throughout the neuropil and around occasional nerve cells (centre). Haematoxylin and eosin ×240. **c** Spongiform change in the cerebellum is characteristically present in the molecular layer with multiple small vacuoles in the neuropil. Confluent spongiform change is uncommon at this site but there is evidence of astrocytosis. Haematoxylin and eosin ×120. **d** Immunocytochemistry for PrP in the cerebellar granular layer shows a single Kuru-type plaque with a dense central core and irregular outline in a case of sporadic CJD. Haematoxylin counterstain ×300

Ridley, 1992). A naturally occurring polymorphism for either methionine or valine exists at codon 129 in the PrP gene; in normal Caucasian individuals around 50% are heterozygous at this locus, around 40% are methionine homozygotes and the remainder are valine homozygotes (Baker and Ridley, 1992; Goldfarb et al., 1994). However, in sporadic CJD

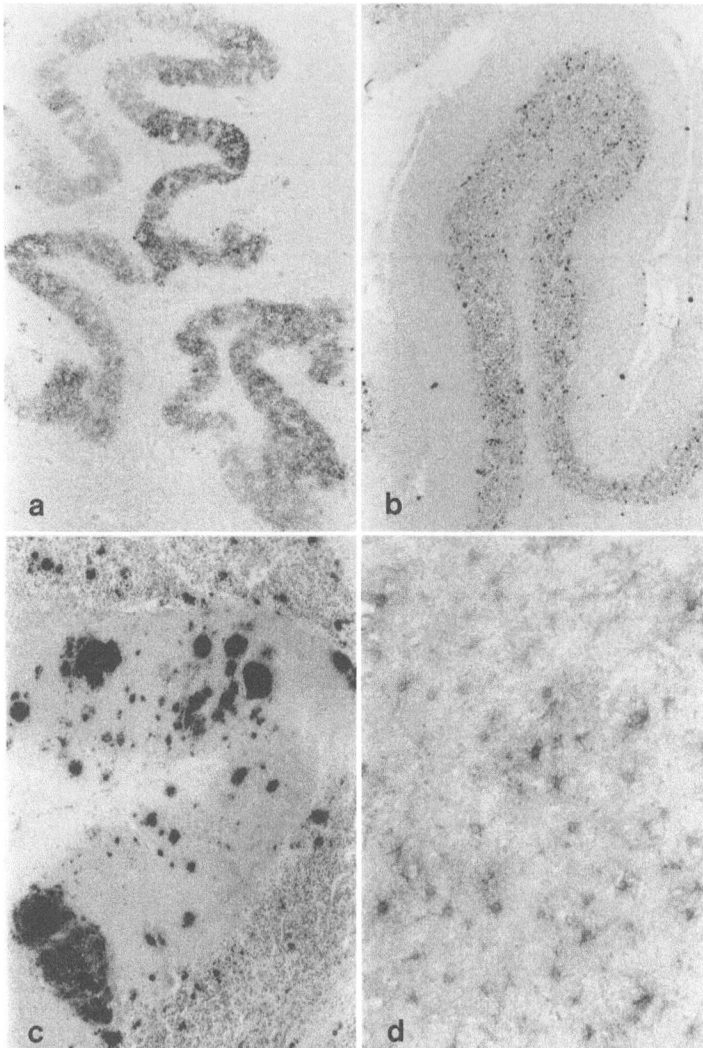

Fig. 2. **a** Immunocytochemistry for PrP in the inferior olivary nucleus in a case of sporadic CJD shows a ribbon-like synaptic pattern of positivity. Haematoxylin counterstain ×80. **b** Immunocytochemistry for PrP in the cerebellum in the case of growth hormone-associated iatrogenic CJD shows cerebellar atrophy with numerous dark plaque-like deposits within the molecular and granular layers. Haematoxylin counterstain ×40. **c** Immunocytochemistry for PrP in the cerebellum in the case of GSS shows numerous large multicentric plaques which give an intense dark staining reaction in the molecular and granular layers. Haematoxylin counterstain ×120. **d** Immunocytochemistry for glial fibrillary acidic protein in the dorsomedial nucleus of the thalamus in a case of FFI shows widespread astrocytosis with no evidence of spongiform change. Haematoxylin counter stain ×240

the incidence of homozygosity at both loci is increased to 90%; similar findings have been described in cases of accidental iatrogenic transmission of CJD by either central or peripheral inoculation. Codon 129 therefore appears to influence susceptibility to both sporadic and iatrogenic CJD

Table 2. Neuropathological changes in human prion diseases

— Classical changes	spongiform change
	neuronal loss
	astrocytosis
	PrP plaques
— Other changes	status spongiosus
	swollen neurones
	abnormal neuritic dendrites
	neuritic dystrophy around PrP plaques
	microgliosis
	Aβ amyloid angiopathy
	white matter necrosis and cavitation
	tubovesicular structures

(Collinge et al., 1991). Recent clinicopathological studies have identified a second effect of codon 129 genotype on pathology, with PrP plaques occurring at a higher frequency in individuals who are heterozygotes or homozygous for valine (de Silva et al., 1994). Apart from PrP genotype, there is current evidence to suggest that ApoE genotype may influence disease onset and pathology in sporadic CJD, although larger studies are required to confirm these preliminary findings (Amouyel et al., 1994; Pickering-Brown et al., 1995).

A new variant of sporadic CJD

An apparently new variant of CJD has been identified recently in ten patients in UK. This variant is characterised by an early age of onset or death (average 27.6 years), a prolonged duration of illness (average 13 months) with a predominantly psychiatric presentation followed by a progressive cerebellar syndrome, forgetfulness and memory disturbance, and myoclonus in the late stage of the illness. Four patients presented with dysaesthesiae in the hands and face. Dementia was not a common feature in the early stages of the illness and none of the patients showed the typical EEG appearances of sporadic CJD. Neuropathologically, the changes in the brain are relatively uniform and are characterised by numerous kuru-type amyloid plaques surrounded by vacuolation, which are present in a wide distribution throughout the cerebral cortex and in the cerebellum. Spongiform change is most evident in the basal ganglia and thalamus, but occurs in a patchy distribution throughout the cerebral cortex and in the cerebellar molecular layer. Immunocytochemistry for PrP shows extensive deposition of prion protein, particularly in the cerebellum where numerous small plaque-like structures and pericellular deposits are identified in addition to the larger kuru-type plaques.

Molecular genetic studies have identified no mutations in the PrP gene in these patients, all of whom were methionine homozygotes at codon 129. Review of previous cases of CJD in young patients in UK has not identified

Table 3. Relationship between pathology and PrP genotype

Pathology	PrP gene
CJD	No mutation in open reading frame 129 met/met met/val 178 Asp → Asn 129 Val 180 Val → Ile 200 Glu → Lys 210 Val → Ile 219 Glu → Lys 232 Met → Arg Octapeptide repeat region (codons 51–91): 48 bp insert 96 bp insert 120 bp insert 144 bp insert 168 bp insert 192 bp insert 216 bp insert
CJD with PrP plaques	129 Met/Val Val/Val
GSS	102 Pro → Leu 105 Pro → Leu 117 Ala → Val 145 Tyr → stop (TAG)
GSS with neurofibrillary tangles	198 Phe → Ser 217 Gln → Arg
FFI	178 Asp → Asn 129 Met
Atypical prion dementia	Octapeptide repeat region (codons 51–91): 144 bp insert

any similar cases in the past. Further studies are required both in UK and in other countries to establish both retrospective and prospective epidemiological data on similar cases. It has been suggested that this disorder may be related to exposure of the population in UK to the bovine spongiform encephalopathy agent, but this suggestion cannot be proven until appropriate strain-typing experiments have been completed.

Familial

Historical studies have suggested that CJD occurs as a familial disorder in around 10–15% of all patients with this disease (Richardson and Masters, 1995). Molecular genetic studies have tended to confirm this figure, and an ever-increasing range of abnormalities in the PrP gene have been described including mutations, deletions and insertions (Table 3), most of which are pathogenic and associated with familial prion disease (Baker and Ridley, 1992; Goldfarb et al., 1994). Interestingly, one of the cases originally described by Jakob has recently been shown to carry a 129val 178asn PrP genotype

Table 4. Comparison between sporadic and growth-hormone (GH) — associated iatrogenic CJD

	Sporadic CJD	GH iatrogenic CJD
Number of cases	20	12
Mean age at death	68 y	28 y
Duration of illness	8 m	11 m
Ataxia on presentation	33%	100%
Dementia on presentation	67%	0%
Typical EEG	65%	0%
Cortical spongiform change	+ + +	+
Cerebellar atrophy	+	+ + +
PrP plaques	15%	100%
Spinal cord PrP depostion	20%	100%

(Brown et al., 1994) which has been found in other cases of familial CJD (Nieto et al., 1991). The term "atypical prion dementia" has been used to describe cases of dementia occurring in a family with a 144 bp insertion in the PrP gene in whom the neuropathological features did not allow a diagnosis of spongiform encephalopathy to be made by standard criteria although PrP accumulation was demonstrable on immunocytochemistry in sections of the cerebellum (Collinge et al., 1990). Other affected family members with a similar genetic abnormality displayed classical clinical and neuropathological features of CJD.

Iatrogenic

Accidental transmission of CJD has occurred following a variety of medical and surgical procedures (Brown et al., 1992). The transmissible agent responsible for this disorder is remarkably resistant to standard methods of microbiological decontamination (Brown et al., 1990; Bell and Ironside, 1993b). In the UK it is now recommended that neurosurgical instruments used on patients either with or at risk of developing CJD or GSS are destroyed in order to eliminate the possibility of subsequent accidental transmission (Metters, 1990; Advisory Committee on Dangerous Pathogens, 1994). Iatrogenic cases of CJD with central inoculation of the transmissible agent, e.g. in dura mater grafts (Martinez-Lage et al., 1994), tend to show clinical and pathological features similar to those of sporadic CJD, with a short duration of illness. Conversely, the clinical course in patients with peripheral inoculation, e.g. in growth hormone or gonadotrophin recipients, is often prolonged (Brown et al., 1992) and the patients usually present with cerebellar dysfunction followed by myoclonus, extrapyramidal signs and ultimately dementia (see Table 4). The pathological features of CJD in pituitary hormone recipients are also distinct from that of sporadic CJD, with predominant cerebellar involvement, marked changes in the basal ganglia and relatively minor cortical abnormalities (Bell and Ironside, 1993a). PrP immunocytochemistry in these cases usually demonstrates a heavy accumulation of PrP in the cerebellum, with numerous plaque-like structures present throughout the cerebellar cortex (Fig. 2b). Recent studies on the spinal cord in patients with growth hormone-associated CJD has demonstrated an accumulation of PrP in the substantia gelatinosa and ascending fibres, suggesting that the transmissible agent may spread from the periphery to the brain via ascending spinal pathways (Goodbrand et al., 1995).

Gerstmann-Sträussler-Scheinker syndrome

This extremely uncommon autosomal dominant disorder is characterised by progressive cerebellar ataxia and dementia with an onset in middle age (Gerstmann et al., 1936). A range of other neurological abnormalities have been described in this disorder, and in contrast to sporadic CJD the symptoms tend to progress slowly over a period of years (Bastian, 1991). Myoclonus is uncommon, but pyramidal signs are present in most patients. This disease is characterised pathologically by the accumulation of large multicentric PrP plaques throughout the brain, being most numerous in the cerebellum (Fig. 2c). These large plaques are frequently associated with abnormal neuritic processes and astrocytosis (Bell and Ironside, 1993a). Spongiform change occurs to a variable degree in GSS, and neuronal loss is most conspicuous in the cerebellum, but in cases with a long clinical duration a more widespread neuronal loss occurs throughout the brain. This disorder is characterised by a codon 102leu mutation in the PrP gene (Hsiao et al., 1989); this abnormality has also been discovered in several other similarly affected families. A recent study on the original family reported by Gerstmann, et al. (1936) has revealed that phenotypic expression in terms of clinical features and neuropathology is variable even within the context of a constant genetic mutation (PrP 102leu) and heterozygosity at codon 129 in the PrP gene (Hainfellner et al., 1995). Recent studies have demonstrated other mutations in the PrP gene which can produce a GSS-like clinical picture (see Table 3). In some cases the pathology is similar to that of classical GSS, although neurofibrillary tangles (similar to those seen in Alzheimer's disease) have been found in cases with codon 145, 198 and 217 mutations. Aβ protein deposition has been reported at the periphery of PrP plaques in these cases (Bugiani et al., 1993).

Fatal familial insomnia

This rare condition was first described in 1986 and is characterised by disturbances of sleep and autonomic function, motor and endocrine systems, while intellectual and cognitive functions remain relatively well preserved (Lugaresi et al., 1986). Subsequent molecular genetic studies have demonstrated that this disorder is characterised by a unique PrP genotype 178 and 129 met (Medori et al., 1992). The neuropathology of FFI is characterised by severe neuronal loss and astrocytosis in the dorsomedial and ventral thalamic nuclei (Fig. 2d), with lesser involvement of other thalamic nuclei (Gambetti et al.,

1993). Similar changes are present in the inferior olivary and pontine nuclei, but the cerebral cortex is relatively spared. Spongiform change is not a constant finding, but may be present in the entorhinal cortex. PrP accumulation is demonstrable in the thalamus and the disease is transmissible to transgenic mice (Collinge et al., 1995). The relationship between the thalamic pathology, PrP accumulation and clinical features of this complex disorder await further study.

Kuru

This disorder was confined to the Fore tribe and adjacent tribes in the eastern highlands of New Guinea, affecting females more often than males with a wide age range from 4 years upwards (Gajdusek and Vigas, 1957). Kuru was characterised by cerebellar ataxia and tremor, dysarthria and dysphagia, with intellectual preservation until the final stages of the disease. In children the clinical duration ranged from 3–9 months but in adults the disease followed a longer course of up to 2–3 years. This unique disorder appears to have resulted from transmission of a human prion agent by practices associated with ritualistic cannibalism in which females and children where involved, explaining the epidemiology of the disease (Bastian, 1991). These practices ceased at least 20 years ago, indicating that the incubation period for this disorder can be prolonged, as occasional cases are still being reported.

Kuru was characterised pathologically by cerebellar atrophy, with extensive neuronal loss and the presence of characteristic amyloid plaques comprising a central eosinophilic core and a peripheral halo of radiating filaments (Klatzo et al., 1959). Neuronal loss was evident in a more widesread distribution in the cerebrum, and the kuru-type amyloid plaques were not confined to the cerebellum. Spongiform change was not a prominent feature in the first descriptions of kuru (Klatzo et al., 1959), but was recorded in subsequent reports (Neumann et al., 1965).

Relationship of human prion diseases to other neurodegenerative disorders

None of the classical neuropathological features of human prion diseases are exclusive to this group of disorders. Spongiform change can occur in a restricted distribution in cases of Alzheimer's disease (AD) or Lewy Body disease (Hansen et al., 1989), and neuronal loss with accompanying astrocytosis is a common feature of many neurodegenerative disorders. Amyloid plaque formation occurs in AD, although the precursor protein is encoded by the APP gene on chromosome 21. Recent studies of plaque structure and reactions in CJD and AD have revealed a number of similarities (DeArmond, 1993), including a postulated role for microglia in the processing of the respective precursor proteins into their amyloid forms, the presence of dystrophic neuritic processes in large plaques and the deposition of other

Table 5. Comparison of human prion diseases and Alzheimer's disease

1 Both cases occur primarily as sporadic disorders with a marked difference in incidence
2 Familial forms occur in both disorders as autosomal dominant conditions with specific genetic mutations in 10–15% of cases
3 Neuronal loss and reactive gliosis occur in both disorders; spongiform change is characteristic of prion diseases but can occur focally in Alzheimer's disease
4 Amyloid plaques (Aβ or PrP) are formed in the CNS with associated neuritic and glial components
5 The precursor of the amyloidogenic protein in both disorders is a cell membrane glycoprotein which is expressed in neurones
6 Neurofibrillary tangles are a diagnositc feature in Alzheimer's disease but are rare in most forms of human prion disease
7 Aβ and PrP are deposited in skeletal muscle in inclusion body myositis
8 Aβ protein deposition can be induced in primates by the intracerebral inoculation of Alzheimer brain homogenates: CJD, GSS, FFI and Kuru can be transmitted to primates
9 ApoE gentotype may influence disease onset

proteins including apolipoprotein E. The Aβ protein of AD can be deposited at the periphery of PrP plaques in human prion diseases, although this is a relatively uncommon feature (Bugiani et al., 1993). Other similarities between AD and prion diseases are summarised in Table 5. Prion protein accumulation within the central nervous system appears to be specific for the human prion diseases, although the recent interesting observation that the protease resistant PrP isoform can be detected by immunocytochemistry and molecular biological techniques in cases of progressive subcortical gliosis (which is linked to chromosome 17) raises the possibility of a secondary role for PrP in this disorder (Petersen et al., 1995).

Relationship between bovine spongiform encephalopathy and human prion diseases

Bovine Spongiform Encephalopathy (BSE) is a new disease of cattle which emerged in UK in 1985 and was confirmed neuropathologically the following year (Wells et al., 1987). Since then an epidemic of this disease has occurred in UK, mostly in dairy cattle. Epidemiological studies have shown that cattle suddenly became exposed to a scrapie-like agent in ruminant-derived food in the form of meat and bone meal in 1981–1982 (Bradley and Wilesmith, 1993). The feeding of ruminant-derived protein to ruminant animals has now been banned and bovine offal is no longer fed to animals or birds. Human health has been protected by compulsory slaughter and destruction of suspect animals and a ban on the use of their milk and by prohibiting the use in human food of bovine tissues which in clinically healthy cattle incubating BSE might conceivably harbour infectivity. The epidemic of BSE reached a peak in 1992–1993 of around 3,500 cases per month and is now declining. Newly reported spongiform encephalopathies have occurred in other species in UK, including exotic ungulates (nyala, gemsbok, Arabian oryx, greater kudu and eland), domestic cats, puma and cheetah (Bradley and Wilesmith, 1993). These animals appear to have acquired the infection through the consumption of infected foodstuff, either in the form of meat and bone meal or in the case of felines uncooked tissues including at least the spinal cord from adult animals affected by BSE.

Following the occurrence of BSE the Southwood Committee recommended the reinstitution of epidemiological surveillance in UK of CJD in 1990 as a prospective case-control study. This is carried out by the clinical team led by Dr R G Will in the National CJD Surveillance Unit, Edinburgh, with neuropathological validation in the dedicated laboratory within the unit (Drs. J. W. Ironside and J. E. Bell). Similar studies are being performed in other EU countries, including France, Germany, Italy and the Netherlands. The incidence of CJD in UK has not increased significantly over the surveillance period to date, nor does there appear to be any specific dietary or occupational factors which are associated with an increased risk of developing human prion disease in UK (Will, 1993). Cases of CJD have occurred in three dairy farmers in UK with cases of BSE within their herds (Smith et al., 1995), but statistical studies indicate that this does not represent a selective occurrence (Delasnerie-Laupretre et al., 1995). CJD has not been identified in other occupations which might be exposed to BSE including veterinary workers, butchers and abattoir workers. However, because of the possible implications for human health and the lengthy incubation periods of transmissible prion diseases in man, it is likely that the surveillance project will continue for some time to monitor the incidence of clinical and neuropathological features of CJD and related disorders in UK, particularly the new variant of CJD reported in young patients in UK.

Conclusion

The human prion diseases represent a unique group of fatal neurodegenerative disorders which are characterised by the accumulation of prion protein in the brain. Although the precise nature of the infective agent responsible for this group of disorders is unknown, our knowledge of the biochemistry and molecular genetics of PrP indicate that the protein plays a major role in disease pathogenesis. Investigative techniques to detect the disease-associated protein and accompanying PrP genetic abnormalities have resulted in the recognition of a wider spectrum of human prion diseases than hitherto suspected, with new genetic variants continually being described. However, these diseases as a group remain uncommon and despite earlier predictions that prion diseases might account for as much as 10–15% of all cases of human dementia (Anonymous, 1990), this has not been borne out by recent investigations. The mechanisms of brain damage in prion diseases and the relationships between clinical features, neuropathology, PrP accumulation and host genotype remain to be elucidated. Although a distinctive group of disorders, the human prion diseases share some pathological characteristics with other human neurodegenerative disorders, including Alzheimer's disease. Further research into human prion diseases is likely to yield information applicable to other neurodegenerative disorders.

References

Advisory Committee on Dangerous Pathogens (1994) Precautions for work with human and animal tranmissible spongiform encephalopathies, 1st edn. HMSO, London

Amouyel P, Vidal O, Launay JM, Laplanche JL (1994) The apolipoprotein E alleles as major susceptibility factors for Creutzfeldt-Jakob disease. Lancet 344: 1315–1318

Anonymous (1990) Prion disease — spongiform encephalopathies unveiled. Lancet 336: 21–22

Askanas V, King EW, Alverez RB (1992) Light and electron microscopic localisation of β-amyloid protein in muscle biopsies of patients with inclusion-body myositis. Am J Pathol 141: 31–36

Askanas V, Bilak M, Engel WK, Alvarez RB, Tome F, Leclerc A (1993) Prion protein is abnormally accumulated in inclusion-body myositis. Neuro Report 5: 25–28

Baker HF, Ridley RM (1992) The genetics and transmissibility of human spongiform encephalopathy. Neurodegen 1: 3–16

Bastian FO (ed) (1991) Creutzfeldt-Jakob disease and other transmissible human spongiform encephalopathies. Mosby Year Book, St Louis

Bell JE, Ironside JW (1993a) Neuropathology of spongiform encephalopathies in humans. Br Med Bull 49: 738–777

Bell JE, Ironside JW (1993b) How to tackle a possible Creutzfeldt-Jakob disease necropsy. J Clin Pathol 46: 193–197

Bradley R, Wilesmith JW (1993) Epidemiology and control of bovine spongiform encephalopathy (BSE). Br Med Bull 49: 932–959

Brown P, Wolff A, Gajdusek DC (1990) A simple and effective method for inactivating virus infectivity in formalin-fixed tissue samples from patients with Creutzfeldt-Jakob disease. Neurology 40: 887–90

Brown P, Preece MA, Will RG (1992) "Friendly fire" in medicine: hormones homografts and Creutzfeldt-Jakob disease. Lancet 340: 24–27

Brown P, Crevenakova L, Boellaard JW, Stavrou D, Goldfarb LG, Gajdusek DC (1994) Identification of a PRNP gene mutation in Jakob's original Creutzfeldt-Jakob disease family. Lancet 344: 130–131

Budka H, Aguzzi A, Brown P, Brucher J-M, Bugiani O, Gullotta F, Haltia M, Hauw J-J, Ironside JW, Jellinger K, Kretzschmar HA, Lantos PL, Masullo C, Scholte W, Tateishi J, Weller RO (1995) Neuropathological diagnostic criteria for Creutzfeldt-Jakob disease (CJD) and other human spongiform encephalopathies (prion diseases). Brain Pathol 5: 459–465

Bugiani O, Giaccone G, Verga L, Pollo B, Frangione B, Farlow MR, Tagliavini F, Ghetti B (1993) βPP participates in PrP-amyloid plaques of Gerstmann-Sträussler-Scheinker disease, Indiana kindred. J Neuropathol Exp Neurol 52: 66–70

Collinge J, Owen F, Poulter M, Leach M, Crow TJ, Rossor MN, Mullan MJ, Janota I, Lantos PL (1990) Prion dementia without characteristic pathology. Lancet 336: 7–9

Collinge J, Palmer MS, Dryden AJ (1991) Genetic predisposition to iatrogenic Creutzfeldt-Jakob disease. Lancet 337: 1441–42

Collinge J, Palmer MS, Sidle KCL, Gowland I, Medori R, Ironside JW, Lantos P (1995) Tranmission of fatal familial insomnia to laboratory animals. Lancet 346: 569–570

Creutzfeldt HG (1920) Über eine eigenartige herdförmige Erkrankung des Zentralnervensystems. Z Ges Neurol Psychiat 57: 1–18

De Silva R, Ironside JW, McCardle L, Esmonde T, Bell JE, Will RG, Windle O, Dempster M, Estibeiro P, Lathe R (1994) Neuropathological phenotype and "prion protein" genotype correlation in sporadic Creutzfeldt-Jakob disease. Neurosci Lett 179: 50–52

DeArmond SJ (1993) Alzheimer's disease and Creutzfeldt-Jakob disease: overlap of pathogenic mechanisms. Curr Opin Neurol 6: 872–881

Delasnerie-Laupretre N, Poser S, Pocchiari M, Wientjens DPW, Will R (1995) Creutzfeldt-Jakob disease in Europe. Lancet 346: 898

Frasier SD, Foley Jr TP (1994) Creutzfeldt-Jakob disease in recipients of pituitary hormones. J Clin Endocrinol Metabol 78: 1277–1279

Gajdusek DC, Zigas V (1957) Degenerative disease of the central nervous system in New Guinea. The endemic occurrence of "kuru" in the native population. N Engl J Med 257: 974–978

Gajdusek DC, Gibbs CJ, Alpers MP (1966) Experimental transmission of a kuru-like syndrome in chimpanzees. Nature 209: 794–796

Gambetti P, Peterson R, Monari L, Tabaton M, Autillo-Gambetti L, Cortelli P, Montagna P, Lugaresi E (1993) Fatal familial insomnia and the widening spectrum of prion diseases. Br Med Bull 49: 980–994

Gerstmann J, Sträussler E, Scheinker I (1936) Über eine eigenartige hereditär-familiäre Erkrankung des Zentralnervensystems, zugleich ein Beitrag zur Frage des vorzeitigen lokalen Alterns. Z Neurol Psych 154: 736–762

Gibbs CJ, Gajdusek DC, Asher DM, Alpers MP, Beck E, Daniel PM, Matthews WB (1968) Creutzfeldt-Jakob disease (subacute spongiform encephalopathy): transmission to the chimpanzee. Science 161: 388–389

Goldfarb LG, Brown P, Cervenakova L, Gajdusek CJ (1994) Molecular genetic studies of Creutzfeldt-Jakob disease. Mol Neurobiol 8: 89–97

Goodbrand IA, Ironside JW, Nicolson D, Bell JE (1995) Prion protein accumulation in the spinal cords of patients with sporadic and growth hormone associated Cruetzfeldt-Jakob disease. Neurosci Lett 183: 127–130

Hainfellner JA, Brantner-Inthaler S, Cercenakova L, Brown P, Kitamoto T, Tateishi J, Diringer H, Liberski PP, Regele H, Feucht M, Mayr N, Wessely P, Summer K, Seitelberger F, Budka H (1995) The original Gerstmann-Sträussler-Scheinker family of Austria: divergent clinicopathological phenotypes but constant PrP genotype. Brain Pathol 5: 201–213

Hansen LA, Masliah E, Terry RD, Mirra SS (1989) A neuropathological subset of Alzheimer's disease with concomitant Lewy body disease and spongiform change. Acta Neuropathol 78: 194–201

Hayward PAR, Bell JE, Ironside JW (1994) Prion protein immunocytochemistry: the development of reliable protocols for the investigation of Creutzfeldt-Jakob disease. Neuropathol Appl Neurobiol 20: 375–383

Hsiao KK, Doh-ura K, Kitamoto T, Tateishi J, Prusiner SB (1989) A prion protein amino acid substitution in ataxic Gerstmann-Sträussler syndrome. Ann Neurol 26: 137

Jakob A (1921) Über eigenartige Erkrankungen des Zentralnervensystems mit bemerkenswertem anatomischen Befunden (Spastische Pseudosklerose-Encephalomyelopathie mit disseminierten Degenerationsherden). Z Ges Neurol Psychiat 64: 147–228

Jendroska K, Hoffmann O, Schelosky L, Lees AJ, Poewe W, Daniel SE (1994) Absence of disease related prion protein in neurodegenerative disorders presenting with Parkinson's syndrome. J Neurol Neurosurg Psychiatry 57: 1249–1251

Kitamoto T, Shin RW, Doh-ura K, Tomokane N, Miyazono M, Muramoto T, Tateishi J (1992) Abnormal isoform of prion protein accumulates in the synaptic structures of the central nervous system in patients with Creutzfeldt-Jakob Disease. Am J Pathol 140: 1285–129

Klatzo I, Gajdusek DC, Vigas V (1959) Pathology of kuru. Lab Invest 8: 799–847

Lugaresi E, Medori R, Montagna P, Baruzzi A, Cortelli P, Lugaresi A, Tinuper P,

Zucconi M, Gambett P (1986) Fatal familial insomnia and dysautonomia with selective degeneration of thalamic nuclei. N Engl J Med 315: 997–1003

Martinez-Lage JF, Poza M, Sola J, Tortosa JG, Brown P, Crevenakova L, Esteban JA, Mendoza A (1994) Accidental transmission of Creutzfeldt-Jakob disease by dural cadaveric grafts. J Neurol Neurosurg Psychiatry 57: 1091–1904

Masters CL, Richardson EP (1978) Subacute spongiform encephalopathy (Creutzfeldt-Jakob disease). The nature and progression of spongiform change. Brain 101: 333–334

Masters CL, Gajdusek DC, Gibbs CJ (1981) Creutzfeldt-Jakob disease: virus isolates from the Gerstmann-Sträussler syndrome. Brain 104: 559–588

Medori R, Tritschler JH, LeBlanc A, Villare F, Manetto V, Ghen HY, Xuf R, Leal S, Montagna P, Cortelli P, Tinuper P, Avoni P, Mochi M, Baruzzi A, Hauw JJ, Ott J, Lugarest E, Autilio-Gambettia L, Gambetti P (1992) Fatal familial insomnia, a prion disease with a mutation at codon 178 of the prion protein gene. N Engl J Med 7: 444–449

Metters JS (1990) Neuro and ophthalmic surgery procedures in patients with or suspected to have or at risk of developing CJD or GSS. Letter PL(92)CO/4 to Consultants and Health Managers, Department of Health, London

Neumann MA, Gajdusek DC, Vigas V (1965) Neuropathologic findings in exotic neurologic disorders among natives of the highlands of New Guinea. J Neuropathol Exp Neurol 18: 486–507

Nieto A, Goldfarb LG, Brown P, McCombie WR, Trapp S, Asher DM, Gajdusek DC (1991) Codon 178 mutation in ethnically diverse Creutzfeldt-Jakob disease families. Lancet 337: 622–623

Petersen RB, Tabaton M, Chen SG, Monari L, Richardson SL, Lynches T, Manetto V, Lanska DJ, Markesbery WR, Currier RD, Autilio-Gambetti L, Wilhelmsen KC, Gambetti P (1995) Familial progessive subcortical gliosis: presence of prions and linkage to chromosome 17. Neurology 45: 1062–1067

Pickering-Brown SM, Mann DMA, Owen F, Ironside JW, de Silva R, Roberts DA, Balderson DJ, Cooper PN (1995) Allelic variations in apolipoprotein E and prion protein genotype related to plaque formation and age of onset in sporadic Creutzfeldt-Jakob disease. Neurosci Lett 187: 127–129

Prusiner S B (1994) Biology and genetics of prion disease. Ann Rev Microbiol 48: 655–686

Richardson EP Jn, Masters CL (1995) The nosology of Creutzfeldt-Jakob disease and conditions related to the accumulation of PrP^{CJD} in the nervous system. Brain Pathol 5: 33–41

Smith PEM, Zeidler M, Ironside JW, Estibeiro P, Moss TH (1995) Creutzfeldt-Jakob disease in a dairy farmer. Lancet 346: 898

Wells GAH, Scott AC, Johnson CT, Gunning RF, Hancock RD, Jeffrey M, Dawson M, Bradley R (1987) A novel progressive spongiform encephalopathy in cattle. Vet Rec 121: 419–420

Westaway D, DeArmond SJ, Cayetano-Canlas J, Groth D, Foster D, Yang S, Torchia M, Carlson GA, Prusiner SB (1994) Degeneration of skeletal muscle, peripheral nerves and the central nervous system in transgenic mice overexpressing wild-type prion proteins. Cell 76: 117–129

Will RG (1991) The spongiform encephalopathies. J Neurol Neurosurg Psychiatry 54: 761–763

Will RG (1993) Epidemiology of Creutzfeldt-Jakob disease. Br Med Bull 49: 960–970

Will RG, Ironside JW, Zeidler M, Estibeiro K, Alperovitch A, Poser S, Pocchiari M, Hofman A, Smith PG (1996) A new variant of Creutzfeldt-Jakob disease in the UK. Lancet 347: 921–925

Author's address: Dr. J. W. Ironside, Neuropathology Laboratory, Department of Pathology, The University of Edinburgh, Western General Hospital, Crewe Road, Edinburgh, EH4 2XU, United Kingdom.

J Neural Transm (1996) [Suppl] 47: 247–258

The survival response of mesencephalic dopaminergic neurons to the neurotrophins BDNF and NT-4 requires priming with serum: comparison with members of the TGF-β superfamily and characterization of the serum-free culture system

K. Krieglstein[1], D. Maysinger[2], and K. Unsicker[1]

[1]Departments of Anatomy and Cell Biology, University of Heidelberg,
Heidelberg, Federal Republic of Germany
[2]Pharmacology, McGill University, Montreal, Quebec, Canada

Summary. The neurotrophins, brain-derived neurotrophic factor (BDNF) and neurotrophin-4 (NT-4), are established survival promoting molecules for dopaminergic (DAergic) neurons cultured from the fetal rat midbrain floor. We have cultured and compared the survival of embryonic day (E) 14 mesencephalic cells in fully defined, serum-free medium, with serum-primed cultures (one hour during dissociation). Cultures were characterized using antibodies against neuron-specific enolase (NSE), tyrosine hydroxylase (TH), vimentin, glial fibrillary acidic protein (GFAP), and the antigen A2B5. The absolute absence of serum did not reduce the survival of TH-positive DAergic neurons nor alter the percentages of cells staining for the above markers. Transforming growth factor-β3 (TGF-β3) and glial cell line-derived neurotrophic factor (GDNF), two members of the TGF-β superfamily, both promoted the survival of TH-positive cells (TGF-β3: 2-fold; GDNF: 1.6-fold) over the 8-day culture period. Survival mediated by TGF-β3 and GDNF was independent of whether or not the cells had been initially exposed to serum. In contrast, the survival promoting effects of BDNF and NT-4 were crucially dependent on serum priming. RT-PCR for the full-length trkB high affinity neurotrophin receptor revealed its presence in both culture systems. We conclude that priming with serum is important to make DAergic neurons fully responsive to BDNF and NT-4. Underlying mechanisms might be sought at the level or distal of trkB receptor expression, without excluding the possiblity that serum elicits production of growth factors that synergistically act with neurotrophins in these cultures.

Introduction

Dopaminergic (DAergic) neurons located in the substantia nigra of the mesencephalon and projecting to the striatum are important for the control and performance of movements. Their degeneration in Parkinson's disease (PD) is the cause for most of the prevailing symptoms in this frequent neurodegenerative disorder. Among a variety of putative mechanisms currently being discussed for the etiology of PD (see Edwards, 1993; Gerlach et al., 1994; Götz et al., 1994, for review), oxidative stress, mitochondrial dysfunction, and insufficient coping of cells with free radicals occupy central positions (Reichmann and Riederer, 1994; Cohen and Werner, 1994; Schapira, 1995). The capacity of neurons to counteract the adverse effects of free radicals depends, in part, on the availability and effectiveness of trophic factors. Nerve growth factor (NGF), the longest known member of the neurotrophin family of trophic factors (Levi-Montalcini, 1987), has been the first neurotrophic molecule with a marked protective role for neurons impaired by free radicals (Jackson et al., 1990; Zhang et al., 1993). More recently, similar roles have been demonstrated for several other growth factors including fibroblast growth factor-2 (FGF-2), transforming growth factor-β (TGF-β), insulin-like growth factors, and the neurotrophins brain-derived neurotrophic factor (BDNF) and neurotrophin-3 (NT-3) (Mattson and Scheff, 1994).

In cell culture and following various types of in vivo lesions, midbrain DAergic neurons respond to a variety of growth factors with improved survival (see Unsicker, 1994; Beck, 1994, for review). The neurotrophins BDNF, NT-3, and NT-4/5 (Hyman et al., 1991, 1994; Beck et al., 1993; Hynes et al., 1994), as well as the TGF-βs 1, 2, 3 (Krieglstein and Unsicker, 1994; Poulsen et al., 1994; Krieglstein et al., 1995), and glial cell line-derived neurotrophic factor (GDNF; Lin et al., 1993; Beck et al., 1995; Tomac et al., 1995; Hoffer et al., 1994) have been shown to prevent the death and loss of differentiation of axotomized and toxically impaired DAergic neurons raising hopes that these molecules could be developed into effective drugs to supplement the classic therapeutic paradigm in PD which is based on the substitution of the nigrostriatal transmitter DA. An important prerequisite towards this goal is the understanding of the cellular and molecular bases of actions of these factors, both in the culture system with its multitude of different cell types in various states of differentiation, and in the complex in vivo situation.

With regard to BDNF, NT-3, and NT-4/5, there is apparent consent that these factors directly affect DAergic neurons (Lindsay et al., 1993; Hyman et al., 1994; Hynes et al., 1994), without requiring non-neuronal cells mediating the effects, nor any other synergistically acting growth factors. Presence of high affinity receptors for each of the neurotrophins on DAergic neurons in the adult rat S. nigra (Lindsay et al., 1993; Hyman et al., 1994) and retrograde transport from the striatum to the substantia nigra (Mufson et al., 1994) apparently support this notion. In the present study, we show that the survival promoting effect of BDNF and NT-4/5 on DAergic cultured from the E14 rat midbrain floor requires an initial priming event with serum, whereas TGF-β and GDNF exert their effects in the absolute absence of serum.

Materials and methods

Mesencephalic cell culture

The ventral midbrain floor of four litters, at a time, was dissected from E14 rat (Wistar) fetuses according to Shimoda et al. (1992). Tissue pieces were collected in ice-cold calcium-magnesium free Hanks' balanced salt solution. Tissues were enzymatically dissociated in 0.25% trypsin (ICN) for 15 min at 37°C. An equal volume of either ice cold 1% BSA (Sigma) and 1 mg/ml DNase (Boehringer Mannheim) (referred to as serum-free) or FCS and 1 mg/ml DNase (referred to as serum-primed) were added prior to trituration by five strokes with wide- and narrow-bored siliconized fire-polished Pasteur pipettes. Undissociated tissue pieces were allowed to settle for 5 min, the supernatant was collected, and the dissociation procedure repeated once. Single cell suspension was then washed with Dulbecco's modified Eagle's medium (DMEM)-F12 medium (1:1; Bio-Whittaker) containing N1 supplements, 0.25% BSA, 2 mM L-glutamine (Sigma), 100 units/ml penicillin, 50 μg/ml streptomycin, 100 μg/ml neomycin (Gibco), 33 mM glucose (Sigma), and seeded at 100 μl on polyornithine-laminin-coated glass coverslips at a density of 200.000 cells /cm^2 (as described by Krieglstein et al., 1995). Cells were allowed to attach for approx. 2 hours, then coverslips were transferred to 24-well plates containing 750 μl of the above mentioned culture medium. On the next day, and subsequently every 3 days, 500 μl of the medium was replaced and growth factors were added at the final (saturating) concentrations of 2 ng/ml for TGF-β3 (kindly provided by Drs Sporn and Flanders, NIH, Bethesda), 10 ng/ml for GDNF, 50 ng/ml for BDNF, and 10 ng/ml for NT-3 (IC Chemikalien). Cultures were processed for RNA isolation or for immunocytochemisty at time points indicated.

Immunocytochemistry

For visualization of neurons (using neuron specific enolase, NSE, as a marker), DAergic neurons (using tyrosine hydroxylase, TH, as a marker), or glial progenitor cells (using A2B5 as a marker), cells were fixed with 4% parafornealdehyde for 10 min, permeabilized with acetone at −20°C (10 min) and washed in phosphate buffed saline (PBS). For characterization of astrocytes (using GFAP as a marker) or glio- or neuroblasts (using vimentin as a marker), cells were fixed and permeabilized with acetone at −20°C (20 min) and washed with PBS. After blocking with 1% H$_2$O$_2$ in PBS, washing and blocking with horse serum, coverslips were stained with a mouse monoclonal antibody to rat TH (1:200; Boehringer Mannheim), to A2B5 (1:100; Boehringer Mannheim), to vimentin (1:25, clone Vim 3B4; Boehringer Mannheim), to GFAP (1:200; Sigma) or with a rabbit polyclonal antibody to NSE (1:1000; Polyscience), for 1 h at 37°C, following by anti-mouse or anti rabbit, respectively, Vectastain ABC kit (Vecto Labs) detection.

Evaluation of cell numbers and statistics

Survival of DAergic neurons was evaluated by counting all TH-positive neurons over one diameter of the coverslip (corresponding to 12% of the total area) using 100-fold magnification. Quantification was done in triplicate and in at least two independent experiments. Total cell numbers and the numbers of GFAP-, NSE-, vimentin-, A2B5-positive cells were assessed likewise. The data were analysed by a one-way ANOVA, and the significance of intergroup differences were determined by applying Student's t-test. Differences were considered significant at **$P < 0.01$, ***$P < 0.001$.

RT-PCR of trkB

Total RNA was isolated by using TRIZOL TM Reagent (Gibci BRL) according to the manufacturers instructions. The quality of RNA was checked by agarose electrophoresis and spectrophotometrically by determining the ratio of absorbance A260/A280nm. Total RNA was then reverse transcribed into cDNA. The reaction was carried out in a total volume of 20μl (thin tubes; Perkin Elmer): first 11μl consisting of 1μg total RNA, 25mM oligo(dT) 12–18 primer (Gibco) and sterile RNAse-free water was incubated for 10min at 70°C, subsequently 10mM dithiothreitol (Gibco), 5mM dNTPs (Gibco), 20 units of RNase inhibitor (Boehringer) and 200 units Superscipt II RNase H- reverse transcriptase and the supplied buffer (Gibco) was added. Tubes were gently mixed and incubated at 37°C for 1 hour. Reaction mixtures were stored at −20°C. As a control for genomic contamination, duplicate samples were treated identical, however substituting buffer for reverse transcriptase. PCR was carried out in a total volume of 25μl containing cDNA (made from 250ng total RNA), 20mM Tris-HCl (pH 8.4), 50mM KCl, 5mM $MgCl_2$, 0.2mM dNTPs, 1μM 5′ and 3′ primers and 1.25 units Taq DNA polymerase (Gibco BRL), employing the hot start method, in order to initially separate primer from cDNA and Taq DNA polymerase, using Ampliwax according to manufacturers instructions (Perkin Elmer). The amplification steps involved 30 cycles of denaturation at 94°C for 1min, annealing at 55°C for 2min and extention at 72°C for 3min using a thermocycler (Model 9600, Perkin Elmer). The trkB primers used corresponded to bp 2384–2405 and 3047–3072 and are therefore specific for the kinase containing form of rat trkB (Middlemas et al., 1991). 5μl aliquots of PCR samples were analyzed by electrophoresis in 1.2% agarose gels and bands were identified by ethidium bromide (0.5μg/ml). PCR products were of the expected size of 689bp.

Results

Cultured DAergic neurons survive in the absolute absence of serum

We first explored whether DAergic neurons isolated from the E14 rat mesencephalon floor could survive in dissociated cell cultures in the absolute absence of serum and without having been exposed to serum during the dissociation procedure. NSE and GFAP were employed as markers for neurons and astroglial cells, respectively. DAergic neurons were recognized by their TH immunoreactivity. TH serves as a reliable marker for DAergic neurons in these preparations, since other catecholaminergic neurons can be excluded from the cultures by restricting the dissection to a one cubic-millimeter piece of the mesencephalon floor (Shimoda et al., 1992). As shown in Fig. 1, cultures processed for NSE, TH, and GFAP at DIV2 and DIV8 contained NSE-positive cells as the dominating cell population, virtually no GFAP-immunoreactive cells, and substantial numbers of TH+ DAergic neurons. Counts of TH+ cells in serum-free cultures on DIV 1, 3, 6, and 8 revealed stability of cell numbers until DIV3 and a subsequent decline resulting, at DIV8, in the maintenance of approximately 25% of the TH+ cells present at DIV1 and DIV3 (Fig. 2). As shown in Figs. 3A and 3B, numbers of DAergic neurons surviving at DIV8 in serum-free and serum-primed cultures were not significantly different. As studied in more detail below, Fig. 2 shows that TGF-β3 (2ng/ml) augmented survival of DAergic

DIV 2   **DIV 8**

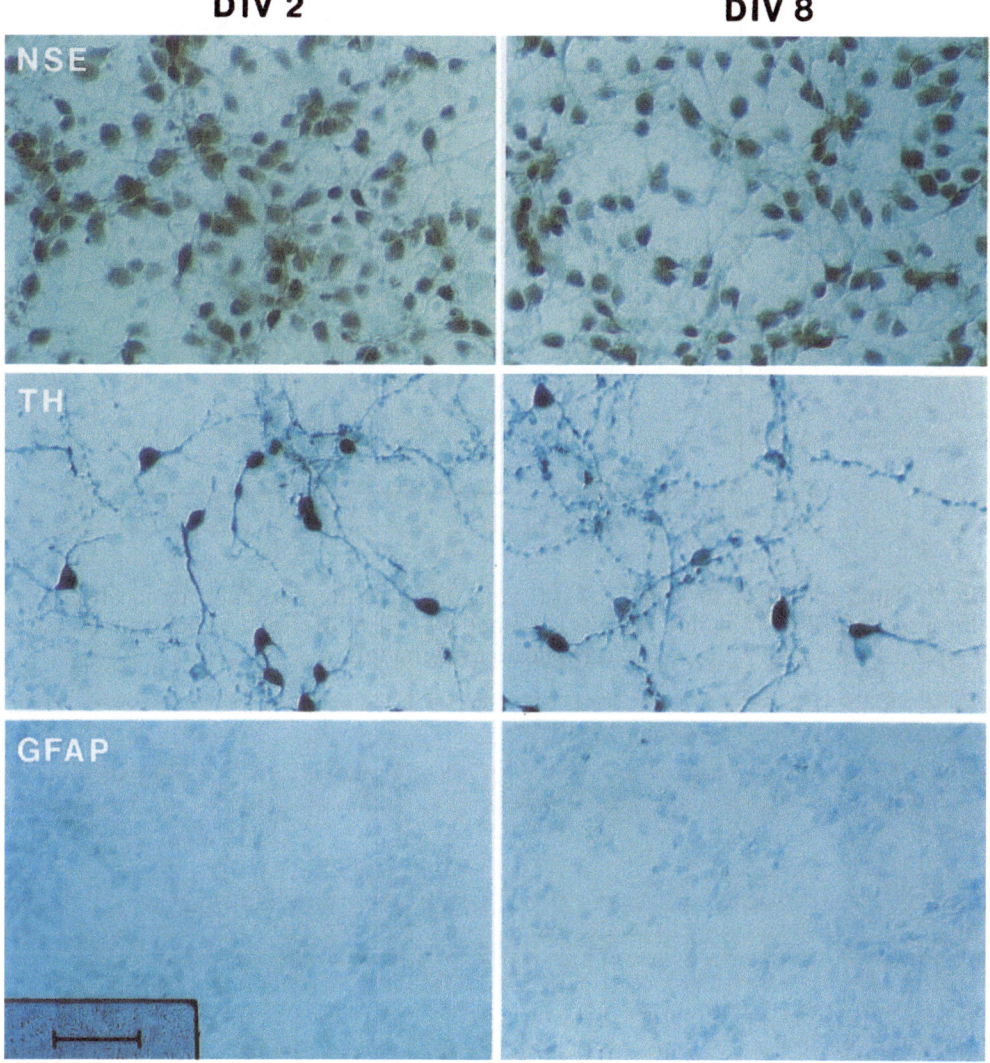

Fig. 1. Photomicrographs of dissociated serum-free cultures of rat E14 mesencephalon floor after 2 (left panels) and 8 days (right panel) in vitro, stained for NSE, TH or GFAP. Bar = 50 μm

neurons above control levels in serum-free cultures. TGF-β3 reduced neuron losses at DIV8 to about 50%, as compared to 75% in the absence of TGF-β3. We therefore conclude that absolute serum-free culture conditions permit survival of DAergic neurons.

The cellular composition of serum-free and serum-primed cultures is not significantly different

Table 1 presents the quantitative results of the cell counts performed at DIV2 and DIV8 in serum-free and serum-primed cultures. In addition to the above

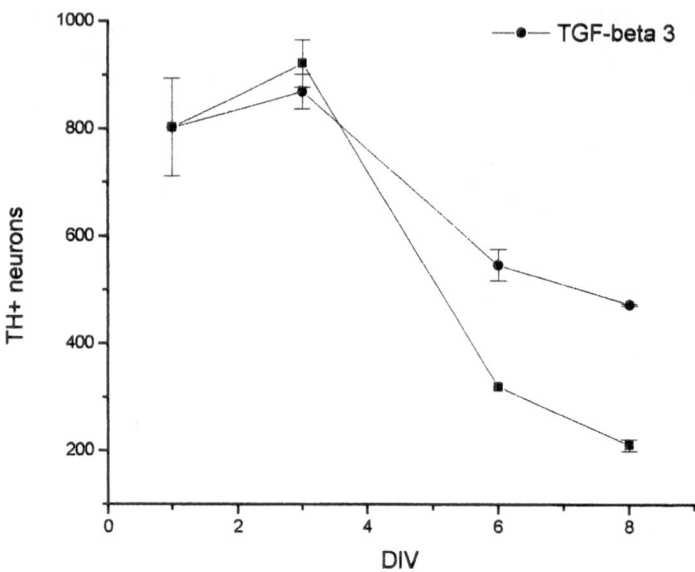

Fig. 2. Time course of survival of TH+ neurons in serum-free cultures in absence or presence of TGF-β3 (2 ng/ml). Results are mean +/− SEM of triplicate determinations, of two replicate experiments

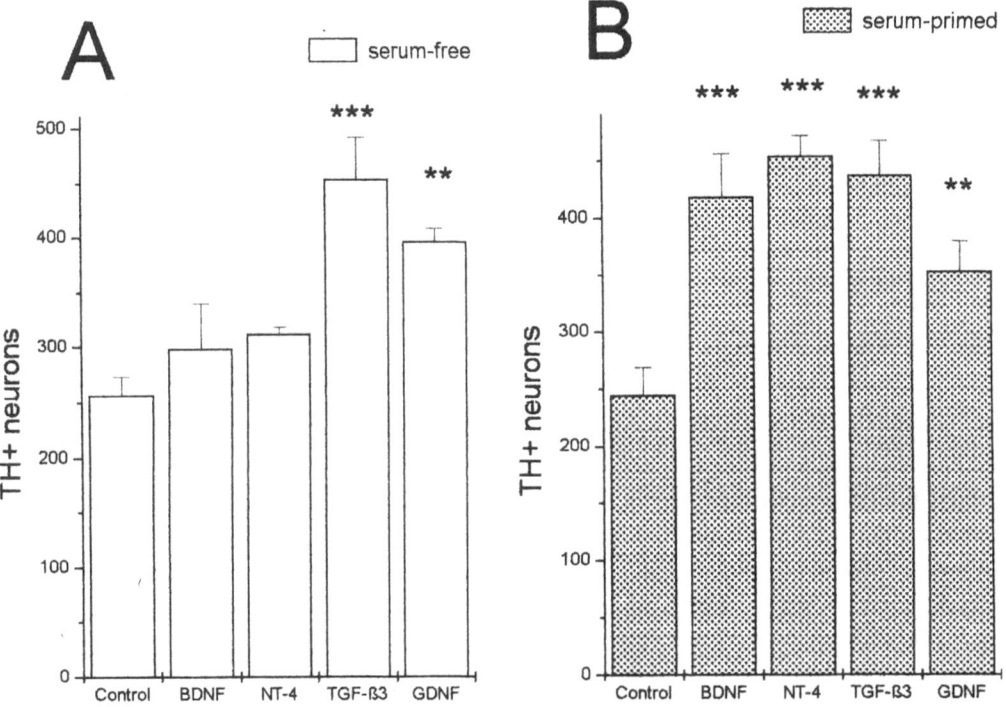

Fig. 3. Numbers of surviving TH-immunoreactive neurons of mesencephalic cultures (E14) at the end of the eight-day culture period under serum-free (**A**) and serum-primed (**B**) conditions. The effects of BDNF (50 ng/ml), NT-4 (10 ng/ml), TGF-β3 (2 ng/ml) and GDNF (10 ng/ml) are shown. Results are mean +/− SEM of triplicate determinations, of two replicate experiments. **P < 0.01, ***P < 0.001

Table 1. Characterization of serum-free culture of embryonic midbrain floor at day two and eight in vitro (DIV)

Marker	DIV2		DIV8	
	serum-free	serum-primed	serum-free	serum-primed
NSE+	>95%	>95%	>95%	>95%
TH+	16–20%	16–20%	16–20%	16–20%
NSE−	<5%	<5%	<5%	<5%
GFAP+	<0.1%	<0.1%	<1%	<1%
Vim+	<5%	<5%	<5%	<5%
A2B5+	<0.1%	<0.1%	<0.1%	<0.1%

markers, cultures were also stained for vimentin, as a marker for immature cells, i.e. neuroblasts or glioblasts, and A2B5 immunoreactivity, as a marker for O2A progenitor cells giving rise to oligodendocytes or type II astrocytes. The majority of cells were neurons (>95%) regardless of the culture conditions chosen. DAergic neurons represented about 16–20% of the cells. Less than 5% showed staining for vimentin. These data are in good agreement with those published by others (Shimoda et al., 1992; Takeshima et al., 1994).

The survival promoting effects of BDNF and NT-4, but not those of TGF-β3 and GDNF, are affected by priming cells with serum

Figure 4 demonstrates in a qualitative fashion that NT-4 and TGF-β3 augmented numbers of TH+ DAergic neurons surviving at DIV8. However, a comparison of serum-free and serum-primed cultures revealed that the survival promoting effect of NT-4 was reduced, if cells had not initially been primed with serum. The quantitative evaluation of these data shown in Fig. 3 provides evidence that priming with serum triggers responsiveness of DAergic neurons to BDNF and NT-4 TGF-β3 and GDNF applied at the saturating concentrations of 2ng/ml and 10ng/ml, respectively, increased DAergic neuron survival to the same extent irrespectively of whether cells had been primed with serum or not.

trkB, the high affinity receptor for BDNF and NT-4, is expressed in serum-free and serum-primed cultures

Using reverse transcription-polymerase chain reaction (RT-PCR) we then investigated whether putative differences in trkB expression might underlie the distinct responsiveness of DAergic neurons to the trkB ligands BDNF and NT-4 in serum-free and serum-primed cultures. As shown in Fig. 5 trkB mRNA was clearly detectable both in serum-free and serum-primed cultures after 24 hours. These data indicate that differences between serum-free and

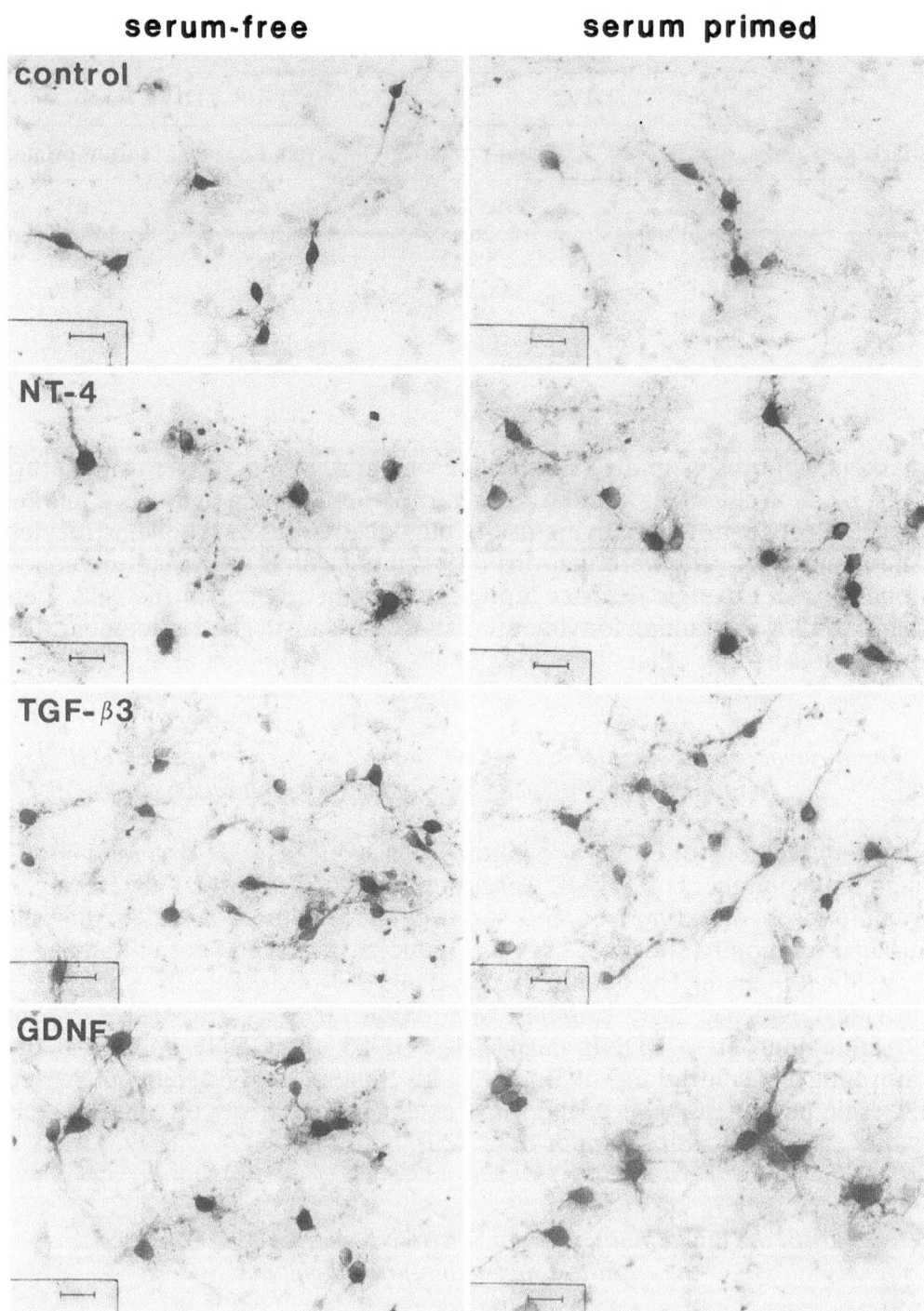

Fig. 4. Photomicrographs of dissociated serum-free (left panel) or serum-primed (right panel) cultures of rat E14 midbrain floor after 8 days in culture stained for TH. Cultures shown are control cultures and cultures treated with NT-4 (10ng/ml), TGF-β3 (2ng/ml) and GDNF (10ng/ml). Bar = 50μm

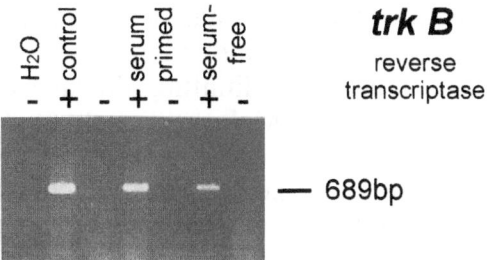

Fig. 5. Expression of trkB in rat mesencephalic cell cultures after 24h under serum-free or serum-primed conditions, detected by RT-PCR. − lanes represent controls, in which total RNA was not transcribed, + lanes represent cDNA, lane marked H_2O shows amplification of H_2O instead of cDNA, and as a control RNA extracted from rat striatum was used. A positive signal for the amplified kinase containing trkB message has 689 bp and is detected after 30 cycles of amplification in serum-free as well as in serum-primed cultures

serum-primed DAergic neurons in their responsiveness to BDNF and NT-4 are likely to exist at levels distal of the trkB receptor rather at the level of trkB mRNA. Another possible explanation might be serum-dependent production of growth factors, which synergistically act with BDNF and NT-4 in the regulation of DAergic neuron survival.

Discussion

The present data indicate that the absolute absence of serum does not impair survival of DAergic neurons cultured from the E14 rat mesencephalon floor. Omission of serum even excluded its application during the dissociation procedure or coverslip pretreatment. Essentially all studies that have addressed survival promoting activities of growth factors on cultured DAergic neurons have employed serum, at least during the initial phases of tissue dissociation and culturing (cf. Engele and Bohn, 1991; Hyman et al., 1991; Beck et al., 1993; Lin et al., 1993; Hynes et al., 1994; Krieglstein and Unsicker, 1994; Takeshima et al., 1994). We show now that the efficacy of the neurotrophins BDNF and NT-4, in contrast to that of TGF-β3 and GDNF, in the promotion of DAergic neuron survival is crucially dependent on at least brief exposure, for appoximately 1 hour, to serum. The mechanism(s), by which serum priming increases the efficacy of the trkB ligands, have been addressed in part, but require future studies. There are several distinct possibilities: (i) serum may interfere with the affinity of BDNF or NT-4 binding to neurotrophin receptors. High affinity binding of neurotrophins apparently requires the concerted actions of p75 and trk receptors (Bothwell, 1995; Hantzopoulos et al., 1994). Onset of expression and presence of trkB and p75 proteins on identified DAergic neurons prior to or at E14 has not been studied as yet. Brief exposure to serum may trigger p75 and/or trkB on DAergic neurons thus contributing to make a high affinity receptor system. Treatment of human neuroblastoma cells with retinoic acid has been shown to induce biological responiveness to BDNF through the induction of trkB (Kaplan et al., 1993). (ii) serum might also induce rate-limiting down-stream components of the signal transduction pathways (Malarkey et al., 1995). (iii) serum might induce production of growth factors synergistically acting with neurotrophins in supporting survival of DAergic neurons. Factors that can act with neurotrophins in augmenting DAergic neuron survival have not been determined as yet.

In conclusion, this first demonstration of the implications of serum priming for neurotrophin-mediated DAergic neuron survival emphasizes the need to employ fully defined culture systems excluding unidentified cocktails such as serum at any time point. Moreover, our data suggest that functions and mechanisms of actions of neurotrophins in the nigrostriatal DAergic system are not yet fully understood.

Acknowledgements

This work was supported by grants from DFG and BMBF. D.M. is the recipient of a fellowship from the Alexander von Humboldt-Foundation. We thank B. Brühl, J. Fey, U. Hinz, and M. Scharpff, for excellent technical assistance.

References

Beck KD (1994) Functions of brain-derived neurotrophic factor, insulin-like growth factor-1 and basic fibroblast growth factor in the development and maintenance of dopaminergic neurons. Prog Neurobiol 44: 497–451

Beck KD, Knüsel B, Hefti F (1993) The nature of the trophic action of brain-derived neurotrophic factor, des(1-3)-insulin-like growth factor-1, and basic fibroblast growth factor on mesencephalic dopaminergic neurons developing in culture. Neuroscience 52: 855–866

Beck KD, Valverde J, Alexi T, Poulsen K, Moffat B, Vandlen RA, Rosenthal A, Hefti F (1995) Mesencephalic dopaminergic neurons protected by GDNF from axotomy-induced degeneration in the adult brain. Nature 373: 339–341

Bothwell M (1995) Functional interactions of neurotrophins and neurotrophin receptors. Annu Rev Neurosci 18: 223–253

Cohen G, Werner P (1994) Free radicals, oxidative stress, and neurodegeneration. In: Calne DB (ed) Neurodegenerative diseases. Saunders, pp 139–161

Edwards RH (1993) Pathogenesis of Parkinson's disease. Clin Neurosci 1: 36–44

Engele J, Bohn MC (1991) The neurotrophic effects of fibroblast growth factors on dopaminergic neurons in vitro are mediated by mesencephalic glia. J Neurosci 11: 3070–3078

Gerlach M, Ben-Shachar D, Riederer P, Youdim MBH (1994) Altered brain metabolism of iron as a cause of neurodegenerative diseases? J Neurochem 63: 793–807

Götz ME, Künig G, Riederer P, Youdim MBH (1994) Oxidative stress: free radical production in neural degeneration. Pharmacol Ther 63: 37–122

Hantzopoulos PA, Suri C, Glass DJ, Goldfarb MP, Yancopoulos GD (1994) The low affinity NGF receptor, p75, can collaborate with each of the trks to potentiate functional responses to the neurotrophins. Neuron 13: 187–201

Hoffer BJ, Hoffman A, Bowenkamp K, Huettl P, Hudson J, Martin D, Lin L-FH, Gerhardt GA (1994) Glial cell line-derived neurotrophic factor reverses toxin-induced injury to midbrain dopaminergic neurons in vivo. Neurosci Lett 182: 107–111

Hyman C, Hoffer M, Barde Y-A, Juhasz M, Yancopoulos GD, Squinto SP, Lindsay RM (1991) BDNF is a neurotrophic factor for dopaminergic neurons of the substantia nigra. Nature 350: 230–232.

Hyman C, Juhasz M, Jackson C, Wright P, Ip NY, Lindsay RM (1993) Overlapping and distinct actions of the neurotrophins, BDNF, NT-3 and NT-4/5, on cultured dopaminergic and GABAegic neurons of the ventral mesencephalon. J Neurosci 14: 335–347

Hynes MA, Poulson K, Armanini M, Berkemeier L, Phillips H, Rosenthal A (1994) Neurotrophin-4/5 is a survival factor for embryonic midbrain dopaminergic neurons in enriched cultures. J Neurosci Res 37: 144–154

Jackson GR, Apffel L, Werrbach-Perez K, Perez-Polo JR (1990) Role of nerve growth factor in oxidant-antioxidant balance and neuronal injury. I. Stimulation of hydrogen peroxide resistance. J Neurosci Res 25: 360–368

Kaplan DR, Matsumoto K, Lucarelli E, Thiele CJ (1993) Induction of TrkB by retinoid acid mediates biologic responsiveness to BDNF and differentiation of human neuroblastoma cells. Neuron 11: 321–331

Krieglstein K, Unsicker K (1994) TGF-β promotes survival of midbrain dopmainergic neurons and protects them against MPP+ toxicity. Neuroscience 63: 1189–1196

Krieglstein K, Suter-Crazzolara C, Fischer WH, Unsicker K (1995) TGF-β superfamily members promote survival of midbrain dopaminergic neurons and protect them against MPP+ toxicity. EMBO J 14: 736–742

Levi-Montalcini R (1987) The nerve growth factor 35 years later. Science 237: 1154–1162

Lin L-FH, Doherty DH, Lile JD, Bektesh S, Collins F (1993) GDNF: a glial cell line-derived neurotrophic factor for midbrain dopaminergic neurons. Science 246:1023–1025

Lindsay RM, Altar CA, Cedarbaum JM, Hyman C, Wiegand SJ (1993) The therapeutic potential of neurotrophic factors in the treatment of Parkinson's disease. Exp Neurol 124: 103–118

Malarkey K, Belham CM, Paul A, Graham A, McLees A, Scott PH, Plevin R (1995) The regulation of tyrosine kinase signalling pathways by growth factor and G-coupled receptors. Biochem J 309: 361–375

Mattson MP, Scheff SW (1994) Endogenous neuroprotection factors and traumatic brain injury: mechanisms of action and implications for therapy. J Neurotrauma 11: 3–33

Middlemas DS, Lindberg RA, Hunter T (1991) TrkB, a neural receptor protein-tyrosine kinase: evidence for full-length and two truncated receptors. GenBank M55291

Mufson EJ, Kroin JS, Sobreviela T, Burke MA, Kordower JH, Penn RD, Miller JA (1994) Intrastriatal infusions of brain-derived neurotrophic factor: retrograde transport and colocalization with dopamine containing substantia nigra neurons in rat. Exp Neurol 129: 15–26

Poulsen KT, Armanini MP, Klein RD, Hynes MA, Phillips HS, Rosenthal A (1994) TGFβ2 and TGFβ3 are potent survival factors for midbrain dopaminergic neurons. Neuron 13: 1245–1252

Reichmann H, Riederer P (1994) Mitochondrial disturbances in neurodegeneration. In: Calne DB (ed) Neurodegenerative diseases. Saunders, Philadelphia, pp 195–204

Schapira AHV (1995) Oxidative stress in Parkinson's disease. Neuropathol Appl Neurobiol 21: 3–9

Shimoda K, Sauve Y, Marini A, Schwartz JP, Commissiong JW (1992) A high percentage of tyrosine hydroxylase-positive cells from rat E14 mesencephalic cell culture. Brain Res 586: 319–331

Takeshima T, Johnston JM, Commissiong JW (1994) Mesencephalic type 1 astrocytes rescue dopaminergic neurons from death induced by serum deprevation. J Neurosci 14: 4769–4779

Tomac A, Lindqvist E, Lin L-FH, Imgren SO, Young D, Hoffer BJ, Olson L (1995) Protection and repair of the nigrostriatal dopaminergic system by GDNF in vivo. Nature 373: 335–339

Unsicker K (1994) Growth factors in Parkinson's disease. Prog Growth Factor Res 5: 73–87

Zhang Y, Tatsuno T, Carney JM, Mattson MP (1993) Basic FGF, NGF, and IGFs protect hippocampal and cortical neurons against iron-induced degeneration. J Cereb Blood Flow Metab 13: 378–388

Authors' address: Dr. K. Krieglstein, Department of Anatomy and Cell Biology, The University of Heidelberg, Im Neuenheimer Feld 307, 2. OG, D-69120 Heidelberg, Federal Republic of Germany.

J Neural Transm (1996) [Suppl] 47: 259–266
© Springer-Verlag 1996

Tau protein and apolipoprotein E in CSF diagnostics of Alzheimer's disease: impact on non Alzheimer's dementia?

N. Rösler*, I. Wichart, C. Bancher, and **K. A. Jellinger**

Ludwig Boltzmann Institute of Clinical Neurobiology, Lainz Hospital,
Vienna, Austria

Summary. Tau protein and apolipoprotein E are suggested to be biochemically related to neurofibrillary tangles and senile plaques in Alzheimer's disease (AD) brains. They can be detected as immunoreactive material (total tau immunoreactivity [TTIR] and apolipoprotein E-immunoreactivity [ApoE-IR]) in the cerebrospinal fluid (CSF).

TTIR and ApoE-IR have been measured in *ex vivo* lumbar and *post mortem* ventricular CSF in AD, other neurological diseases without cognitive impairment, elderly depressive patients, and young and elderly controls.

In lumbar CSF, there was a highly significant increase of TTIR and a minor, insignificant decrease of ApoE-IR in CSF of AD patients. The latter result was also found in ventricular CSF, whereas TTIR showed no significant difference between groups in the rostral CSF compartment.

As depressive periods in the elderly may mimick a dementing process, these findings contribute to the differential diagnosis of these disorders by showing a different neurobiochemical CSF profile. Work in progress will include a variety of non-Alzheimer's dementias and possibly will further increase the value of CSF investigation in neurodegenerative disorders.

Introduction

Alzheimer's disease (AD) is the most frequent cause of dementia in the elderly and shows a relative incidence of 70–80% (Jellinger et al., 1990). The clinical syndrome is characterized by a progressive deterioration of intellectual functions. The *ex vivo* diagnosis using established clinical criteria reaches an accuracy of about 80–90%, but the definite diagnosis remains a neuropathological one based on the (semi)quantitative assessment of neuritic plaques and neurofibrillary tangles (NFT) (Galasko et al., 1994). NFT are composed of bundles of paired helical filaments (PHF), the main component

---

* Present address: Department of Psychiatry, University Medical School, Freiburg, Federal Republic of Germany

of which is the microtubule-associated tau protein in a pathologically hyperphosphorylated form (Goedert, 1993).

Human apolipoprotein E (ApoE) is a 299 amino acid-containing glycoprotein (molecular weight 34kDa) present within the brain where it is synthesized by astrocytes and oligodendrocytes. It plays a role in phospholipid and cholesterol metabolism mainly by interacting with the ApoB/ApoE (low density lipoprotein ([LDL]) receptor hereby mediating the cellular uptake of lipid complexes (Poirier, 1994). ApoE is present within plaques, neurofibrillary tangles and dystrophic neurites of AD brains (Namba et al., 1991); it binds soluble and insoluble forms of β-amyloid with high avidity (Wisniewski et al., 1993), and it has been proposed that ApoE, acting as a molecular chaperone, influences conformational changes of amyloid fibrils during plaque formation (Wisniewski et al., 1992). Genotyping studies have shown an increased frequency of the ApoE-ε4-allele in AD (Strittmatter et al., 1993; Martinoli et al., 1995) suggesting a role of ApoE-ε4 as a susceptibility marker of the disease.

Tau protein and ApoE can be detected as immunoreactive material in the cerebrospinal fluid (CSF). As valid biological markers for the *ex vivo* diagnosis of AD are still lacking, their quantification in the CSF appears of utmost interest.

Patients and methods

Total tau immunoreactivity (TTIR) and total apolipoprotein E-immunoreactivity (tApoE-IR) were measured in a series of 85 *ex vivo* lumbar CSF. In addition, tApoE-IR was measured in the corresponding serum samples. Informed consent was obtained before lumbar puncture. The whole group was subdivided as follows (Table 1):

1. 20 patients with "probable" AD according to the NINCDS-ADRDA criteria; in addition, the Mini Mental Status Examination (MMSE) (Folstein et al., 1975) was performed;
2. 24 patients with other neurological disorders (OND) without cognitive impairment: 1 intracerebral hemorrhage, 8 brain infarctions, 6 multiple sclerosis, 2 myelitis, 2 control taps after viral meningoencephalitis, 2 epilepsy, 2 multisystem atrophies, 1 meningioma;
3. 11 elderly patients with major depression (DEPR) according to ICD-10 and DSM-IIIR;
4. and 5. 18 young and 12 elderly subjects without CNS disease, in whom lumbar puncture was performed for exclusion purposes.

In addition, 28 *post mortem* CSF samples were obtained through ventricular tap, immediately centrifuged and kept at −70°C until analysis. Sixteen patients had neuropathologically confirmed AD, twelve cases (OND/CO) had no or other neurological diesase. Clinical and neurochemical data of these patients are given in Table 2.

Histologic criteria for the diagnosis of AD followed those outlined by the NIH/AARP Working Group (Khachaturian, 1985) and the criteria for "pure" AD (Tierney et al., 1988). Moreover, the cases were evaluated using the staging of Braak and Braak (1991). Six patients met the criteria for limbic stage III–IV, ten had isocortical stage V–VI. Age at onset of dementia, defined as the earliest age at which behavioral changes were noticed, and qualitative assessment of the mental status prior to death were determined from the medical records, showing that all AD patients were severely demented. The

Table 1. Clinical and neurochemical data of patients with "probable" Alzheimer's disease (AD), other neurological disorders (OND), elderly depressed patients (DEPR), and young (COY) and elderly controls (COE)

Intra vitam lumbar CSF	AD	OND	DEPR	COY	COE
n (M/F)	20 (8/12)	24 (12/12)	11 (3/8)	18 (6/12)	12 (6/6)
Age (yr.)	72.1 ± 3.5	59.8 ± 3.5	68.3 ± 4.2	37.5 ± 2.4	72.5 ± 3.6
CSF cell count (/μl)	1.2 ± 0.5	2.2 ± 0.8	1.6 ± 0.4	1.0 ± 0.3	1.2 ± 0.2
Q_{Alb} (×10^{-3})	6.8 ± 0.6	6.7 ± 1.0	6.5 ± 0.4	5.8 ± 0.3	6.7 ± 0.8
Q_{IgG} (×10^{-3})	3.2 ± 0.3	3.0 ± 0.6	3.0 ± 0.4	2.4 ± 0.3	2.8 ± 0.5
LCSF-TTIR (pg/ml)	335.7 ± 23.4***	192.2 ± 15.5	142.1 ± 17.2††	88.4 ± 7.2	117.9 ± 13.8
tApoE-IR Serum (mg/l)	28.1 ± 3.1[b]	22.1 ± 1.8	24.5 ± 2.2	21.6 ± 1.8[a]	28.7 ± 3.1
LCSF-tApoE-IR (μg/10^2 ml)	149 ± 7.0[b]	160 ± 12.0	154 ± 10.0	148 ± 11.0	168 ± 14.0
$Q_{tApoE-IR}$ (Serum/CSF)	18.9	14.1	15.9	14.6	17.1
MMSE (points)	15.9 ± 1.4	—	—	—	—

[a] p = 0.05 vs. COE; [b] not significant (p > 0.05) vs. OND, DEPR, COY, COE; *** p < 0.005 vs. OND, DEPR, COY, COE; †† p < 0.01 vs. COY

Table 2. Clinical and neurochemical data of patients with neuropathologically confirmed Alzheimer's disease (AD) and patients with or without other neurological disease (OND/CO)

Post mortem ventricular CSF	AD	OND/CO
n (M/F)	16 (8/8)	12 (3/9)
Age at onset (yr.)	73.1 ± 3.3	—
Age at death (yr.)	78.9 ± 3.4	79.5 ± 3.8
Duration of illness (yr.)	5.8 ± 0.8	—
Total CSF protein (mg/10^2ml)	136.1 ± 31.2[b]	176.6 ± 32.5
Brain weight (g)	1,150.8 ± 48.3[b]	1,161.8 ± 41.3
Post mortem delay (h)	25.3 ± 3.4[b]	24.3 ± 4.2
VCSF-TTIR (ng/ml)	85.6 ± 16.0[b]	116.9 ± 29.4
VCSF-tApoE-IR (μg/10^2ml)	108 ± 18.7[b]	117 ± 23.9

[b] not significant vs. OND/CO

diagnoses of the OND/CO group were made using current pathological criteria: vascular dementia (2), Parkinson's disease, Lewy body dementia (1), multiple sclerosis (1), acute brain infarctions (2), postanoxic parahippocampal sclerosis (1), Creutzfeldt-Jakob disease (1), and brains of aged subjects showing nothing abnormal (4).

TTIR was measured with a specific sandwich ELISA (Innogenetics, Belgium) (Mercken et al., 1992; Vandermeeren et al., 1993) in a modified version (van de Voorde et al., 1995). Three monoclonal antibodies were employed (AT 120, BT 2, HT 7), which detect different epitopes of the tau protein. AT 120 (coating antibody) and HT 7 (second detecting antibody) detect both normal and hyperphosphorylated tau, whereas BT 2 (first detecting antibody) detects a non-phosphorylated epitope. For detection of antigen binding streptavidin-peroxidase was used, as a chromogen 3,5,3',5'-tetramethylbenzidine (TMB) was used. Absorption was read at 450 nm.

tApoE-IR was measured using a slightly modified specific symmetrical non-competitive sandwich ELISA (Carlsson et al., 1991). Instead of a polyclonal antibody, we used a monoclonal mouse antibody (Boehringer, Mannheim, FRG) as coating and biotinylated detection antibody. Using this technique, problems of sterical hindrance were not observed, and typical standard curves could be obtained. For detection of antigen binding streptavidin-peroxidase was ued, as a chromogen 2,2-Azino-di-[3-ethyl-benz-thiazolin-sulphonic acid] (ABTS) was used. Absorption was read at 410 nm.

Wilcoxon two sample test and Spearman's rank correlation coefficient were used for statistical analysis.

Results

The results of lumbar and ventricular fluid TTIR and ApoE-IR measurements are given in Table 1 and 2. In lumbar CSF (LCSF), there was a highly significant (p < 0.005) increase of tau levels in the AD group compared with the elderly depressive patients, with OND patients, and with young and elderly controls. The elderly depressive subjects had an insignificant increase compared with elderly controls; the difference to young controls was significant (p < 0.01). Elderly controls had no significant difference compared with young controls. OND patients had significantly higher values ($p < 0.005$) than both young and elderly controls. There was a significant negative correlation of MMSE score with total tau levels when all AD patients were included ($r = -0.6204$, $p < 0.01$). However, the correlation remained insignificant ($r = -0.2935$, $p > 0.05$) when testing only patients with MMSE greater than 10/30 points.

As for ApoE in lumbar CSF, there was a tendency to lower levels of ApoE-IR in the AD group, but the difference was not significant when compared with all other groups ($p > 0.05$). The mean lumbar CSF ApoE-IR of all patients investigated was $155\,\mu g/10^2\,ml$, the mean serum concentration of all patients was $24.8\,mg/l$, resulting in a mean serum/lumbar CSF ratio of 16.0. There was no significant correlation ($r = 0.074$, $p > 0.05$) of MMSE scores of AD patients and their ApoE levels in lumbar CSF.

In ventricular CSF (VCSF), there was a striking increase of TTIR in all patient groups compared with the lumbar compartment results. The AD group tended to lower levels of TTIR, but the difference was not significant ($p > 0.05$). As for ApoE, there was, similar to the results in lumbar CSF, a tendency towards lower levels in the AD group, but the difference remained insignificant ($p > 0.05$).

Discussion

To our knowledge, this is the first study investigating CSF tau and ApoE levels which includes *post mortem* samples of autopsy confirmed AD cases. Our study revealed a highly significant increase of lumbar CSF total tau levels in patients with probable AD compared with elderly depressive, OND subjects, and young and elderly controls. It seems plausible that these elevations are the result of enhanced release of tau protein from damaged neurons into the extracellular space, and, as a consequence, into CSF. The observed difference between AD patients and elderly depressive patients confirms a recent study (Hock et al., 1995) and is of particular clinical interest. Depressive periods can be accompanied by a severe impairment of attention, receptivity and concentration which may mimic a dementing process. Thus, early neurochemical identification of a depressive syndrome is of great importance with regard to appropriate therapeutic strategies. The reason for the elevation of tau in depressed patients in comparison to young controls is unknown. On the other hand, the insignificant difference between young and elderly controls leds to the assumption that tau is not merely a marker of aging *per se*. There are contradictory reports regarding the correlation between MMSE and TTIR in lumbar CSF of AD patients (Hock et al., 1995; Tato et al., 1995; Van de Voorde et al., 1995). In our group, there was a significant negative correlation only when including the whole range of scores, which became insignificant when excluding the patients with severe dementia. These results corroborate neuropathological findings which showed a significant correlation between the number of NFT and MMSE scores only when including severely demented patients (Jellinger et al., 1992).

In ventricular CSF, there was a striking increase of TTIR in all patient groups investigated reaching the ng/ml concentration range compared with pg/ml levels in lumbar CSF. Although there was no correlation between TTIR and *post mortem* delay and total protein content, nonspecific *post mortem* effects due to neuronal cell death and membrane breakdown could be the cause for these elevations. On the other hand, neuropathological findings suggest that accumulation of abnormally phosphorylated tau is one of the earliest neuronal alterations in the course of tangle formation in AD. Moreover, immunocytochemistry for tau is the most sensitive method for detection of tangles at earlier stages, but leads to staining of only a minority of end stage tangles (Bancher et al., 1989). As all AD patients in our study were severely demented, they possibly had fewer releasable total tau material than the OND/CO group. Further work measuring only hyperphosphorylated tau in *post mortem* ventricular CSF of AD patients could possibly clarify this point.

As for ApoE, the AD group showed a slight, insignificant decrease of ApoE in both the lumbar and the ventricular compartment. Although the absence of an increase of ApoE in CSF of AD corrobarates recent *in vivo* findings in a heterogenous patient group with degenerative, toxic and metabolic brain disorders (Carlsson et al., 1991), our results are at variance with the findings of another group (Blennow et al., 1994), who detected a significant decrease of lumbar ApoE in AD. Methodological differences could account for the overall higher ApoE levels in their study, but not for the observed difference between controls and AD patients. In the mentioned study, no information is given about the MMSE of the AD patients. In fact, we investigated a broad range of MMSE scores, and no correlation of MMSE with ApoE in lumbar CSF could be observed.

The mean ApoE serum/CSF ratio was 16.0, thus being similar to results of another group (Carlsson et al., 1991) who found a ratio of 1:12. Taking into account the hydrodynamic diameter of ApoE and its molecular weight, it can be assumed that the main portion of CSF ApoE stems from intrathecal synthesis making the use of a quotient unnecessary.

ApoE is involved in the maintenance and regeneration of myelin and neuronal membranes in both the peripheral and central nervous system and has been linked to synaptoneogenesis and, thus, to phenomena of synaptic plasticity (Poirier, 1994). Therefore, our results could reflect poor reinnervation capacity, increased utilization or adsorption of ApoE to senile plaques and neurofibrillary tangles in AD brains.

Taking together lumbar and ventricular CSF findings of tau and ApoE measurements, the diagnostic value of total tau measurements as a single determination seems to be more pronounced in differentiating AD patients from elderly depressive patients and other neurological disorders than measurements of total ApoE. On the other hand, both results could be neurobiologically meaningful as part of neurochemical profiles of different neurodegenerative diseases and conditions which may mimick dementing processes. Therefore, further work is necessary including a variety of non-Alzheimer's dementias, the results possibly further enhancing the value of CSF investigation in neurodegenerative disorders.

Acknowledgement

This study was sponsored by a grant of the Research Inititaive EBEWE.

References

Bancher C, Brunner C, Lassmann H, Budka H, Jellinger K, Wiche G, Seitelberger F, Grundke-Iqbal I, Iqbal K, Wisniewski HM (1989) Accumulation of abnormally phosphorylated tau precedes the formation of neurofibrillary tangles in Alzheimer's disease. Brain Res 477: 90–99

Blennow K, Hesse C, Fredman P (1994) Cerebrospinal fluid apolipoprotein E is reduced in Alzheimer's disease. NeuroReport 5: 2534–2536

Braak H, Braak E (1991) Neuropathological staging of Alzheimer-related changes. Acta Neuropathol 82: 306–315

Carlsson J, Armstrong VW, Reiber H, Felgenhauer K, Seidel D (1991) Clinical relevance of the quantification of apolipoprotein E in cerebrospinal fluid. Clin Chim Acta 196: 167–176

Galasko D, Hansen LA, Katzman R, Wiederholt W, Masliah E, Terry R, Hill LR, Lessin P, Thal LJ (1994) Clinical-neuropathological correlations in Alzheimer's disease and related dementias. Arch Neurol 51: 888–895

Goedert M (1993) Tau protein and the neurofibrillary pathology of Alzheimer's disease. Trends Neurosci 16: 460–465

Hock C, Golombowski S, Naser W, Müller-Spahn F (1995) Increased levels of tau-protein in cerebrospinal fluid of patients with Alzheimer's disease-correlation with degree of cognitive impairment. Ann Neurol 37: 414–415

Jellinger K, Danielczyk W, Fischer P, Gabriel E (1990) Clinicopathological analysis of dementia disorders in the elderly. J Neurol Sci 95: 239–258

Jellinger K, Bancher C, Fischer P, Lassmann H (1992) Quantitative histopathologic validation of senile dementia of the Alzheimer type. Eur J Gerontol 3: 146–156

Khachaturian Z (1985) Diagnosis of Alzheimer's disease. Arch Neurol 42: 1097–1105

Martinoli MG, Trojanowski JQ, Schmidt ML, Arnold SE, Fujiwara TM, Lee VMY, Hurtig H, Julien JP, Clark C (1995) Association of apolipoprotein ε4 allele and neuropathologic findings in patients with dementia. Acta Neuropathol 90: 239–243

Mercken M, Vandermeeren M, Lübcke U, Six J, Boons J, Vanmechelen E, Van de Voorde A, Gheuens J (1992) Affinity purification of human tau proteins and the construction of a sensitive sandwich enzyme-linked immunosorbent assay for human tau detection. J Neurochem 58: 548–553

Namba Y, Tomanaga M, Kawasaki H, Otomo E, Ikeda K (1991) Apolipoprotein E immunoreactivity in cerebral amyloid deposits and neurofibrillary tangles in Alzheimer's disease and kuru plaque amyloid in Creutzfeldt-Jakob disease. Brain Res 541: 163–166

Poirier J (1994) Apolipoprotein E in animals models of CNS injury and in Alzheimer's disease. Trends Neurosci 17: 525–530

Strittmatter WJ, Saunders AM, Schmechel D, Pericak-Vance M, Enghild J, Salvesen GS, Roses AD (1993) Apolipoprotein E: high avidity binding to β-amyloid and increased frequency of type 4 allele in late onset familial Alzheimer disease. Proc Natl Acad Sci USA 90: 1977–1981

Tato RE, Frank A, Hernanz A (1995) Tau protein concentrations in cerebrospinal fluid of patients with dementia of the Alzheimer type. J Neurol Neurosurg Psychiatry 59: 280–283

Tierney MC, Fisher RW, Lewis AJ, Zorzitto ML, Snow WG, Reid DW, Nieuwstraten P (1988) The NINCDS-ADRDA Work Group criteria for the clinical diagnosis of probable Alzheimer's disease. A clinico-pathologic study of 57 cases. Neurology 38: 359–364

Vandermeeren M, Mercken M, Vanmechelen E, Six J, Van de Voorde A, Martin JJ, Cras
    P (1993) Detection of tau proteins in normal and Alzheimer's disease cerebrospinal
    fluid with a sensitive sandwich enzyme-linked immunosorbent assay. J Neurochem
    61: 1828–1834
Van de Voorde A, Vanmechelen E, Vandermeeren M, Dessaint F, Beckman W, Cras P
    (1995) Detection of tau in cerebrospinal fluid. In: Iqbal K, Mortimer JA, Winblad W,
    Wisniewski HM (eds) Research advances in Alzheimer's disease and related disor-
    ders. Wiley, Chichester, pp 189–195
Wisniewski T, Frangione B (1992) Apolipoprotein E: a pathological chaperone protein in
    patients with cerebral and systemic amyloid. Neurosci Lett 135: 235–238
Wisniewski T, Golabek A, Matsubara E, Ghiso J, Frangione B (1993) Apolipoprotein E:
    binding to soluble Alzheimer's β-amyloid. Biochem Biophys Res Commun 192: 359–
    365

Authors' address: Prof. Dr. K. A. Jellinger, Ludwig Boltzmann-Institut für klinische
Neurobiologie, Krankenhaus Wien-Lainz, Wolkersbergenstrasse 1, A-1130 Wien,
Austria.

J Neural Transm (1996) [Suppl] 47: 267–273
© Springer-Verlag 1996

Death of cultured telencephalon neurons induced by glutamate is reduced by the peptide derivative Cerebrolysin®

B. Hutter-Paier, E. Grygar, and **M. Windisch**

Center of Animal Biology, Medical School, University of Graz, Graz, Austria

Summary. Glutamate induced neurotoxicity has been proposed to account for the loss of neurons after ischemia as well as in the cause of neurodegenerative diseases. We have studied the effects of exogenous glutamate on survival of neurons from chick embryo telencephalon, precultured with a peptide derivative for 8 days. The peptide derivative Cerebrolysin® is a drug produced by standardised enzymatic breakdown consisting of 80% peptides and 20% amino acids. Toxic effects of acute glutamate exposure were prevented by Cerebrolysin in a concentration-dependent manner. 20 and 40 µl Cerebrolysin produce distinct neuroprotective effects. However, 80 µl Cerebrolysin/ml nutrition medium more than doubles neuronal viability compared to untreated control cells. These concentration-dependent effects of Cerebrolysin were evident even at the light microscopic level.

Introduction

Glutamate is an important excitatory amino acid at many central nervous synapses (Greenamyre, 1986). Persistent stimulation of glutamate receptors causes neurotoxicity and neuronal death. After a few minutes of exposure, glutamate can induce neurotoxicity in cultured neurons, possible due to an excessive Ca^{2+} influx through N-methyl-D-aspartate (NMDA) receptor activated channels (Choi et al., 1988). Such rapid triggered neurotoxicity might contribute to the acute brain injury associated with cerebral hypoxia-ischemia and cortical spreading depression (Lauritzen and Hansen, 1992). Furthermore, glutamate has been proposed as a key factor in the pathophysiology of several neurologic disorders including Huntington disease (Young et al., 1988), amyotrophic lateral sclerosis (Plaitakis and Caroscio, 1987) and Alzheimer's disease (Maragos et al., 1987).

Recently, Cerebrolysin®, a drug consisting of small peptides and amino acids has been described to prevent neurotoxicity in vivo (Gschanes et al., 1993) and in vitro (Xiong et al., 1995). We report here that Cerebrolysin attenuates injury to cultured chick embryo cortical neurons, resulting from exposure to exogenous glutamate.

Material and methods

Primary neuronal cultures were prepared from 8-day-old white Leghorn chick embryo telencephalons as described by Pettmann et al. (1979). 3×10^6 cells per ml medium were plated in microtiter plates previously coated with poly-D-lysine. Cultures were maintained in Dulbecco's modified Eagle's medium (DMEM; Bio Whittaker) supplemented with 5% (v/v) heat-inactivated fetal calf serum (FCS; Bio Whittaker), 2M glutamine (Bio Whittaker) and gentamycine (0.1mg/ml; Bio Whittaker). Cerebrolysin® (from EBEWE Pharmaceuticals, Austria) was added to the cultures in concentrations of 80, 40, 20 and 10μl/ml medium from the first day onwards. Cerebrolysin is a peptide derivative produced by standardised enzymatic breakdown, consisting of 80% peptides and 20% amino acids. Cultures were kept at 37°C in a humidified atmosphere of 5% CO_2 and 95% air. After 8 days in vitro (DIV 8), cytotoxic ischemia was induced by replacing the nutrition medium by a 1mM L-glutamate solution. After 60 minutes, the glutamate containing medium was aspirated and replaced by their original nutrition medium. Two days later, the percentage of neuronal damage was assessed by means of the MTT assay (Mosmann, 1983). In detail 48 hours after glutamate exposure MTT solution was added to the medium to a concentration of 0.5mg/ml and incubation continued for an other 2 hours. This MTT containing medium was aspirated and 3% SDS was added to lyse cells. After adding Isopropanol / HCl and allowing several minutes for the blue formazane product to solubilize at room temperature, spectrophotometric absorbance was measured at 570nm.

Because of small differences in interpreparation plating densities and according to Skaper et al. (1991), MTT values were scaled to the mean of glutamate treated control cultures (=100). Values are given as means ± s.e.m. For statistical comparison one-way analysis of variance and subsequent Duncan's test were used.

Results

The neuroprotective effect afforded by different concentrations of Cerebrolysin® added to the cortical cultures is shown in Fig. 1 and Fig. 2. Figure 1 shows representative photomicrographs of cortical neuronal cells. Exposure of the neurons to 1mM L-glutamate for 60 minutes was rapidly followed by swelling of the cell bodies. Compared to glutamate-free control cells (Fig. 1F) glutamate injured neurons began to undergo obvious degeneration over the next 48 hours of the recovery period (Fig. 1A). In these ischemic control cultures the vast majority of neurons together with their neurite network had disintegrated, being replaced by debris. The injury induced by exogenous glutamate can be dramatically minimised by the addition of 10 to 80μl Cerebrolysin®/ml nutrition medium (Fig. 1B–E). It is remarkable that at the light microscopic level the addition of 80μl Cerebrolysin®/ml medium attenuates almost complete loss of cortical neurons after glutamate exposure (Fig. 1E).

The results of the MTT viability assay shown in Fig. 2, can be taken as an index for the mitochondrial activity. When neurons were preincubated with Cerebrolysin® for 8 days before acute glutamate exposure, the drug is able to reduce this injury significantly. 10, 20 and 40μl Cerebrolysin®/ml medium significantly increase cell viability according to MTT dehydrogenases activity (p < 0.001). 80μl Cerebrolysin®/ml nutrition medium are able to double the

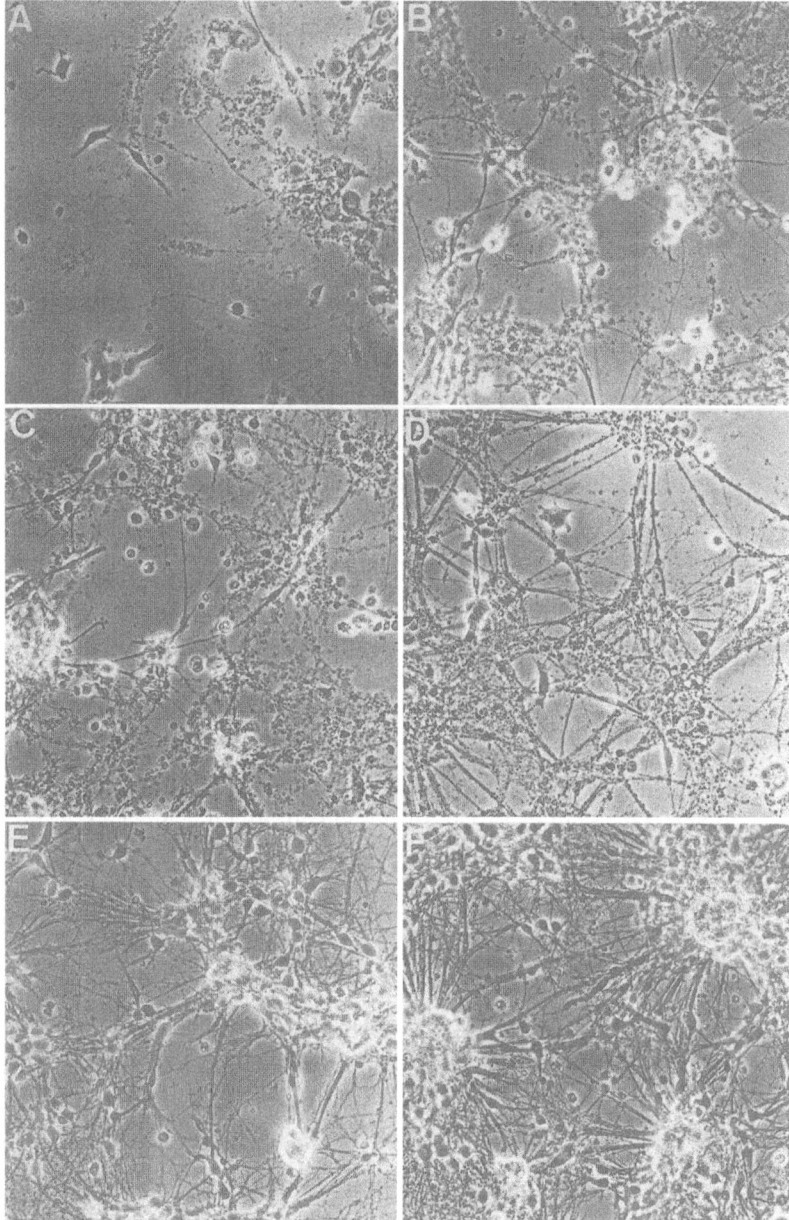

Fig. 1. Neuroprotective effect of Cerebrolysin® on glutamate induced neurotoxicity. In **A–E** cultures were exposed to 1 mM L-glutamate for 60 minutes at the 8th day in vitro followed by a recovery period of 48 hours with the original glutamate free solution. **A** Untreated cells. **B–E** Cells treated for the whole experimental procedure with 10, 20, 40 and 80 μl Cerebrolysin/ml medium respectively. **F** Glutamate untreated cells (controls). Bar 25 μm

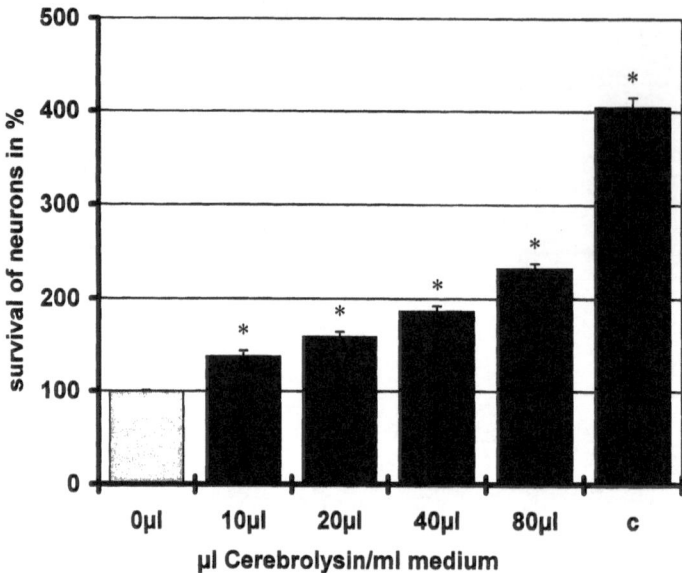

Fig. 2. Cerebrolysin prevents L-glutamate induced injury of cultured neurons from chick embryo telencephalon. After 8 days in culture, neurons were damaged by adding 1 mM L-glutamate for 60 minutes. Cerebrolysin was present in the culture medium during the whole experiment except during the glutamate exposure period. 48 hours after injury, the percentage of surviving neurons was determined using the MTT assay. Values, scaled to the mean of glutamate treated control cultures (=100), are given as means ± s.e.m. from n = seven experiments (2wells on 2plates). Different from L-glutamate treated controls: *p < 0.001 (analysis of variance and subsequent Duncan's test)

amount of surviving cells compared to glutamate exposed controls, which were calculated as 100% (p < 0.001). Although none of the added concentrations of Cerebrolysin® are in able increase the MTT dehydrogenase activity comparable to that of untreated control cultures, Cerebrolysin® clearly protects neurons from cell death induced by large concentrations of L-glutamate in a concentration dependent manner.

Discussion

Glutamate is the main amino acid in the brain but under certain conditions it can become neurotoxic. Excitotoxic mechanisms have been proposed to play a role in the pathogenesis of several chronic neurodegenerative disorders (Meldrum and Garthwaite, 1990). Current thinking holds that an excess of this excitatory transmitter, acting via NMDA receptors, leads to pathologic concentrations of cytosolic free calcium in the postsynaptic neurons (Choi, 1987). It has been clearly established that antagonists of the NMDA receptor prevent neuronal death induced by glutamate, indicating that the sustained increase in Ca^{2+} leads to the death of the neurons (Drian et al., 1991; Olney et al., 1987). This dramatic Ca^{2+} increase occurs in several steps. For example, Ca^{2+} activates several enzymes including proteases, protein kinases and protein phosphatases. One of these activated protein kinases is protein kinase C (Choi, 1990). Although NMDA receptor and ion channel blockade is reported to be effective, such drugs can have adverse consequences for normal NMDA receptors physiology (Morris, 1989).

In the recent study, we present the examination of an alternative cerebroprotective agent, the peptide derivative Cerebrolysin®, on neuronal cell death resulting from exposure to exogenous L-glutamate. Cerebrolysin® is known to stimulate brain metabolism (Piswanger et al., 1990) and exerts beneficial effects on passive avoidance reaction in rats when injected immediately after birth (Paier et al., 1992). These effects do extend to other measures of memory, e.g. the place navigation task of Morris (Gschanes et al., 1993). In this test situation Cerebrolysin® improves the swimming latencies of ischemic rats and facilitates the learning ability in somato-sensory cortex lesioned rats (Windisch et al., 1993). Furthermore, this peptide derivative has been shown to improve neurophysiological deficits in patients suffering from Alzheimer's disease (Rüther et al., 1993). Cerebrolysin® is an agent mainly consisting of small peptides. Since it is known that several peptide growth factors can influence neuronal growth and survival it is speculated that these peptides play a pivotal role in preventing cells from glutamate induced neuronal cell death (Thoenen et al., 1987; Barde, 1989). Matteson et al. (1989) showed that fibroblast growth factors reduce glutamate induced rises in intracellular calcium levels. In addition, neuroprotective effects of an other multifunctional peptide, transforming growth factor-β1 (TGF-β1), was shown to have neuroprotective properties. After glutamate exposure protection of TGF-β1 was indicated by morphological observations as well as by an increase of cell viability (Prehn et al., 1993). In general, peptide growth factors are believed to participate in the regulation of the expression of other growth factors and their receptors (Roberts and Sporn, 1990). It is therefore conceivable that neuroprotection by Cerebrolysin® is a result of a complex interaction between its peptides and hormones, vitamins or peptide growth factors elicited by the neuronal population.

The precise mechanism of the neuroprotective effect of Cerebrolysin® requires further investigation. Nevertheless, this peptide derivative when tested here, attenuated glutamate dependent injury to cortical neurons in an concentration effective fashion.

References

Barde A (1989) Trophic factors and neuronal survival. Neuron 2: 1525–1534
Choi DW (1987) Ionic dependence of glutamate neurotoxicity. J Neurosci 7: 369–379
Choi DW (1990) Methods for antagonising glutamate neurotoxicity. Cerebrovasc Brain Metab Rev 2: 105–147
Choi DW, Koh JY, Peters S (1988) Pharmacology of glutamate neurotoxicity in cortical culture: attenuation by NMDA antagonists. J Neurosci 8: 185–196

Drian MJ, Kamenka JM, Pirat JL, Privat A (1991) Non-competitive antagonist of N-methyl-D-aspartate prevent spontaneous neuronal death in primary cultures of embryonic rat cortex. J Neurosci Res 29: 133–138

Greenamyre JT (1986) The role of glutamate in neurotransmission and neurologic disease. Arch Neurol 43: 1058–1063

Gschanes A, Windisch M, Bures J (1993) Cerebrolysin, a peptidergic drug increases performance of ischemic rats in the Morris water maze. Eur J Neurosci [Suppl 6]: 140

Lauritzen M, Hansen AJ (1992) The effect of glutamate receptor blockade on anoxic depolarisation and cortical spreding depression. J Cereb Blood Flow Metab 12: 223–229

Maragos WF, Greenamyre JT, Penny JB, Young AB (1987) Glutamate dysfunction in Alzheimer's disease: a hypothesis. Trends Neurosci 10: 65–68

Matteson MP, Murrain M, Guthrie PB, Kater SB (1989) Fibroblast growth factor and glutamate: opposing action in the generation and degeneration of hippocampal neuroarcitecuture. J Neurosci 9: 3728–3740

Meldrum B, Garthwaite J (1990) Excitatory amino acid neurotoxicity and neurodegenerative disease. Trends Pharmacol Sci 11: 379–387

Morris RGM (1989) Synaptic plasticity and learning: selective impairment of learning in rats and blockade of long-term potentiation in vivo by the N-methyl-D-aspartate receptor antagonist AP5. J Neurosci 9: 3040–3057

Mosmann T (1983) Rapid colorimetric assay for cellular growth and survival: application to proliferation and cytotoxic assays. J Immunol Methods 65: 55–63

Olney J, Price M, Salles KS, Labruyere J, Friedrich G (1987) MK-801 powerfully protects against N-methyl-D-aspartate neurotoxicity. Eur J Pharmacol 141: 357–361

Paier B, Windisch M, Eggenreich U (1992) Postnatal administration of two peptide mixture affects passive avoidance behaviour of young rats. Behav Brain Res 51: 23–28

Pettmann B, Louis JC, Sensenbrenner LM (1979) Morphological and biochemical maturation of neurons cultured in the absence of glia cells. Nature 281: 378–380

Piswanger A, Paier B, Windisch M (1990) Modulation of protein synthesis in a cell free system from rat brain by Cerebrolysin during development and ageing. In: Lubec G, Rosenthal GA (eds) Amino acids. Escom Sciences Publishers B.V., Leiden, pp 651–657

Plaitakis A, Caroscio JT (1987) Abnormal glutamate metabolism in amyotrophic lateral sclerosis. Ann Neurol 22: 575–579

Prehn JHM, Peruche B, Unsicker K, Krieglstein J (1993) Isoform-specific effects of transforming growth factors-β on degeneration of primary cultures induced by cytotoxic hypoxia or glutamate. J Neurochem 60: 1665–1672

Roberts AB, Sporn MB (1990) The transforming growth factors-β. In: Sporn MB, Roberts AB (eds) Handbook of experimental pharmacology, peptide growth factors and their receptors. Springer, Berlin Heidelberg New York Tokyo, pp 419–472

Rüther E, Ritter R, Apecechea M, Freytag S, Windisch M (1993) Efficacy of the peptidergic drug Cerebrolysin in patients with senile dementia of the Alzheimer's type (SDAT). Pharmacopsychiatry 27: 32–37

Skaper SD, Leon A, Facci L (1991) Ganglioside GM1 prevents death induced by excessive excitatory neurotransmission in cultured hippocampal pyramidal neurons. Neurosci Lett 117: 154–159

Thoenen H, Bantlow C, Heumann R (1987) The physiological function of nerve growth factor in the central nervous system: comparison with periphery. Rev Physiol Biochem Pharmacol 109: 145–178

Windisch M, Gschanes A, Valouskova V (1993) The effects of different growth factors in rats after lesion of the somatosensory cortex. Eur J Neurosci [Suppl 6]: 140

Xiong H, Wojtowicz JM, Baskys A (1995) Brain tissue hydrolysate acts on presynaptic adenosine receptors in the rat hippocampus. Can J Physiol Pharmacol 73: 1194–1197

Young AB, Greenamyre JT, Hollingsworth Z, Albin R, D'Amato C, Shoulson I, Penny JB (1988) NMDA receptor losses in putamen from patients with Huntington's disease. Science 241: 981–983

Authors' address: Dr. B. Hutter-Paier, Center of Animal Biology, Medical School, University of Graz, Roseggerweg 48, A-8036 Graz, Austria.

J Neural Transm (1996) [Suppl] 47: 275
© Springer-Verlag 1996

Molecular regulation of the blood-brain barrier GLUT1 glucose transporter by brain-derived peptides

R. J. Boado

Department of Medicine and Brain Research Institute, UCLA School of Medicine,
Los Angeles, CA, USA

The blood-brain barrier (BBB) GLUT1 glucose transporter represents the limiting step in transport of glucose from blood to brain, and its activity has been shown to be altered in different pathophysiological conditions such as hypoglycemia, brain tumors, development, and Alzheimer's disease. The molecular regulation of the BBB-GLUT1 gene is directed at both transcription and post-transcriptional stabilization of mRNA by brain-derived factors present in a bovine brain homogenate [Boado, et al. (1994) Mol Brain Res 22: 259] and in the brain-derived peptide rich preparation Cerebrolysin® (CL, EBEWE, Austria) [Boado (1994) Eur J Neurosci [Suppl] 7: 58], respectively. Since increased GLUT1 mRNA stability was correlated with augmented GLUT1 immunoreactive protein in hypoglycemia and with the antidiabetic agent pioglitazone, it is possible that Cl increases the translation efficiency of BBB-GLUT1 transcript. Therefore, in order to test this hypothesis, the present investigation studied the effect of CL on the expression of the BBB-GLUT1 gene in brain endothelial cultured cells transfected with a luciferase expression vector containing the complete 171 nucleotides of the 5'-untranslated region of the human GLUT1 mRNA, which possesses the GLUT1 translational control elements. Dose response studies showed that Cl at concentrations of $1-10\,\mu l/ml$ culture media produced a marked increase in the levels of luciferase (122–324% of control), whereas no significant changes were observed with 25 or $50\,\mu l/ml$. Desensitation of the protein kinase (PK) receptor with the phorbol ester TPA ($10^{-6}M$, for 20 hours) had no effect on the increased levels of luciferase induced by Cl. The PK inhibitor H7 stimulated the expression of luciferase in control cells, and this effect was not potentiated by $1\,\mu l$ CL/ml (pg luciferase/60mm dish, mean $\pm$ SE (n = 6): control, 3.06 ± 0.15; Cl, 9.92 ± 0.54; control + H7, 12.77 ± 1.13; CL + H7, 11.75 ± 1.54). On the contrary, staurosporine, another PK inhibitor, had a deleterious effect on the expression of luciferase in control cells, but CL maintained the levels of expression 183% higher than controls. Conclusion: data presented here i) demonstrate that CL increases the translation efficiency of the BBB-GLUT1 transcript in brain endothelial cultured cells, and ii) suggest that this property of CL may be useful in increasing the expression of GLUT1 at the blood-brain barrier. The role of PK and its inhibitors on the CL-induced changes in the BBB-GLUT1 will be discussed.

J Neural Transm (1996) [Suppl] 47: 276
© Springer-Verlag 1996

Cerebrolysin® protects neurons from ischemia-induced loss of microtubule — associated protein 2

B. Hutter-Paier, M. Frühwirth, E. Grygar, and **M. Windisch**

EBEWE-Research Initiative, Center of Animal Biology, University of Graz, Austria

Microtubule — associated protein 2 (MAP2) was studied in cultured neurons from chick embryo hemispheres after neuronal damage caused by cytotoxic ischemia. Cortical cells were pretreated with 0, 10, 20, 40 or 80 μl Cerebrolysin® per ml media. After 8 days in vitro (DIV), ischemia was induced by a 60 minutes incubation with 1 mM L-glutamate. After this toxic stress, cells were allowed to recover from ischemia for 48 hours in a medium again supplemented with Cerebrolysin® in the appropriate concentration. For immunoblot analysis cortical cells were lysed in 1% SDS and the supernatants were assayed for protein content by the method of Lowry. Proteins were then separated and transferred to nitrocellulose (0.5 A for 2h). Western blots were blocked with low fat milk and incubated with the primary monoclonal antibody (Chemicon) reacting with all forms of MAP2 (Map2a, Map2b, Map2c) for 12–14 hours at 4°C. Incubation with the horseradish peroxidase — conjugated secondary antibody lasted for 2h. For detection we used a nonradioactive ECL (enhanced chemiluminescence) system (Amersham).

Western immunoblot analysis shows that there is a significant decrease of MAP2 in glutamate treated control cells. In comparison to that Cerebrolysin® significantly increases MAP2 in a dose-dependent manner. In cortical neurons exposed to glutamate but pretreated with 40 or 80 μl Cerebrolysin/ml medium the amount of MAP2 is almost comparable to the MAP2 concentration in nonischemic control cells. The present results obtained from immunoblot methods strongly provide evidence that Cerebrolysin® is able to protect neurons from ischemia-induced loss of MAP2.

J Neural Transm (1996) [Suppl] 47: 277
© Springer-Verlag 1996

The long-term effect of NGF, b-FGF and Cerebrolysin® on the spatial memory after fimbria-fornix lesion in rats

L. Francis-Turner[1], **V. Valouskova**[2], and **J. Mokry**[3]

[1] International Center of Neurological Restoration, Havana, Cuba
[2] Institute Physiology, Academy of Sciences, Prague, and
[3] Department of Histology and Embryology, Charles University, Hradec Kralove, Czech Republic

Nerve Growth Factor (NGF) and Cerebrolysin® (Cer) can support the function of neurons affected by unilateral fimbria-fornix lesion in short term experiment, while no short-term influence of Fibroblast Growth Factor (FGF) was found.

After unilateral lesion of fimbria-fornix the rats were treated with NGF (groups NGF, 11 mg/ml and ngf 0.5 μg/ml), with b-FGF (group FGF, 0.2 μg/ml) or with Cer (group CER, 2.5 ml/kg). Group NGFCER was formed by rats treated with NGF and Cer. The animals were divided in two subgroups according to a prolongation of the treatment: 2 or 4 weeks (subgroups 2w or 4w, respectively). Lesioned (LES) and intact (INT) animals served as control groups. Six moths after the lesion, 99 rats (9 moths old, 550–650 g) from short-term experiment were tested again in the Morris water maze for their ability to retrieve the old position of the platform (1 day, 8 trials). Next day the rats were trained to find the platform replaced to a new position (3 days, 8 trials/day). The length of trajectory was compared.

No significant differences were found among the groups in retrieval test. Groups of subgroup 2w were found to differ only during the last day of training. INT was significantly better than group LES. No one of the experimental groups significantly differed from LES, although groups FGF, NGF and INT were statistically comparable. Prolonged treatment with Cer significantly improved rat's performance and groups CER, NGFCER and FGF from subgroup 4w used similar length of trajectory as group INT.

It is concluded that NGF in higher concentration protects the brain against spatial memory impairment, while FGF supports a long-term restoration of the spatial memory. The effect of Cerebrolysin is dependent on a time of treatment and only prolonged (4 weeks) administration lead to a permanent restorative changes in the damaged brain. Histological changes of the brains are currently evaluated.

J Neural Transm (1996) [Suppl] 47: 278
© Springer-Verlag 1996

The influence of Cerebrolysin® and E021 on spatial navigation of young rats

A. Gschanes and **M. Windisch**

Research Initiative Ebewe, Graz, Austria

In the present study the effects of early administration of Cerebrolysin® or E021 (enriched peptide concentrate) were investigated. Rat pups received either the drugs or saline as control (2.5ml/kg, subcutaneous) on postnatal days 1–7. Rats were tested in the Morris water maze (MWM) on day 28 after birth for six consecutive days (day 1–6). Eight trials were done on each day.

In order to prevent finding of the hidden platform by chance, the rigid underwater platform was replaced with a collapsible island, resting at the bottom of the pool. A computerized videosystem stored the rat's movement across the pool. The platform was raised when the animal stayed in the target area for a predetermined time.

Both, Cerebrolysin® and E021 treated rats showed significant shorter escape latencies to find the hidden collapsible platform than control animals on day 1 to day 6. In addition, sex differences were observed. During day 1–6 Cerebrolysin caused a significant better performance in females when compared to controls of the same sex. In contrast, E021 had positive influence on females on day 1, day 2 and day 6. Cerebrolysin® or E021 treated males showed a significantly better performance than control animals only on day 3, day 4 and day 5. Additional Cerebrolysin® had a more positive effect when compared to controls on day 6.

Summarizing, the application of Cerebrolysin® or E021 improved spatial memory in young rats. Cerebrolysin® lead to shorter escape latencies in both males and females, whereas the effects of E021 were less pronounced.

J Neural Transm (1996) [Suppl] 47: 279

Effects of Cerebrolysin® on cytoskeletal proteins after focal ischemia in rats

M. Schwab[1], **I. Antonow-Schlorke**[1], **U. Dürer**[2], and **R. Bauer**[1]

[1] Institute of Pathological Physiology, Klinikum, Friedrich-Schiller-University, and
[2] Institute of Molecular Biotechnology, Beutenberg Campus, Jena,
Federal Republic of Germany

In previous studies it was shown that Cerebrolysin® has cerebroprotective effects after moderate global ischemia in rats. In order to investigate mechanisms of these effects, we studied the influence of Cerebrolysin® on dynamics of neurodegeneration of cytoskeletal proteins (MAP2 and alpha-tubulin) after focal brain ischemia in adult male Thomae rats. We used different combinations of ischemia/reperfusion-intervals (2 hrs/90 min and 3 hrs/15 min). Ischemia was induced by a reversible occlusion of the middle cerebral artery by insertion of a nylon monofilament thread. Spreading depressions, ischemic depolarisation, and ECoG were recorded above the core and penumbra of the infarct. CBF (cortical blood flow) was measured in the same regions by a two channel Laser Doppler flowmeter. After fixation procedure and paraffin embedding, the brains were sectioned in 24 slices, each 0.5 mm thick. Slices (5 µm) from each plane were used for immunohistochemical staining against MAP2 and alpha-tubulin. The size of the infarction zone and the penumbra was calculated morphometrically. First results indicate that Cerebrolysin® may stabilize cytoskeletal structures. More details will be presented.

J Neural Transm (1996) [Suppl] 47: 280
© Springer-Verlag 1996

The short-term influence of b-FGF, NGF and Cerebrolysin® on the memory impaired after fimbria-fornix lesion

V. Valouškova[1] and **L. Francis-Turmer**[2]

[1]Institute of Physiology, Academy of Science of Czech Republic,
Prague, Czech Republic
[2]Center of Neurological Restoration, Havana, Cuba

Neurotrophic factors were shown to prevent degeneration and to facilitate regeneration in damaged CNS. In an attempt to compare the effect of b-FGF, NGF and the nootropic drug Cerebrolysin® (Cer) (EBEWE Arzneimittel), naive 3-month-old rats (Long Evans strain) were trained to escape from water in the Morris pool to a hidden platform (3 consecutive days; D1, D2, D3; 8 trials/day). Next day, fimbria-fornix (FF) was unilaterally removed by suction. A needle connected to a micro-osmotic pump filled by b-FGF (0.2 µg/ml) or NGF (11 µg/ml or 0.5 µg/) was placed into the lateral ventricle ipsilateral to the lesion., Cer was applied via intraperitoneal injection (2.5 ml/kg/day). One group was treated by Cer and NGF (11 µg/ml)(group NGFCER). As control groups served intact (INT) and lesioned only rats (LES). After the 14-day-treatment (D19) rats were tested for their ability to remember the position of the platform. During the next 3 days (D20, D21, D22) rats were trained to find the platform placed in a opposite quadrant of the pool. The length of trajectory and escape latency were recorded and speed of swimming was calculated.

Groups LES, NGF, and FGF were similary impaired in their ability to retrieve the old position of the platform. Groups CER, NGF and NGFCER did not differ from the intact animals. Groups LES and FGF learned the new position of the platform (D20–22) very slowly and were significantly impaired when compared to D1–3. Performance of lesioned rats receiving Cer and NGF on D20–22 was similar to their performance on D1–3.

It is concluded that retrograde amnesia elicited by the fimbria-fornix lesion can be shortened by NGF and/or Cer, while anterograde amnesia is absent only in rats treated by Cer. No short-term effect of b-FGF was found. Similar effect of Cerebrolysin® was found in the same behavioral experiment performed with rats with excitotoxic lesion of substantia innominata.

J Neural Transm (1996) [Suppl] 47: 281
© Springer-Verlag 1996

Brain tissue hydrolysate, Cerebrolysin®, acts on presynaptic adenosine receptors in the rat hippocampus

J. M. Wojtowicz, H. Xiong, and **A. Baskys**

Department of Physiology, University of Toronto, Toronto, Ontario, Canada

Adenosine is a potent inhibitory modulator in the brain. It suppresses glutamatergic synaptic transmission and possibly acts as an endogenous brain neuroprotective agent. In this study we have examined the effects of a clinically used porcine brain tissue hydrolysate, Cerebrolysin®, on synaptic transmission in the CA1 area of the rat hippocampus. Hippocampal slices were prepared for in vitro experiments using standard procedures and perfused with artificial cerebrospinal fluid at 32°C and pH = 7.4. Field potentials were evoked by stimulating the Schaffer collateral/commissural afferents and recorded in the stratum radiatum of CA1 field. Cerebrolysin® or other pharmacological agents were dissolved in the perfusate prior to applications. The application periods were usually 5–15 minutes, sufficiently long to obtain steady state effects on synaptic transmission. A major effect of Cerebrolysin® at 10 µl/ml was a depression of synaptic transmission at the Schaffer collateral/commissural pathway. Detailed analysis showed that the inhibition is presynaptic and can be reduced by a specific blocker of A1 adenosine receptors, 8-cyclopentyltheophylline (100 nM). Since Cerebrolysin does not contain a detectable amount of adenosine, the effect on adenosine receptors must be indirect, perhaps by release of an endogenous agonist. This action of Cerebrolysin® is consistent with the putative neuroprotective action underlying its clinical usage. Supported by EBEWE Initiative.

Subject Index

α-B crystallin 5, 19, 37
Achromatic neurons 48
Adrenergic receptor binding 79
AIDS associated encephalopathy 56
AIDS complex 147, 150
Alzheimer's disease 1, 2, 4, 7, 9, 10, 31, 32, 38, 56, 61, 62, 65, 66, 68, 73, 103, 108, 112, 133, 139, 158, 169, 187, 196, 199, 200, 210, 221, 241, 259, 275
– apolipoprotein E allele frequencies 209
– atypical presentation 109
– cognitive deficit 104
– language disorder 109
– Lewy body variant 10
– morphological diagnosis 7
– neurofibrillary predominant type 9
– neurochemical changes 73
– non-amnestic deficits 108
– plaque-only type 9
– synaptic pathology 10
– white matter changes 145, 146
Amnesia 65
Amnesic syndrome 65
Amyloid deposits 7
– plaques 240
– precursor protein 8
Amyotrophic complex 138
Amyotrophic lateral sclerosis 220
Anomia 111, 135, 137
Anterograde episodic memory 105
Antidepressive pharmacotherapy 197
– with clomipramine 200
Apilipoprotein E (APO E) 259, 260, 263
– allele 205, 210
– binding 207
– frequency 211
– gene 205, 206, 241
– genetics 213
– genotype 213
– homozygotes 211
– immunoreactivity 259
– protein 213

APO E ε2 206, 211
APO E ε3 206
APO E ε4 206, 260
Argyrophilic grains 138
Aspartate 82
Astrocytic plaques 32, 42, 43
Atypical prion dementia 233, 237

Balint's syndrome 109
Ballooned cells (neurons) 34, 37, 39, 40, 42, 43, 55, 56, 133
Benzodiazepine receptor binding 82
Binswanger's disease 74, 144
Biogenic amines 76
Blood-brain barrier 275
Boston Diagnostic Aphasia Examination 104
Bovine spongiform encephalopathy 231, 242
– epidemic 242
– occurrence 242
– surveillance project 242
Braak staging 8, 260
Bradyphrenia 200
Brain derived peptides 275
β-amyloid peptide 206, 212

CA2/3 neurites 37
CERAD criteria 8, 14
Cerebellar ataxia 239
Cerebral glucose metabolism 186
– oxygen 157
Cerebrolysin® 271, 275–280
– cerebroprotective effects 279
– neuroprotective effect 268
Cerebrospinal fluid 259, 260
– APO E 259, 260
– ventricular 263, 264
– tau 263
Cerebrovascular amyloid 206
Cholecystokinin 85
Choline acetyltransferase 74, 205, 210

Cholinergic activity 213
– systems 14, 74, 75
Choreoacanthocytosis 6
Chromogranin A 5, 85
Codon 102 phenotype 225
Codon 129 225, 235, 240
Codon 145 240
Codon 178 226
Codon 200 226
Cognitive decline 109
– symptoms 195
Comprehensive Psychiatric Rating Scale 116
Computerized tomography 143
Consortium of dementia with Lewy bodies 11
Cortical hypometabolism 157
Corticobasal degeneration 1, 4, 5, 6, 15, 31, 33, 38, 39, 56, 66, 133, 160, 161
Creutzfeldt-Jakob disease 6, 56, 139, 147, 219, 231, 233, 234
– age at onset 221
– clinical characteristics 220
– corneal transplant 224
– dura mater grafts 224
– duration of illness 222
– familial disease 224
– gonadotrophin 224
– growth hormone 224
– human growth hormone 223
– iatrogenic cases 224
– mean incubation period 223
– myoclonus 234
– neuropathological features 234
– neurosurgery 224
– sporadic 234
– stereotactic EEG 224
– with PrP plaques 238
Cultured telencephalon neurons 267
Cytoplasmic tau 19
Cytoskeletal pathology 2, 31
– proteins 279
Cytotoxic ischemia 276

Degenerative dementia 178
Dementia 11, 61, 138, 139, 162, 178, 186, 189, 200, 207, 213
– alcohol 207
– cortical 156
– differential diagnosis 178
– global 109
– metabolic ratio 186
– prevalence 2

– pugilistica 38
– scores 8
– severity 186, 188
– subcortical 156
– thalamic 6
– vascular type 73
– with argyrophilic grains 16
Dementia lacking distinctive histopathology 16, 48, 138, 139
– cortical variant 48
– thalamostriatal variant 48
– leukogliotic variant 48
Dementia of frontal type 49, 62, 110, 125
– delusions, halluzinations 117
– diagnosis 112, 113
– elevated mood 117
– epidemiology 110
– intellectual symptomatology 117
– neurobehavioural features 111
– neuropsychology 113
– neurotic symptomatology 117
– psychiatric symptomatology 115
Dementia syndrome of depressive disorder 196, 197
Dementia with Lewy bodies 10, 12
– clinical diagnosis 13
Dentatorubropallidoluysian atrophy 6, 19, 20
Depression 200, 260
– agitated 115
Depressive dementia 137
Depressive disorder 193, 196
– cognitive symptoms 196
– psychometric testing 196
Depressive pseudo-dementia 193, 199, 201
– description 195
– history 194
– myth 194
– nosology 195
– psychometric diagnosis 195
– subjects 262
– symptoms 116, 194, 195
Depressive syndrome 263
Diffuse Lewy body disease 31, 33, 65, 67, 156, 159
Disinhibition phenomenon 137, 138
Dopamine 76
– D1 receptor binding 79
– D2 receptor binding 79
– receptors 160
Dopaminergic neurons 247
– system 76, 78

Down's syndrome   207–209, 211–213
– APO E ε4 frequencies   211
Dvorak dimension   171, 178
Dynamic aphasia   111
Dysexecutive syndrome   16, 19
Dystrophic neurites   19, 36, 42

Early onset AD   207
– APO E ε4   211
Echolalia   111
EEG fractal dimension   169
EEG recording   170
– bandpower   170
– coherence   170
Energy metabolism   85–87
Entorhinal region   8
Excitatory amino acid   82, 83

F-dopa uptake   162
Familial progressive subcortical gliosis   6, 18, 55
Fatal familial insomnia   6, 219, 226, 231, 233, 240
Fibroblast growth factor   248, 277
Fimbria-fornix lesion   280
– cognitive changes   61
Focal ischemic rats   279
Fractal dimension   178
Frontal dementia   133
– lobe degeneration   48, 110, 128
Frontal lobe dementia   38, 54, 103, 125, 126, 133, 137, 138, 169
– clinical features   103, 125, 136
– diagnostic criteria   47
– Dvorak dimension   176
– Grassberger-Procaccia dimension   175, 178
– motor neuron disease   130, 134
– nosology   47
– pathological findings   126
Frontal lobe dysfunction   125, 126, 131
– dementia   18, 49, 110, 125, 134
– lobe degeneration   18, 57, 110
Fuld Object Memory Evaluation   198
Functional neuroimaging   131

GABAergic system   81, 82
GABA receptor   82
Ganser state   201
Geriatric Mental State schedule   118
Gerstmann-Sträussler-Scheinker syndrome   6, 219, 231, 233, 239
– with neurofibrillary tangles   238

Glial cytoplasmic inclusions   43
– plaques   138
Gliofibrillary tangles   15, 31, 38
Global brain attractor   176
Global ischemia   279
GLUT1 glucose transporter   275
Glutamate   82, 267, 270
– dehydrogenase   85
– receptor   82
Glutathione transferase   87
Grassberger-Procaccia dimension   171, 177
Growth hormone   223
Guam parkinsonism-dementia   15, 38

Hachinski score   184
Hallervorden-Spatz-disease   148
Heat shock protein   37
Hemiparkinsonian patients   157
Hemorrhagic dementia   144
Hereditary dysphasic dementia   138
High affinity receptor   253
Hippocampal formation   8, 108
HIV encephalopathy   150
Human growth hormone   222
Human prion disease   231, 232, 234, 241
– APO E genotype   237
– classification   233
– familial   237
– neuropathological changes   234, 237
Huntington's disease   6, 7, 19, 65, 67, 148, 161
– CAG repeat length   20
– dementia   161
– dopaminergic system   162
– gene   20
– gene carriers   162
– IT15   20
– metabolic studies   161
– PET findings   162
– striatal glucose metabolism   161
Hydrocephalus   151
Hypometabolism   183
Hypofrontality   160
Hypoxic encephalopathy   152

Iatrogenic CJD   221, 233
Immunocytochemistry   33
Inclusion body myositis   232
Infectious cerebral amyloidosis   7
Insulin-like growth factor   248
IT-15 gene   19

Joseph disease   56

Klüver-Bucy syndrome 109, 111
Kuru 219, 231, 233, 240, 241
– type amyloid plaques 241
– type morphology 234

Lacunes 144
Language dysfunction 111
Late-onset Alzheimer's disease 210, 212
Leukoaraiosis 145, 186
Leukodystrophies 146
Lewy body 10, 31, 37, 43, 156, 207, 213
Lewy body dementia 6, 205, 207–209, 213
Lewy body disease 5, 10, 38, 156, 157
– activation studies 158
– resting metabolic studies 157
Linguistic perturbations 67
Lobar atrophy 1, 16, 62, 63, 68
– differential diagnosis 16
Logopenia 137
Lumbar CSF 263, 264
– Apo E 263
Lund and Manchester Group 51, 54, 112,
    134

Machado-Joseph disease 6, 19, 20
Magnetic resonance spectroscopy 155
MAO-B 87
Mattis' Dementia Rating Scale 104
Melancholia cum delirio 198, 199, 201
Mesencephalic cell culture 249
Mesocorticolimbic dementia 55
Metabolic pathology 186
Metabolism, cortical 162
– frontal 189
– glucose 157
Microtubule-associated protein 276
Midbrain 248
Mini Mental State Examination 8, 104,
    186, 260
Mixed type dementia 73, 118
Monoamine oxidase 87
Motor neuron disease 125, 126
– classic 130
Motor neuron disease type of dementia 18,
    38, 55
Multiinfarct dementia 74, 118
– encephalopathy 144
Multisystem atrophy 19, 43, 66, 67, 148
– cytoplasmic inclusions 19
Multisystem degeneration 38
Muscarinic receptors 76

National Adult Rating Scale 104

Nerve growth factor 248, 277
Neuritic plaques 7, 41, 65
Neurochemistry 73
Neurodegenerative disorders, classification
    6, 38
Neurofibrillary tangles 7, 31, 34, 47, 65,
    206, 207, 210, 240, 259, 260
Neurofilament 34, 37
– antibodies 34
– epitopes 5
– immunocytochemistry 43
Neuron survival 255
Neuronal inclusions 5
Neuropeptides 84, 85
Neurophil threads 7, 15, 40
Neurotoxicity 267
Neurotrophic factor 247, 280
Neurotrophin brain-derived neurotrophic
    factor 248
Neurotrophin receptor 255
Nicotinic binding 76
NMDA receptor 267, 270, 271
Non-Alzheimer's degenerative diseases
    68
– cognitive deficits 61
Non-Alzheimer's dementia 2, 6, 31, 147,
    205, 259, 264
– functional imaging 155
– MR-imaging 143
Non-Pick frontal atrophy 56
Noradrenergic system 79, 80
Normal pressure hydrocephalus 152
Nucleus basalis of Meynert 10, 14, 157

Oligodendroglial inclusions 138
Olivopontocerebellar atrophy 6, 19, 43
Oxidative stress 85–87

Parietal syndrome 109
Pallidal degeneration 6
Parkinson's disease 1, 6, 10, 35, 65–67,
    156, 207–209, 211, 213, 248
– APO E allele 205
– dementia 147, 156
– mental impairment 11
Parkinsonism 138
Pathological aging 8
Phosphor MR-spectroscopy 151
Pick bodies 1, 16, 31, 43, 47–49, 56, 110,
    128, 138
– cells 47–49, 56, 110, 128
– complex 138, 139

Pick's disease 4, 6, 15, 16, 18, 31, 33, 38, 47, 62, 63, 110, 128, 133, 138, 139, 149, 160, 169
– atypical 18
– EEG 169
Positron emission tomography (PET) 155, 157, 183, 188
Postencephalic parkinsonism 6, 15, 38
Posterior cortical atrophy 63, 109
Present State Examination 118
Primary degenerative dementia 189
Primary progressive aphasia 6, 18, 55, 63, 133, 135
– neuroimaging 135
– pathological features 138
Prion diseases 6, 7, 54, 56, 231
Prion protein 231, 232
– biochemistry 232
– genotype 238
– iatrogenic 238
– molecular genetics 232
Progressive amnestic dementia 64, 65, 103
Progressive aphasia 134, 138
Progressive language disorder 133
Progressive multifocal leukencephalopathy 147, 151
Progressive/visuospatial dysfunction 64
Progressive subcortical gliosis 56, 160, 233
Progressive supranuclear palsy (PSP) 1, 4, 6, 15, 32, 38, 56, 65, 67, 159
– atypical 15
– caudate ^{18}F-dopa uptake 160
– cerebral glucose metabolism 161
– metabolic studies 159
– PET studies 160
– pharmacologic studies 160
– striatal ^{18}F-dopa uptake 160, 161
– typical 15
Propentofylline 189
Proton MR-spectroscopy 147, 151
Pseudo-dementia 197, 201
Psychomotor retardation 198, 200
Psychopathological Rating Scale 119
Pure amnesic syndrome 109
Pyruvate dehydrogenase 85

Quantitative EEG 169

Rat mesencephalon 255
Resting glucose metabolism 158
Retrograde amnesia 280
– memory 107

Reverse transcription-polymerase chain reaction 253
Rey Complex Figure Test 104

Scrapie 231
Second messenger system 82, 86
Semantic aphasia 135, 139
– deficit 107
– memory 105, 107, 108
Senile plaques 36, 42, 206, 210, 259
Serotonergic systems 76, 77, 87
Serotonin receptor binding 76
Shy-Drager syndrome 6, 19
Silver impregnation techniques 32
Single photon emission tomography (SPECT) 155, 187
– diagnostic accuracy 187
Somatostatin 87
– receptor 85
Spatial memory 277, 278
– navigation 278
Speech disturbances 62
Spinecho MR-imaging 151
Spongiform encephalopathy 6, 231, 232, 237
– changes 54
Sporadic familial AD 206
– APO E ε4 allele 206
Staurosporine 275
Steele-Richardson-Olszewski syndrome 159
Stereotactic electroencephalography 221
Strategic infarct dementia 144
Striatal D_2 sites 162
– metabolism 162
Striato-frontal dysfunction 12
Striato-frontal loops 19
Striatonigral degeneration 6, 19, 43, 66
Subcortical arteriosclerotic encephalopathy 144
– gliosis 55
– infarcts 186
Subcortico-frontal dementia 68
Substance P 85
Substantia innominata 280
Survival promoting effect 247, 253
Superficial siderosis 147
Superoxide dismutase activity 87

Tau protein 7, 15, 18, 37, 38, 207, 212, 259, 263
Temporal lobe degeneration 103
Temporo-parietal dysfunction 67

Thalamic atrophies 55
Token Test 104
Topographical ANOVA 172, 173
– band power 172
– coherence 173
Transforming growth factor 247, 248, 271
Transmissible cerebral amyloidosis 219
– contamination 223
– corneal grafts 223
– dura mater grafts 223
– familial forms 225
– growth hormone 223
– incubation period 223
Transcortical motor aphasia 63
Transentorhinal region 108
Tufted astrocytes 38
Tubuline 5

Ubiquitin 5, 19, 36, 37, 42

Unusual Views Matching Test 104

Vascular dementia   2, 74, 144, 183, 184,
    187, 207
– diagnosis 184
– effects of therapy 183
– frequency 183
– hypometabolism 184
– metabolic disturbances 183
– neuroimaging 184
– positron emission tomography 184
– SPECT 187
Vasopressine 85
Verbal short-term memory 108

Wernicke's aphasia 135
White matter lesions 151
Wilsons disease 148
Working memory 107, 111

SpringerNeurology

Peter Riederer, Wolfgang Wesemann (eds.)

Parkinson's Disease:
Experimental Models and Therapy

1995. 121 figures. XI, 466 pages.
Soft cover DM 240,–, öS 1680,–
Reduced price for subscribers to "Journal of Neural Transmission":
Soft cover DM 216,–, öS 1512,–
ISBN 3-211-82749-8
Journal of Neural Transmission, Supplement 46

Current research on Parkinson's disease is aimed at the goal of determining the underlying cause of this terrible disease and of developing adequate treatment strategies to deal with it. This volume focuses on models that mirror the progression of the symptoms of Parkinson's disease (iron, MPTP, 6-hydroxydopamine, "TaClo", etc.) while other topics are the evaluation of oxidative stress, calcium, excitotoxicity, nitric oxide, or nerve growth factors as possible pathophysiological candidates or causal parameters. Further topics are the interplay between exogenous and endogenous toxins, the potential of brain imaging by PET, MRI and SPECT, as well as promising therapeutic drug strategies. This volume represents a comprehensive survey of the state of the art for neurologists, biochemists, neuropharmacologists and toxicologists.

Springer Wien New York

P.O.Box 89, A-1201 Wien • New York, NY 10010, 175 Fifth Avenue
Heidelberger Platz 3, D-14197 Berlin • Tokyo 113, 3-13, Hongo 3-chome, Bunkyo-ku

SpringerNeurology

Kurt A. Jellinger, Gernot Ladurner,
Manfred Windisch (eds.)

New Trends in the Diagnosis
and Therapy of Alzheimer's Disease

1994. 33 figures. VII, 146 pages.
Soft cover DM 118,–, öS 826,–
ISBN 3-211-82620-3
Key Topics in Brain Research

Alzheimer's Disease (AD), the most frequent cause of mental decline in the elderly represents one of the major health problems facing modern society. Despite considerable progress in the clinical diagnosis, epidemiology, structural basis, biochemistry, molecular genetics, and pharmacological aspects of AD, its etiology, molecular backgrounds, and treatment challenges are still poorly understood. This volume based on the 2nd International Symposium of EBEWE Research Initiative in October 1993 in Salzburg, Austria, is conceived as a review of our current knowledge of morphology, diagnostic clinical and imaging techniques, methodological approaches of cognitive assessment, trial designs, outcome variables and possibilities of therapy of AD and other neuro-degenerative disorders. The book's coverage is broad and it should be of interest for investigators, clinicians, and researchers involved in the problems of AD.

SpringerWienNewYork

P.O.Box 89, A-1201 Wien • New York, NY 10010, 175 Fifth Avenue
Heidelberger Platz 3, D-14197 Berlin • Tokyo 113, 3-13, Hongo 3-chome, Bunkyo-ku